Heart Failure

Pathophysiology, Molecular Biology, and Clinical Management

SECOND EDITION

Heart Failure

Pathophysiology, Molecular Biology, and Clinical Management

Arnold M. Katz, MD, DMed (Hon.)

Professor of Medicine and Cardiology Division Chief Emeritus
University of Connecticut School of Medicine

Visiting Professor of Medicine and Physiology
Dartmouth Medical School

Marvin A. Konstam, MD

Professor of Medicine
Tufts University School of Medicine

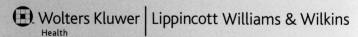 Wolters Kluwer | Lippincott Williams & Wilkins
Health
Philadelphia • Baltimore • New York • London
Buenos Aires • Hong Kong • Sydney • Tokyo

Acquisitions Editor: Frances R. DeStefano
Project Manager: Jennifer Harper
Manufacturing Manager: Benjamin Rivera
Marketing Manager: Kimberly Schonberger
Graphic Designer: Steve Druding
Production Services: Aptara Corporation

© 2009 by Lippincott Williams & Wilkins, a Wolters Kluwer business

530 Walnut Street
Philadelphia, PA 19106 USA
LWW.com

First edition, © 2000 by Lippincott Williams & Wilkins, Philadelphia

Printed in the USA

Library of Congress Cataloging-in-Publication Data

Katz, Arnold M.
  Heart failure : pathophysiology, molecular biology, and clinical management / Arnold M.
Katz, Marvin A. Konstam. — 2nd ed.
    p. ; cm.
  First ed. lacks subtitle.
  Includes bibliographical references and index.
  ISBN 978-0-7817-6946-4 (alk. paper)
  1. Heart failure. I. Konstam, Marvin A. II. Title.
  [DNLM: 1. Heart Failure—physiopathology. 2. Heart Failure—genetics. 3. Heart
Failure—therapy. WG 370 K195h 2009]
  RC685.C53K38 2009
  616.1'29—dc22   2008025849

To purchase additional copies of this book, call our customer service department at (800) 638-3030 or fax orders to (301) 223-2320. International customers should call (301) 223-2300.

Visit Lippincott Williams & Wilkins on the Internet: at LWW.com. Lippincott Williams & Wilkins customer service representatives are available from 8:30 am to 6 pm, EST.

10 9 8 7 6 5 4 3 2 1

Disclosure: Dr. Konstam has served as a consultant and/or received research support from the following companies: Otsuka, Merck, Astra-Zeneca, Novartis, Wyeth, Cardiokine, Nitromed, Biogen, Boehringer-Ingelheim. He has received salary support and stock options, serving as Medical Director of Orqis Medical.

*For Phyllis
and
Varda*

CONTENTS

Despite the dramatic advances in the care of patients with cardiovascular diseases that have occurred in the past half century, these conditions remain—by far—the most common causes of death in developed nations. Moreover, the prevalence of cardiovascular diseases is now rising rapidly in developing nations as well. It has been projected that within 20 years, cardiovascular disease will, for the first time in human history, be the most common cause of death worldwide.

As the treatment of most cardiovascular disorders—acute myocardial infarction and other acute coronary syndromes, hypertension, valvular disease and many congenital cardiac disorders—improves, early mortality is reduced. However, these patients are rarely "cured," but instead they often develop myocardial disease and ultimately heart failure. Thus, heart failure has become the most frequent "final common pathway" to death or serious disability in cardiovascular diseases and might be considered to be the price paid for successful early management of these disorders. In the United States, heart failure is also the most frequent hospital discharge diagnosis of patients 65 years of age or older. It is, therefore, mandatory that physicians involved in the care of patients with this very common and serious condition understand its pathogenesis, clinical features, and the mechanisms underlying various therapies. Of equal importance, investigators of heart failure, be they basic or clinical scientists, have a great need to understand the relation between abnormalities at the molecular, cellular, organ, and clinical levels.

Heart failure is actually a much more complex condition than it was thought be 20 years ago. At that time, the pathophysiology of heart failure had been well described, but the responsible alterations in cellular biochemistry and biophysics were just being elucidated. The underlying genetic alterations were a total mystery.

Heart Failure: Pathophysiology, Molecular Biology and Clinical Management provides important insights into this important condition. Comprehensive medical texts on complex subjects are usually multiauthored because few individuals possess the understanding and perspective to do justice to fields as enormous as heart failure. Drs. Katz and Konstam have, by themselves, successfully tackled this Herculean task. In this magnificent book, they have not only reviewed all relevant aspects of this vast subject, but have provided a "grand vision" of how molecular biology provides explanations of the abnormalities of myocardial contraction and relaxation and how abnormalities of myocyte function affect the performance of the cardiac pump. Furthermore, they carefully describe the links between the disturbed pathobiology and both the clinical manifestations and treatment of heart failure. The breadth and depth of understanding provided by these two authorities, who uniquely span the disciplines of genetics, molecular biology, cardiac biochemistry, physiology, clinical cardiology, and therapeutics, are matched by their extraordinary ability to relate these fields to one another and to explain complex concepts clearly, both in words and diagrams.

This book is truly a joy to read and study. It will be equally useful to clinicians, scientists, and their trainees. It will surely stand as a landmark in the field.

Eugene Braunwald, MD
Boston, Massachusetts

Knowledge of the pathophysiology and treatment of heart failure has expanded rapidly since the first edition of this text was published in 2000. Discoveries in the basic sciences, notably molecular biology, are increasing the importance of pathophysiology for those who manage this common syndrome and revolutionizing the way we treat these patients. At the same time, new clinical information, by focusing attention on the mechanisms responsible for death and disability in heart failure, is drawing basic science and clinical practice toward one another. Because this expansion is making it increasingly difficult for a single individual to provide informed views of the many important features of this syndrome, this second edition has two authors: Arnold Katz, whose focus is on basic science, and Marvin Konstam, whose chapters describe patient management.

The goal of this text remains unchanged: to describe the molecular mechanisms that cause hearts to fail; the hemodynamic and other functional abnormalities that disable these patients; the neurohumoral and proliferative responses, both adaptive and maladaptive, that modify these disabilities; the clinical manifestations caused by these abnormalities; and therapeutic strategies for patient management.

This second edition covers more information than the first, but the text has been shortened to clarify our descriptions of disease mechanisms and therapeutic strategies. Achieving these goals in a concise text precludes inclusion of many details, so that readers seeking more exhaustive discussions are referred to standard textbooks of medicine and cardiology, reviews (many of which are cited in the present text), and original articles.

A number of changes have been made in this second edition. The historical overview in Chapter 1 includes discoveries made in the 20th century. All of the other chapters have been reorganized. Chapter 2 describes the hemodynamic basis for the clinical manifestations of this syndrome, while Chapter 3 reviews the neurohumoral responses evoked by impaired cardiac performance and key signaling pathways that mediate the functional responses. Chapter 4 describes the proliferative responses in failing hearts, as many of these have been recognized to play a central role in determining long-term prognosis in these patients and so are becoming targets for new therapy. The mechanisms by which cellular and molecular abnormalities impair the performance of failing hearts are reviewed in Chapter 5. Chapter 6 discusses the rationale for the many therapeutic approaches to this syndrome, and Chapter 7, which concludes this text, integrates the material covered in the earlier chapters to describe the management of specific groups of heart failure patients.

The goal of this text remains to aid physicians and other health professionals, along with students of medicine, basic science, nursing, and other fields related to cardiology, in understanding the pathophysiology and treatment of heart failure. We hope that this second edition will explain the pathophysiological mechanisms that are the basis of modern strategies for managing patients with this syndrome, and provide an overview for scientists who seek to apply basic concepts to this important clinical problem.

Arnold M. Katz, MD, DMed (Hon.)
Norwich, Vermont

Marvin A. Konstam, MD
Boston, Massachusetts, and Bethesda, Maryland

ACKNOWLEDGMENTS

We are indebted to our wives, Phyllis Katz and Varda Konstam, and our children, Paul, Sarah, Amy, and Laura (Katz), and Amanda and Jeremy (Konstam), for providing us with perspective and balance, without which our ability to write this book would have been merely half-fulfilling.

We thank Frances DeStefano and Chris Potash, our editors at Lippincott Williams and Wilkins, for their help in organizing this text, Cindy Fullerton at Aptara for her many forms of assistance in production, and Beth Douglass for her tireless and expert secretarial assistance.

Heart Failure

Pathophysiology, Molecular Biology, and Clinical Management

SECOND EDITION

CHAPTER 1

Definition, Historical Aspects

Arnold M. Katz • Marvin A. Konstam

Heart failure has become epidemic in the developed world. In the United States, this syndrome is now the most common hospital discharge diagnosis in the population over age 65, accounting for more than 1,000,000 discharges in 2003, and the estimated cost of caring for these patients in 2006 is ~$30 billion (American Heart Association [AHA] Statistical Update, 2006). Heart failure can be diagnosed in ~5% of individuals between the ages of 65 and 74, and in ~10% of the population over the age of 75. Furthermore, this syndrome carries a worse prognosis than most malignancies; for example, mean survival for patients with heart failure, which in the late 1990s was 3–5 years, is about the same as that for stage 3B breast cancer (chest wall metastases and/or extensive lymph node metastases) (Woodward et al., 2003).

What is heart failure? This apparently simple question, which must be addressed in any book about this condition, presents a surprisingly difficult challenge. In the first place, heart failure is not a disease, but instead is a syndrome that can be viewed as a final common pathway by which various etiologies damage the heart to cause disability and premature death. These include coronary disease, systemic and pulmonary hypertension, valvular abnormalities, and abnormalities in heart muscle, called cardiomyopathies. Definitions traditionally focus on hemodynamics, highlighting the clinical signs and symptoms that result from impaired pumping of blood from the veins to the arteries. The consequences, increased venous pressures and reduced cardiac output, are often viewed as the primary manifestations of this syndrome. However, the clinical picture in heart failure is commonly dominated by abnormalities involving other organs. Accumulation of fluid in the lungs behind a failing left ventricle increases the work of breathing and impairs gas exchange; along with reduced cardiac output, these abnormalities lead to shortness of breath. Low cardiac output also signals the kidneys to retain salt and water, which adds to the clinical disability and, when severe, can cause renal and hepatic failure. The profound weakness noted by many of these patients is due mainly to a skeletal muscle myopathy. These and other abnormalities in the lungs, kidneys, liver, skeletal muscle, and other organs can dominate the clinical picture, even though these tissues are the victims of disorders that originate in the heart.

Heart failure can be defined in several ways. Because the most obvious abnormality is impaired pump function, this syndrome was initially viewed simply as a hemodynamic disorder. Emphasis on pump malfunction was heightened because, until the mid-20th century, the most common causes of this syndrome were structural, notably rheumatic valvular disease. At the beginning of the 19th century, various types of cardiac enlargement were recognized to play an important role in determining prognosis. In the 1960s and 1970s, the focus of cardiovascular physiology shifted to myocardial contractility and its regulation, which led heart failure to be viewed largely as a hemodynamic syndrome characterized by depressed contractility; later, in the 1970s, when relaxation was found also to be impaired, definitions began to include decreased lusitropy. However, it was not until the late 1980s, when long-term clinical trials revealed the dismal prognosis in patients with heart failure, that definitions began to include progressive deterioration of the failing heart and the shortened life expectancy. The latter made it clear that, in addition to the hemodynamic abnormalities caused by impaired pump performance, definitions of heart failure must also recognize the abnormalities that cause the heart to deteriorate.

The following definition, which considers both the hemodynamic abnormalities and progressive deterioration of the failing heart, states that heart failure is *a clinical syndrome in which heart disease reduces cardiac output, increases venous pressures, and is accompanied by molecular and other abnormalities that cause progressive deterioration of the failing heart.*

HISTORICAL ASPECTS

Our modern understanding of heart failure has evolved through studies of clinical, physiological, anatomical, and biochemical abnormalities seen in this syndrome; more recently, efforts to understand this syndrome have come to consider molecular abnormalities seen in the failing heart (Table 1-1). Some, but not all, of these transitions exemplify *paradigm shifts,* as described by Thomas Kuhn (1970). According to Kuhn, a paradigm is a coherent tradition of scientific research that, while "sufficiently unprecedented to attract an enduring group of adherents away from competing models of scientific theory [is] sufficiently open-ended to leave all sorts of problems for the redefined group of practitioners to resolve." Inability of an established paradigm to explain new knowledge leads to a "crisis" that is resolved when the older paradigm is replaced by a new paradigm. This process, which Kuhn called a paradigm shift, is "revolutionary" because the new paradigm provides a radical approach to the unresolved problems that invalidates the earlier paradigm. The evolution of our understanding of heart failure summarized in Table 1-1 includes at least one clear Kuhnian paradigm shift; this occurred when Harvey's discovery that the heart is a pump that circulates the blood invalidated the ancient view that the heart generates and distributes heat by an ebb and flow. However, most other major advances in our understanding of heart failure have added to, rather than invalidated, earlier concepts; examples include identification of anatomical causes of heart failure by postmortem examinations, and recognition that abnormal calcium fluxes within cardiac myocytes contribute to the depressed contractility in failing hearts. Similarly, the recent ability of molecular biology to explain the progressive deterioration of the failing heart does not represent a Kuhnian paradigm shift because this

TABLE 1-1
Evolution of Our Understanding of Heart Failure
Heart failure as a clinical syndrome
Abnormal physiology (hemodynamics)
Abnormal anatomy (architecture)
Abnormal biochemistry
Molecular abnormalities

new knowledge, although revolutionary, is not irreconcilable with earlier views of the pathophysiology of heart failure (Katz, 1988; Katz and Katz, 1991).

Heart Failure as a Clinical Syndrome

Descriptions of patients who may have suffered from heart failure can be found in ancient Greek and Roman writings, but because the signs and symptoms in these patients are not diagnostic, most of these illnesses cannot be attributed to the syndrome we now recognize as heart failure. The severity of various clinical manifestations (Table 1-2) depends on whether the predominant abnormality is accumulation of blood behind the failing ventricle (backward failure) or reduced forward flow (forward failure), and whether the underlying cause affects primarily the right or left side of the heart (see Chapter 2). In patients with right heart failure, where the principal clinical manifestations are generally related to backward failure, accumulation of blood in the systemic veins elevates systemic venous pressure; this causes edema that, because of the effects of gravity, is greatest in the lower extremities. Backward failure of the right heart also causes the body cavities to fill with fluid—in the spaces surrounding the lungs as pleural effusions, in the peritoneal cavity as ascites, and as pericardial effusion in the sac that surrounds the heart. Together, these manifestations of backward failure of the right heart represent a syndrome called dropsy or anasarca. In backward failure of the left heart, accumulation of fluid in the pulmonary veins stiffens the lungs and leads to fluid transudation into the pulmonary

---

TABLE 1-2

Common Clinical Manifestations Noted in Early Descriptions of Heart FAILURE

Right Heart (Backward) Failure: Accumulation of blood "behind" the right heart elevates systemic venous pressure:

Edema: Painless soft swelling caused when fluid accumulates in the soft tissues. This is often referred to as "pitting edema" because a depression remains after removal of a finger slowly pressed into the swelling. This differs from edema due to infection, which is generally painful, inflamed, and indurated. Cardiac edema is most prominent in the ankles and legs, where gravity helps force fluid out of the capillaries into the soft tissues.

Dropsy, anasarca: Accumulation of fluid in the pleural spaces (pleural effusion), peritoneal cavity (ascites), and pericardium (pericardial effusion). This fluid, which is usually thin and colorless, differs from the yellow or green purulent fluid found when these cavities are infected and the bloody fluid usually found in malignant effusions.

Left Heart (Backward) Failure: Accumulation of blood "behind" the left ventricle elevates pulmonary venous pressures:

Dyspnea: Shortness of breath, typically worsened by effort. When severe, this can cause pulmonary edema (once called "acute dilatation") that can drown the patient.

Orthopnea: Shortness of breath that worsens when the patient lies down.

Paroxysmal nocturnal dyspnea: Episodes of shortness of breath that occur suddenly during sleep.

Low Output (Forward) Failure: Reduced cardiac output:

Weakness, fatigue, dyspnea: When severe, blood pressure decreases and tissue perfusion is reduced. This leads to weakness, confusion, cool and sweaty skin, dyspnea, and failure of various organs, notably the kidneys.

lymphatics and interstitium. These abnormalities cause patients to become short of breath (dyspnea) by increasing the work of breathing and impairing oxygen exchange across the alveolar membranes. When severe, backward failure of the left heart causes transudation of fluid into the air spaces, which results in pulmonary edema that can literally drown a patient. The clinical findings associated with forward failure (reduced cardiac output), which occur in both right and left heart failure, include weakness and fatigue.

The signs and symptoms described in the preceding paragraph occur in various diseases other than heart failure and so are not diagnostic. Edema, dropsy, anasarca, and dyspnea, the most common clinical manifestations of heart failure mentioned in early writings, have other causes. Edema in heart failure, which is typically soft, painless, and dependent, differs from that caused by infection or phlebitis, where the swelling is hard (indurated) and accompanied by pain and inflammation. However, liver and kidney failure, along with malnutrition, can also cause soft, painless, dependent edema, and patients with any of these conditions can develop dropsy and anasarca. Dyspnea, the major symptom of left heart failure, also occurs in lung disease, notably pneumonia and pulmonary tuberculosis, which, until the 20th century, were common causes of dyspnea. Weakness and fatigue, which are associated with low cardiac output, are also nonspecific. For these reasons, it was difficult—and often impossible—to identify patients with heart disease until the 16th and 17th centuries, when understanding of the circulation coupled with postmortem examinations made it possible to correlate clinical findings with pathophysiology.

The Hippocratic Writings

There is no doubt that a physician named Hippocrates (c. 460–370 B.C.E.) had achieved considerable renown in ancient Greece (Fig. 1-1). However, the many books included in the Hippocratic corpus represent a collection from a number of ancient sources. These medical texts include several clinical case histories, of which

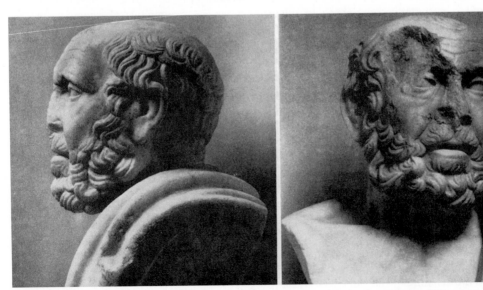

Figure 1-1: Roman copy of a Greek bust, found at the Roman port of Ostia, that may be of Hippocrates.

a few probably represent descriptions of heart disease (Katz and Katz, 1962). The latter include examples of dropsy that may have been due to right heart failure, and dyspnea that might have been caused by left heart failure; however, many of these patients could have suffered from diseases such as liver failure, kidney failure or phlebitis (edema and dropsy), and pneumonia or tuberculosis (dyspnea).

The Hippocratic corpus describes rales, the fine crackling sounds commonly heard in the lungs of patients with left heart failure: "When the ear is held to the chest, and one listens for some time, it may be heard to seethe inside like the boiling of vinegar" (*Diseases* II, LXI, tr. by the author from Littré, 1839–1861). The "succussion splash," heard when the ear is pressed against the chest of a patient with a large pleural effusion who is shaken vigorously (*Coan Prognostics*, 424), allowed the Hippocratic physician to localize and then drain this fluid:

> Incise over the third rib, down to the bone, then drill through the rib with a trephine. The perforation completed, remove a little water and after the evacuation, put in a plug of raw flax, and over this a soft sponge; you must then apply a bandage so that the plug does not fall out. You must take off the water over a period of twelve days, once daily; after the twelve days, on the thirteenth, evacuate all of the water. For the remaining time if more water forms, you must remove it (*Internal Afflictions* XXIII, tr. by AMK from Littré, 1839–1861).

However, there was no understanding of pathophysiology, as is apparent when dyspnea was attributed to the passage of "phlegm" (the cold humor) from the brain to the heart: "when the phlegm descends cold to the lungs and heart the blood is chilled; and the veins . . . beat forcefully against the lungs and heart, and the heart palpates, so that under this compulsion difficulty of breathing and orthopnea result" (*The Sacred Disease* IX, tr. Jones, 1923–1931).

Heart failure caused by rheumatic mitral valve disease probably explains the findings in a patient who:

> [I]n the fourth or fifth month of her pregnancy, had watery swellings in her legs, swellings in the hollows of her eyes, and her whole body puffed up. Besides these she had a dry cough, sometimes orthopnea, dyspnea and suffocation. Sometimes she was so near suffocation that she was obliged to sit up in bed without being able to lie down; and if she tried to sleep it was in a sitting position. Yet there was not much fever (*Epidemics* VII, tr. by AMK from Littré, 1839–1861).

As is common in this condition, the symptoms improved after the patient delivered her child.

The Hippocratic writings distinguish soft pitting edema, such as is seen in chronic heart failure (as well as hepatic and renal failure), and the indurated edema that is characteristic of phlebitis and cellulitis:

> Swellings that are painful . . . and hard indicate a danger of death in the near future; such as are soft and painless, yielding to the pressure of the finger, are of a more chronic character" (*Prognostics* VII, tr. Jones, 1923–1932),

and describe the wasting (cachexia) seen in end-stage heart failure:

> Dropsy is usually produced when the patient remains for a long time with impurities of the body following a long illness. The flesh is consumed and becomes water . . . the abdomen fills with water, the feet and legs swell, the shoulders, clavicles, chest and thighs melt away (*Affections* XXII, tr. by AMK from Littré, 1839–1861).

However, some of these patients probably suffered from malaria or nephritis, rather than heart disease.

Ancient physicians were unable to define the causes of these clinical syndromes because the heart's function as a pump was not understood; furthermore, early attempts to explain pathophysiology and provide treatment were based on a philosophy that viewed health as a balance between competing humors, a concept that had just emerged from Greek mythology (Katz and Katz, 1995).

The Alexandrians

In the third century B.C.E. the center of medical science shifted to Alexandria, in Egypt, where Herophilus (325–280 B.C.E.) and Erasistratus (c. 304–250 B.C.E.) practiced human dissection and carried out physiological experiments. Unfortunately, virtually all of their writings have been lost, so that most of what we know of these physicians comes from later citations of their work. Largely through Galen (see subsequent text) we learn that Erasistratus, who is sometimes called the "father of physiology," had come close to discovering the circulation. Galen tells us that Erasistratus described contraction and expansion of the heart and recognized the function of the semilunar valves, but held that the arteries contain *pneuma* (air) and that blood flows from the right ventricle into the veins. Although a few of these concepts presage modern circulatory physiology, they had no impact on the understanding of heart failure.

Roman Medicine

The poet Horace (65–8 B.C.E.) describes a man with what might be heart failure; the patient, who had "carried elaborate opulence almost to the point of decadence," developed dropsy along with intense thirst, which led Horace to write:

> Dire dropsy swells by feeding, and thirst
> is not quenched until the disease's cause
> has fled from the veins and watery dullness
> from the pallid flesh (*Odes*, Book II, 2, tr. Shepherd, 1983).

Celsus (25 B.C.E.–50 C.E.), a Roman aristocrat, may have been describing heart failure in a medical text that he compiled when he wrote:

> [W]hen dyspnoea [is severe] the patient can hardly draw in his breath unless with the neck outstretched . . . Blood-letting is the remedy unless anything prohibits it. Nor is that enough, but also the bowels are to be relaxed by milk, the stool being rendered liquid . . . as the body becomes depleted by these measures the patient begins to draw his breath more readily. Moreover, even in bed the head is to be kept raised (*De Medicina* IV. 8, tr. Spencer, 1938).

A century later, Aretæus of Cappadocia (2nd–3rd century C.E.) described the effects of gravity on the distribution of edema:

> When in an erect posture, [the patients] become swollen in their feet and legs, but when reclining, in the parts they lay upon; and if they change their position, the swelling changes accordingly, and the course of the cold humor [edema] is determined by its weight (tr. Adams, 1856).

Galen

Galen (c. 130–200 C.E.), the most influential of the Roman physicians, used palpation of the arterial pulse, which had been performed millennia earlier by the Egyptians (Saba et al., 2006), for prognostication. Galen described "complete irregularity or unevenness [of the pulse], both in the single beat and in the succession of beats" that almost certainly represents atrial fibrillation. He tells of Antipater, a physician, who after observing that he had an asymptomatic irregularity of the pulse, developed increasingly severe dyspnea followed by sudden death:

> Everybody knows what happened to Antipater, who practiced medicine with great renown in Rome. As a man less than 60 but more than 50 years of age, Antipater suffered from a short fever of unknown cause. It happened that he felt his pulse after the fever's decline in order to know what to do about himself. Antipater was at first shocked when he found a complete irregularity of his arterial pulse. . . .
>
> Antipater met me one day and stretched his arm out and, laughing, asked me to feel his pulse. Smiling in my turn I said: 'What is the riddle you want me to solve?'. . . Feeling his pulse I found complete irregularity . . . and asked him if he had any difficulties in breathing. He answered that he did not feel any difficulties. I observed him very frequently for six months to see if any change occurred, by feeling his radial pulse. . . .
>
> After a six months lapse . . . he experienced some but not a great deal of dyspnea with short-lasting palpitations of the heart; first once, then twice and three times a day. Then suddenly the respiration became very agitated; then it stopped and he died very suddenly (*De locis affectis*, 4, ii, tr. Siegel, 1968).

It has been suggested that Antipater suffered from rheumatic mitral valve disease (Siegel, 1968; Harris, 1973), but the appearance of atrial fibrillation in an otherwise asymptomatic middle-aged man who subsequently died after developing acute respiratory distress is more consistent with the natural history of untreated hypertension complicated by acute pulmonary edema and ventricular fibrillation.

Galen's failure to recognize the circulation of the blood is puzzling because he (like Erasistratus five centuries earlier [see previous discussion]) had recognized that contraction of muscular fibers in the walls of the heart decreases ventricular volume during systole, and was aware of the functions of the heart's valves:

> [The aortic and pulmonary valves] prevent any of the contents of the heart which are going outwards from returning back into it, and [the valves] in the mouths of the vessels bringing matter in [mitral and tricuspid valves] prevent matter from flowing back out of it (*De usu partium* II, K.iii.459–460, tr. Harris, 1973).

Galen also provided a lucid description of ventricular "suction" during diastole:

> Now the heart has every kind of power of attraction that one could imagine, and receives the [blood] quickly into the hollows of its ventricles, seizing it, and, as it were, sucking in the matter that is pouring into it (*De usu partium* VI.15.K.iii 480–481, tr. Harris, 1973).

Although Galen viewed the heart as the source of arterial pulsations, he did not realize that it is a pump, as evidenced by his statement:

> [T]he arteries are not filled like an inflated wineskin by the heart's squeezing the pneuma out; but because they are attached to the heart and grow from it, they share the same power as the whole organ. And that the whole body of the heart pulsates, expanding and contracting of itself (*Of Hippocrates and Plato* VI 7.7–8, tr. De Lacy, 1984).

In describing the function of these pulsations, he states:

> By their dilatations the arteries draw into the body the outside air through the openings that extend to the skin, for three purposes: to cool, to fan, and to generate psychic pneuma. Then by their contraction the arteries squeeze out as much of the humors in them as has become sooty and smoky (*Of Hippocrates and Plato* VIII 8.7–8, tr. De Lacy, 1984).

Galen's failure to appreciate that the heart is a pump (Fig. 1-2) may have been due in part to his misinterpretation of an experiment carried out to explain the arterial pulse. After ligating a hollow tube within an artery, Galen observed that distal pulsations were abolished even though blood continued to flow through the artery. He interpreted these findings to mean that "the power of dilatation of the arteries [the pulse] is communicated to their coats by the heart, and not by matter flowing through the tube" (*De Sang. in art*, K733, tr. Harris, 1973). Today, we would attribute the absent distal pulsations to the increased resistance to flow caused when the tube reduced luminal diameter.

Galen's view that the heart generates pulsations that are transmitted along the walls of the arteries, rather than by pulsatile flow through the lumen, dominated thinking about the pathophysiology of dyspnea, edema, and dropsy until Harvey described the circulation more than 1,500 years later.

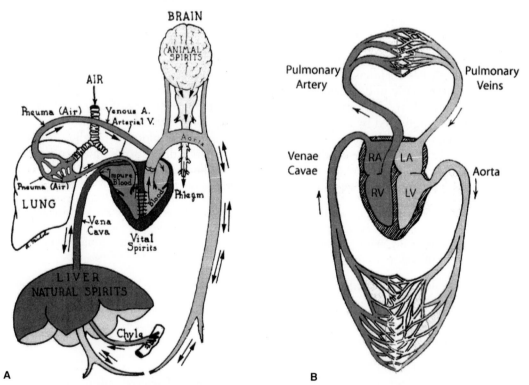

Figure 1-2: Two views of the circulation. **A:** Galen's view. Pneuma derived from air reaches the heart from the lungs via the venous artery (pulmonary artery) and arterial vein (pulmonary veins). Natural spirits that enter the heart from the liver, along with vital spirits (heat) generated in the left ventricle, are distributed throughout the body by an ebb and flow in the arteries. Animal spirits transported from the brain through nerves as phlegm contribute to formation of pleural effusions. Modified from Major RH (1954). *A History of Medicine*. Springfield IL, CC Thomas. **B:** The view after Harvey. Deoxygenated blood is darkly shaded; oxygenated blood is lightly shaded. Modified from Starling EH (1926). *Principles of Human Physiology*. Philadelphia, Lea & Febiger.

Medieval Clinical Observations

Avicenna (980–1037), one of the great Arab physicians who had access to Greek and Roman medical texts, along with Persian and Indian texts, noted the effect of posture on dyspnea and the use of accessory muscles of respiration in patients with dyspnea:

> [P]ernicious suffocation hastens to stop the breathing; when the patient lies down, his breathing is hindered completely, and when he is not recumbent his breathing is difficult also. In addition, he himself keeps extending his neck in contriving to breathe. He is restless and wants to stand erect and cannot lie down (*Canon of Medicine* iii.11.1.9, tr. Jarcho, 1980).

Even though Avicenna did not appreciate the pathophysiological connection between heart disease and dyspnea, he was aware that pericardial tamponade impairs ventricular filling:

> For fluids are very often found between [the bulk of the heart and its membrane]. And it is known that when they are abundant they restrain the heart from diastole (*Canon of Medicine* iii.11.1.2, Jarcho, 1980).

The ability of a pericardial effusion to prevent the heart from filling, which was recognized shortly after Harvey described the circulation, provided the first link between impaired cardiac pumping and clinical heart failure (see subsequent text).

The Fasciculus Medicinae of Johannes de Ketham (Fig. 1-3), published in 1491 shortly after Gutenberg's invention of movable type, represents a medical guide that combined "various rules, graphic diagrams and schemes that were in actual daily use by medical men" (Sudhoff K, in Singer, 1988). The author/compiler Johannes de Ketham (Johan von Kircheim, active 1455–1470) defined dropsy as "an error of the nutritive faculty" and carditis as "the disease by which the heart palpitates." de Ketham's proposal that carditis is caused "from great warmth and from overabundant blood" echoes the ancient view that the heart is the source of the body's heat.

To treat dropsy, de Ketham recommended that the physician "take scabwort and grind and squeeze its juice through a cloth, collect in an eggshell and temper with honeycomb; give the patient daily a full shell of the juice, do this for eleven days when the moon is waning because also man wanes in his abdomen" (Singer, 1988). For carditis, de Ketham's treatment includes aromatic ointments made of roses, violets, and flax, or from cinnamon, clove-gilly flowers, cubeb, aloe wood, anise and violets, and the bone of stag's heart, along with phlebotomy from the left hand" We should resist the temptation to laugh at these treatments because medieval physicians had no knowledge of the pathophysiology of heart disease; humility is also appropriate because it is only recently that inotropic therapy for heart failure was recognized to do more harm than de Ketham's herbal remedies (see Chapter 7).

Autopsy Findings before Harvey's Description of the Circulation

Early in the 16th century, clinical investigations began to be carried out by physicians who observed their patients until they died, after which they (or someone whom they supervised) performed an autopsy in an effort to identify the cause of the patient's illness. However, these early autopsies were performed at a time when there was little or no knowledge of hemodynamics, which made it impossible to identify the pathophysiological basis for the clinical manifestations of heart failure. This is apparent in

Figure 1-3: Detail of a drawing of the anatomy of a pregnant woman showing the heart in the left chest giving rise to a single vessel that connects to the throat. The words in the left heart are "cough of lung" and "sanguineness"; those in the right heart are "cardiac ailment." At the base of the "aorta" is written "Asthma." (Reprinted with permission from Singer C (1988). *The Fasciculus Medicinae of Johannes de Ketham.* Birmingham AL, The Classics of Medicine Library, Gryphon Editions, 1988.)

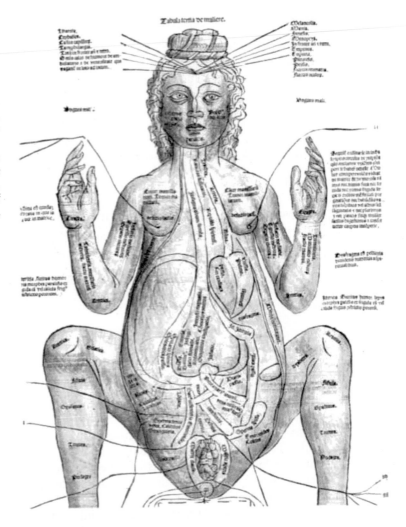

the *Sepulchretum,* a collection of early autopsy reports published in 1679 by Théophile Bonet; most consist of "two or three lines of symptomatology and four or five lines of gross autopsy findings" (White, 1957). A few of these patients appear to have had heart disease, including a man with calcific aortic stenosis who died suddenly, a patient with dyspnea who had a diseased heart, and the following patient who appears to have developed acute pulmonary edema caused by coronary artery disease:

> A very fat poet who for a long time had suffered from asthma and frequency of urination and for some little time also from dull pain in the left side, spent a convivial evening at dinner with friends and relatives reciting to them all manner of odes, both hilarious and sad, including even a funeral lamentation. At nine o'clock he rose from his seat and as he made the effort of mounting the stairs he was seized with an increasing difficulty in drawing his breath. Aided by his secretary, with great effort he reached his couch, reclined, accepted absolution, and expired. The next day when his abdomen was opened, everything was found loaded with fat. . . . The heart was rather large and the coronary blood vessels were unexpectedly and extensively bony with thin membranes covering the bone on both sides, and in two places the bony walls were so contiguous that not even the point of a fine needle could enter. The lungs were large (White, 1942).

Hieronymus Capivaccius, a Professor at the University of Padua who died in 1589—less than 40 years before Harvey's discovery of the circulation—accepted the ancient view that the heart is the source of the body's warmth. He did, however, provide an excellent description of what we would recognize today as manifestations of the neurohumoral response to a fall in cardiac output (see Chapter 3):

> In general this disease is recognized by the fact that the pulse becomes small and weak in all dimensions . . . It is recognized also by the fact that the face is pale because the spirit, and with the spirit the blood, is recalled to the heart; for the same reason the external structures are cold. It is recognized also by sweat and dewy moisture, especially in the forehead . . . and the skin is cold because the heat has been recalled (*Opera Omnia* 2.9.433, tr. Jarcho, 1980).

Ludovicus Mercatus (Luiz Mercado, c. 1520–c. 1606), a Spanish physician, recognized the relationship between dyspnea and dropsy in describing the origins of pleural effusion. However, he followed earlier views that can be traced back to Hippocrates when he referred to the " . . . thin, serous fluid, which either rushes down copiously by reason of its thinness from the brain through the trachea and lungs, or from the rest of the body or from the abdominal cavity in dropsical persons, and reaches there through hidden ducts" (*De internorum morborum curatione* 2.4.175–182, tr. Jarcho, 1980).

Carolus Piso (Charles le Pois, 1563–1633), who like Harvey studied at the University of Padua, provided an elegant description of paroxysmal nocturnal dyspnea:

> [A] nobleman somewhat more than eighty years old . . . gradually began to be oppressed by severe difficulty in breathing, which manifested itself especially at night. After he had first fallen asleep as usual, a suffocation would suddenly excite the old man and interrupt his sleep, so that against his will he was obliged to get out of bed and rush at once to the windows of his bedroom in order to breathe fresh air through dilated nostrils. The old man could be seen, with inflamed face, drawing breath deeply, and with his shoulders trembling. He could not remain quietly in one place and especially could not stand the fireplace but exposed himself even in a severe winter. Gradually and inevitably as the day advanced he would be relieved of his oppression, especially in the afternoon, but during the next sleep the affection returned and troubled the old man again. . . .
>
> Having carefully observed the gasping and having reflected for hours on the causes of such obstinate oppression, which made a daily cycle, I concluded finally that the fluid which was occupying his bronchi and the lung itself, or which more probably was stagnating in the middle of his chest, was of the kind that at the time of sleep through return of the vital spirit flowing back into the precordia received a certain new fervor, so that while bubbling in this way it could not be kept within its own space as formerly and it would necessarily compress the lungs and block their free motion. However, when this fervor gradually became spontaneously quiescent and the spirit flowed again out of the precordia into the body generally, as is the case of persons who are awake, then the lungs could more freely regain their space and the patient could breathe without such great oppression (*Selectiorum observationum et consiliorum de praetervisis hactenus morbis affectibusque praeter naturam, ab aqua seu serosa colluvie et diluvie ortis*, 214–216, tr. Jarcho, 1980).

A postmortem examination performed on this patient by a surgeon "who was bolder in dissecting the dead patient than in striking and opening him while he was alive, found the lung and precordia floating in a large amount of water which was enclosed within the walls of the thorax" (*Selectiorum*, 216, tr. Jarcho, 1980).

This autopsy confirmed Piso's view that accumulation of fluid in the chest caused the progressive dyspnea, but because Piso did not know that the heart is a pump, it remained for others to identify the connection between "dropsy of the thorax" and heart disease.

Abnormal Physiology (Hemodynamics)

Harvey's Discovery of the Circulation

William Harvey (1578–1657) (Fig. 1-4) provided the first clear description of the circulation in his *De Motu Cordis* (*Movement of the Heart*), published in 1628. Harvey's proof included a calculation showing that the amount of blood flowing from the heart is much greater than could be derived from the foodstuffs metabolized in the liver. His conclusion, which was to revolutionize cardiology, is stated forcefully and succinctly:

> I am obliged to conclude that in animals the blood is driven round a circuit with an unceasing, circular sort of movement, that this is an activity or function of the heart which it carries out by virtue of its pulsation, and that in sum it constitutes the sole reason for that heart's pulsatile movement (*Movement of the Heart and Blood in Animals*, Chapter 14, tr. Franklin, 1957).

Even though Harvey was a physician, he did little to clarify the link between an impaired cardiac pump and the signs and symptoms of heart failure. He did note that obstruction of the return of blood to the heart causes edema, that application of a ligature sufficiently tight to obstruct venous but not arterial flow causes tissue swelling, and that weak cardiac contraction causes a weak pulse:

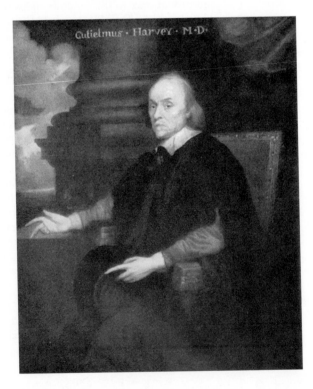

Figure 1-4: William Harvey. State portrait at the Royal College of Physicians, painted when Harvey was in his late 60s.

[W]hen the heart beats over-languidly [*languidius* = weak], it is not only in the fingers but also in the wrist and temples that I have failed to detect a pulse; this I have experienced in cases of fainting, of onset of hysterical symptoms, and of asphyxia, also in over weak subjects and in those about to die (*De Motu Cordis,* Chapter 17, tr. Franklin, 1957).

Although Harvey's concept of the circulation (Fig. 1-2) provided the key to understanding the hemodynamic basis for clinical heart failure (see subsequent text), the views of Galen and others persisted; for example, Melchior Sebezius, Jr., in a text published in 1661, attributed hydrothorax to the cold humor:

[I]n some patients the water of dropsy travels through imperceptible and hidden channels into the thoracic cavity and then into the bronchi of the lungs, even though these channels are unknown to us. . . . For when the lung is strongly chilled by food, drink, medicine, air and other causes, it is likely that it can produce a large amount of serum and water, and this is properly regarded as a cause of dropsy (*Manualis, sive speculi medicinae practici* .3.1.815–818, tr. Jarcho, 1980).

Early Descriptions of the Hemodynamics of Heart Failure

The relationship between the clinical manifestations of heart failure and anatomic abnormalities of the heart was recognized on postmortem examination within decades after Harvey pointed out that the heart is a pump. Because medical advances were widely discussed among authorities, and because case reports were generally collected in books that often appeared after the author's death, it is difficult to assign priority for 17th and 18th century discoveries. Furthermore, as is true for most discoveries, the circulatory causes for heart failure were recognized almost simultaneously by several individuals (Fig. 1-5), so that it is not possible to credit a single individual with the first description of the hemodynamic basis of heart failure.

Lazare Rivière (1589–1655) (Fig. 1-6), an early advocate of Harvey's view of the circulation, described the hemodynamic consequences of left ventricular outflow obstruction in a patient who died from what was probably aortic stenosis complicated by infectious endocarditis. This case report appeared in Rivière's *Opera omnia*, published in 1723, almost 50 years after his death. Rivière described a patient who, after several days of palpitations, increasing dyspnea, bloodstained

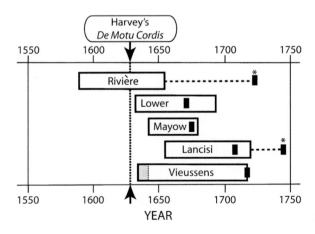

Figure 1-5: Time lines showing events at the time of publication of Harvey's *De Motu Cordis* (*vertical dotted line*) and the births and deaths of Rivière, Lower, Mayow, Lancisi, and Vieussens (*rectangles;* the *shaded area* for Vieussens reflects uncertainty regarding the date of his birth). Dates of key publications (see text) are shown by the *thick vertical rectangles;* posthumous publications are indicated by *asterisks.* Modified from Katz AM (2004). Raymond Vieussens and the 'first' pathophysiological description of heart failure. Dialogues Cardiovasc Med 9:179–182.

Figure 1-6: Lazare Riviére. Frontispiece to his *Practice of Physick*. Reprinted from Major RH (1945). *Classic Descriptions of Disease,* 3rd ed. Springfield IL, CC Thomas.

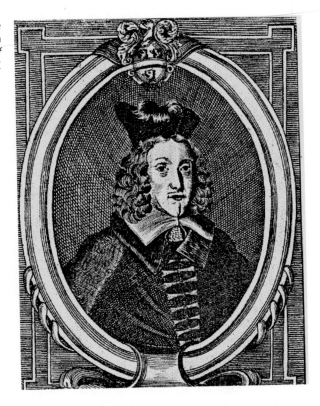

sputum, and swollen legs, worsened until "no pulse appeared at the wrist, and when the hand was applied over the heart, a most rapid, weak, and irregular palpitation was felt." The patient soon died and the autopsy demonstrated "round carbuncles . . . which resembled a cluster of hazelnuts & filled up the opening of the aorta" (Major, 1945). Rivière's understanding of the hemodynamic consequences of impaired left ventricular ejection is apparent in his statement: "[T]he ventricle was filled with a blood mass and the whole lung was filled with much blood from which the suffocation of the natural beat spread to each part. . . . For the blood ascending continually by the vena cava . . . to the heart overflowed in the lung and filled it up" (Major, 1945). However, this case description concludes with an echo of Galen's view that the heart is a furnace when Rivière speculates that the carbuncles "were caused by the excessive blood which the marked heat of the ventricle hardened & in this manner changed its substance" (Major, 1945).

The link between heart disease and dropsy was described by Richard Lower (1631–1691) (Fig. 1-7), who was one of a remarkable group of Oxford scientists that included Robert Hooke, Christopher Wren, Robert Boyle, Thomas Willis, and John Mayow (see subsequent text). Lower, in his *Tractus de Corde, item de motu, et colore sanguinis et chili in eum transitu,* published in 1669, stated that when the heart lacks the strength to "[preserve] a constant circulation of the blood [by] driving this fluid everywhere in regular sequence and in due quantity through the vessels, [the movement of the blood is] feeble and slow." He noted that this can occur when "the parenchyma of the heart . . . is too heavily laden with fat, or suffers from inflammation, ulcer, abscess, or a wound, so that it is unable to pulsate and contract without great difficulty or hardship" (Gunther, 1932). Lower identified the role of pericardial tamponade as a cause of impaired cardiac function:

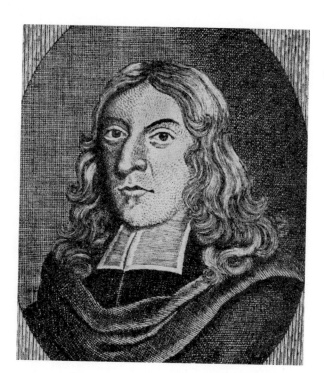

Figure 1-7: Richard Lower at age 55. Reprinted from Major RH. (1945) *Classic Descriptions of Disease,* 3rd Ed. Springfield IL, CC Thomas.

[T]he walls of the [heart] are compressed on all sides by the surrounding fluid to such an extent, that they are unable to dilate sufficiently to receive the blood, the heart-beat diminishes greatly, until at length it is completely suppressed...and syncope and death result (Gunther, 1932).

One of Lower's few case reports describes the pathophysiology of constrictive pericarditis:

[T]he wife of a certain citizen of London, aged 30, healthy and active enough previously, [who] became very dejected and melancholy during the last three years of her life, suffered from breathlessness on the least exertion, had a small and often intermittent pulse, and complained almost continually of attacks of pain and of great physical discomfort in the precordium. She had at last become subject to frequent fainting fits, and to loss of consciousness and chilling of the extremities on the gentlest movement of the body . . . her strength at length slowly exhausted [and] she died (Gunther, 1932).

At autopsy Lower found the patient's lungs to be "healthy enough" but the pericardium was "closely attached all over the surface of the heart [and] had become thick, opaque, and hard, instead of being thin and transparent as it should naturally have been. Hence, as there was no space for the free movement of the heart, and no fluid for moistening its surface, it is little wonder that she complained all the time of these ills" (Gunther, 1932).

John Mayow (1634–1679) (Fig. 1-8), a contemporary of Lower at Oxford, described how obstruction of blood flow into the aorta or pulmonary artery causes the arterial pulse to be "quite languid" and why, in mitral stenosis, the right ventricle becomes dilated:

Figure 1-8: John Mayow. Frontispiece to his *Tractus Quinque*. Reprinted from Major RH (1954). *A History of Medicine.* Springfield IL, CC Thomas.

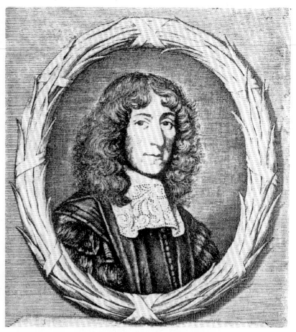

[T]he blood could not, on account of the obstruction, pass into the left ventricle of the heart [so that] the pulmonary blood-vessels and also the right ventricle were necessarily distended with blood (*Tractus Quinque*, tr. East, 1958).

Mayow postulated that the "asthmatic paroxysm [was caused by] blood stagnating in the pulmonary vessels." He was among the first to recognize the pathophysiology of overload-induced hypertrophy, stating that because the right ventricle in this patient was "forced to contract violently so as to propel the mass of the blood as much as possible through the lungs into the left ventricle . . . this also accounts for the great thickness and strength of the right ventricle since muscles accustomed to more violent exercise increase more than others" (*Tractus Quinqu*, tr. East, 1958).

Giovanni Maria Lancisi (1654–1720) (Fig. 1-9), who was educated in Rome and became physician to several popes, described the hemodynamic consequences of obstruction to blood flow through the heart in his *De subitaneis mortibus*, which was published in 1707. He described a young man with shortness of breath and a "buried strangling over the precordia" who died suddenly and was found at autopsy to have aortic "obstruction," and suggested that the "oppression and . . . heaviness of the precordia from which the patient ultimately died [occurred because] the left ventricle . . . was prevented from propelling readily the larger amount of blood into the obstructed aorta. This delay of blood, to be sure, brought about the oppression of the precordia and ultimately the deadly suffocation and syncope" (*De subitaneis mortibus*, 185–195, tr. Jarcho, 1980).

Lancisi, in *De Aneurysmatibus*, published in 1745, 25 years after his death, stated that aortic valve narrowing causes blood to be "driven into the left cavity and . . . retarded in the pulmonary vein as far as the vena cava," and that this results in dyspnea and dilation of the chambers behind the obstruction. He related dependent edema to backward failure of the right heart and stated that "dilatation of the right cavities of the heart" could be diagnosed when the jugular veins "are in turn

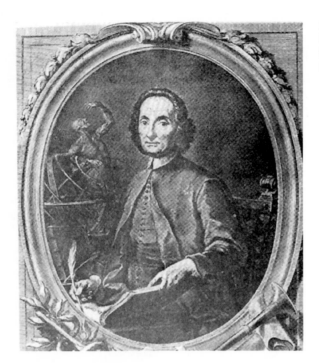

Figure 1-9: Giovanni Maria Lancisi. Etching by Sebastian Conra. Reprinted from Major RH (1954). *A History of Medicine.* Springfield IL, CC Thomas.

dilated, undulate, are agitated in a remarkable manner and collapse." He described the hemodynamics of tricuspid insufficiency, noting that "incompletely closed valves at the mouth of the vena cava [cause blood] to be driven back again through gaping chinks of the valves and forced back along the whole path of the superior vena cava; then from that path it flows straight on into the jugulars" to cause dilatation of the neck veins. He also identified the hemodynamic cause for the large "v" waves and rapid "y" descent seen in tricuspid insufficiency, noting that "when the systole of the heart ceases, the blood without delay flows back downward from the jugulars into the vena cave; hence the jugulars cease to swell and in their turn collapse" (*Aneurysmatibus* Proposition LVII, tr. Wright, 1952).

Lancisi also described what appears to have been familial arrhythmogenic right ventricular cardiomyopathy in a "family of high rank," of which four male members—great-grandfather, grandfather, father, and son—suffered from palpitations. At autopsy, all three who died had "aneurysm" of the right ventricle. Lancisi concludes: "It may well be that what I have so far observed only in the right cavities of the heart can also occur in other channels of the blood as well" (*Aneurysmatibus*, Proposition XLVII, tr. White, 1952). As noted in the subsequent text, Lancisi also described architectural abnormalities in failing hearts.

Raymond Vieussens (c. 1633–1641 to 1715) (Fig. 1-10), who was educated in Montpelier, provided the most complete of the early descriptions of the pathophysiology of heart failure. Vieussens also described the anterior medullary velum between the cerebellar peduncles (valve of Vieussens), a mass of white matter within the cerebral hemispheres (centrum ovale or Vieussens' centrum), a small space sometimes found within the septum pellucidum beneath the corpus callosum (fifth ventricle or Vieussens' ventricle), the celiac ganglia (ganglia of Vieussens), and a loop of sympathetic fibers linking the middle and inferior cervical ganglia (ansa subclavia or Vieussens' loop). In the heart, he described collateral vessels connecting the

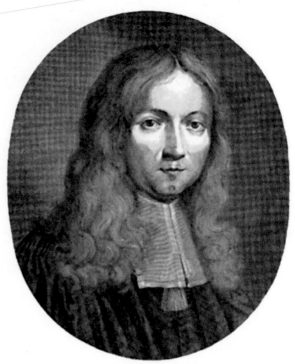

Figure 1-10: Raymond Vieussens as a young man. Reprinted from Major RH (1954). *A History of Medicine.* Springfield IL, CC Thomas.

left anterior descending and right coronary arteries (circle of Vieussens), a fold of endothelium at the junction of the great cardiac vein and coronary sinus ostium (Vieussens' valve), and a depression along the margin of the fossa ovalis (limbus fossae ovalis or Vieussens' annulus); he may also have been the first to describe small communications, now generally called thebesian vessels, that connect coronary vessels to the ventricular cavities.

In his *Traité nouveau de la structure et des causes du movement naturel du coeur,* published in 1715 (the year he died), Vieussens discussed the pathophysiological basis for dyspnea and pleural effusions in a patient with mitral stenosis. He began by describing the clinical syndrome in a patient who, a week before he died:

> [W]as lying in bed with his head very high. It seemed to me that his breathing was very difficult. His heart was burdened by a violent palpitation. His pulse seemed very small, weak and altogether irregular. His lips had the color of lead, his eyes showed great dejection, and his legs and thighs were swollen and were cold instead of warm.

At autopsy the thoracic cavity was found to be filled with yellowish serum, the heart was huge, approaching the size of an ox heart, the right atria and ventricle were "excessively large," and the tricuspid valve annulus was dilated. Vieussens then described the stenotic mitral valve (Fig. 1-11):

> [T]he entrance of the left ventricle appeared to be extremely small and . . . looking for the cause of such a surprising fact I discovered that the [mitral valve leaflets] were truly bony [and] that the [mitral valve] had shrunk greatly. . . . The entry of the left ventricle having become greatly contracted and its margin having lost all its natural suppleness, the blood could not pass freely and as abundantly as it should into

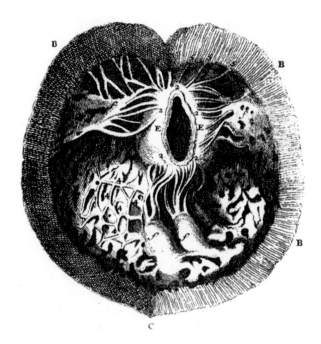

Figure 1-11: Vieussens' illustration of the narrowed mitral valve, viewed from below, illustrating the typical fish mouth appearance of rheumatic mitral stenosis. Reprinted from Major RH (1954). *A History of Medicine.* Springfield IL, CC Thomas.

the cavity of this ventricle. As soon as the circulation became impeded by this, it began to expand to an extraordinary extent the trunk of the pulmonary vein, because the blood remained there too long and accumulated there in too large an amount. The blood had no sooner begun to stay too long in the trunk of this vein than it delayed the [flow] of the blood in all the blood vessels of the lung, so that the branches of the pulmonary artery and vein, spread by all the tissue of this organ, were always too full of blood and hence so dilated that they compressed the [lung parenchyma] enough to prevent the air from entering freely and leaving just as freely. This is why the patient always breathed with great difficulty. Since the blood in the lung thickened considerably during its long sojourn in the blood vessels, part of its serum separated little by little and fell into the thoracic cavity (*Traité nouveau de la structure et des causes du movement naturel du cœur,* 105–106, tr. Jarcho, 1980).

Vieussens then commented: "The smallness, the weakness, and the irregularity of his pulse were caused by the excessive smallness of the amount of blood that the left ventricle furnished to the aorta."

In another case report in *Traité nouveau*, Vieussens described the hemodynamics of aortic insufficiency in a patient whose pulse was so strong "that the artery of each arm struck my fingertips just as a strongly stretched and violently shaken cord would have done. The patient's pulse, of which I have never seen and never hope to see the like, convinced me that he was suffering from a violent palpitation of the heart." A few days later the patient died, and at autopsy the left ventricle was found to be "dilated to an extraordinary extent" and the aortic valves "greatly stretched and cut off at the end" so that during diastole "the aorta...sent back into the left ventricle a part of the blood that it had just received" (tr. Jarcho, 1980).

Vieussens' use of clinical and postmortem data to explain the hemodynamic basis for the signs and symptoms of heart failure in these two cases, which was made possible by Harvey's discovery of the circulation, ranks among the monumental achievements in cardiology.

Later 17th and 18th Century Descriptions of Heart Failure

The hemodynamic causes of signs and symptoms of heart failure were noted by several other 17th century physicians, including Marcello Malpighi (1628–1694), whose discovery of the capillaries completed Harvey's description of the circulation. Malpighi proposed that dyspnea is caused by "particles" that impede blood flow through the lungs:

> [W]hen blood reaches the heart and lungs, the dregs ["acid particles" arising from poorly digested food] with which the ends of the veins are supplied alter the entry of blood into the heart. As a result the respiration and pulse are changed, for when blood in the lungs has been delayed, their weight is increased. This causes dyspnea (*Marcelli Malpighi, et Jo: Marie Lancisii consultationum medicarum*, Consultation 2, tr. Jarcho, 1980).

Malpighi's writings provide a surprisingly modern view of the role of fluid transudation in causing dyspnea, which he suggested is caused by "impeded passage of blood through the lungs" (*Marcelli Malpighi, et Jo: Marie Lancisii consultationum medicarum*, Consultation 29, tr. Jarcho, 1980). He also stated that edema occurs "when the veins were not resorbing the fluid pushed forth by the arteries" (*Marcelli Malpighi, et Jo: Marie Lancisii consultationum medicarum*, Consultation 29, tr. Jarcho, 1980).

The conservatism that resists scientific progress is illustrated in an attack on Malpighi's work by a former pupil, Paolo Mini, who wrote:

> No wise man will deny that Almighty God has prepared a wonderful domicile in the body for the most noble human soul. But it is our firm opinion that the anatomy of the exceedingly small, internal conformation of the viscera, which has been extolled in these very times, is of use to no physician (Andelmann, 1966).

Sadly, Mini's skepticism regarding the practical value of basic research, is still found today.

Georgio Baglevi (1668–1706), in a text published in 1696, rejected the Hippocratic view that dyspnea is caused by descent of the cold humor from the brain. Instead, he proposed that pulmonary edema is caused by the accumulation of blood and lymph in the lungs:

> Next is to be considered a dangerous disease of the lungs, which is called suffocative catarrh. It is caused chiefly by stagnation of sudden coagulation of blood in the lungs and about the precordium. . . . In this kind of catarrh the patient has a cold, and pain in the chest, and difficulty in breathing; also interrupted speech, anxiety, cough, stertor, a widely spaced slow pulse, foam at the mouth, and the like. . . . The foam at the mouth is caused by impaired circulation of blood about the lungs and consequent circulation of the lymph in the upper parts of the body near the face; hence this [kind of] catarrh comes from sudden stagnation of blood in the vicinity of the heart and lungs, and not from phlegm running down from the head as the ancients believed to be the condition in this disease . . . An instant remedy for this disease during the paroxysm is repeated bloodletting. . . . The disease is very precipitous; unless phlebotomy is done immediately the blood coagulates more and stagnates. Thus the opportunity for cure is lost (*De praxi medica*, tr. Jarcho, 1980).

Although virtually every physician since antiquity had practiced phlebotomy, the urgency of Baglevi's recommendation suggests that he appreciated the ability of reduced blood volume to alleviate the severity of acute pulmonary edema.

A less physiological view of dropsy, which echoes 2,000-year-old Hippocratic writings, was published in 1769, almost 150 years after *De Motu Cordis,* by William Buchan (1729–1805), who described dropsy as:

[A] preternatural swelling of the whole body, or some part of it, occasioned by a collection of watery humour. . . . I have often known the dropsy occasioned by drinking large quantities of cold, weak, watery liquor when the body is heated by violent exercise. A low, damp, or marshy situation is likewise a frequent cause of it, hence it is also a common disease in moist, flat, fenny countries. It may also be brought on by a long use of a poor watery diet, or of viscous aliment that is hard of digestion. It is often the effect of other diseases, as the jaundice, a [cirrhosis] of the liver, a violent ague of long continuance, a diarrhœa, a dysentery, an empyema, or a consumption of the lungs. In short, whatever obstructs the circulation of the blood, or prevents its being duly prepared, may occasion a dropsy (Buchan, 1774, Ch. XXXVII, 43).

William Withering (1741–1799), who in 1783 identified digitalis leaf as the active ingredient in a remedy used to treat dropsy by "an old woman of Shropshire," recognized that digitalis "has a power over the motion of the heart, to a degree yet unobserved in any other medicine, and that this power may be converted to salutary ends." However, Withering viewed the drug primarily as a diuretic, as is apparent in his description of the effects of digitalis on a woman in her 40s who was:

[N]early in a state of suffocation; her pulse extremely weak and irregular, her breath very short and laborious, her countenance sunk, her arms of a leaden colour, clammy and cold. She could not lye down in bed, and had neither strength nor appetite but was extremely thirsty. Her stomach, legs and thighs were greatly swollen; her urine very small in quantity, not more than a spoonful at a time, and that very seldom. It had been proposed to scarify her legs, but the proposition was not acceded to . . . [Administration of five doses of digitalis] made her very sick, and acted very powerful upon the kidneys, for within the first twenty-four hours she made upwards of eight quarts of water. The sense of fullness and oppression across her stomach was greatly diminished, her breath was eased, her pulse became more full and regular, and the swellings in her legs subsided (Major, 1945, 442).

Although we do not know the diagnosis in this patient, Withering stated that she was alive 9 years later. In a woman with atrial fibrillation and heart failure, this history is consistent with rheumatic tricuspid and/or mitral stenosis, where slowing of the heart can lead to long-lasting improvement.

Architectural Anatomy (Architecture): Concentric and Eccentric Hypertrophy (Dilatation)

The prognostic implications of different patterns of cardiac enlargement attracted attention at the end of the 18th century, when physicians began to relate various architectural changes in diseased hearts to specific clinical syndromes. Subsequently, throughout the 19th century, efforts were made to understand the prognostic implications of different patterns of cardiac enlargement, and to determine whether cardiac hypertrophy is a compensatory (adaptive) response to a hemodynamic overload or whether the enlargement contributed to clinical deterioration. At the same time, distinction between eccentric hypertrophy (dilatation) and concentric hypertrophy (usually referred to simply as "hypertrophy") led to questions regarding the prognostic significance of these different types of cardiac enlargement.

Distinctions between Eccentric Hypertrophy (Dilatation)
and Concentric Hypertrophy

Lancisi (see previous discussion) was among the first to distinguish between eccentric hypertrophy, which he called *dilatationem* (dilatation) and *augmento molis* (concentric hypertrophy):

> So varied and so serious are the maladies of the heart that we often discover that it has suffered from an increase of its own bulk [*augmento molis*]. . . . Nor do I mean here by increased *dilatationem* of the cavities only, but thickening of the fibers and increase of density [which] makes the base of the heart larger and heavier than is normal (*Aneurysmatibus*, Proposition XLVIII, tr. Wright, 1952).

He also recognized that dilatation weakens the heart:

> [T]he left ventricle, on account of the lessened force because of the dilatation, was prevented from propelling readily the larger amount of blood into the aorta (*De subitaneis mortibus*, 193, tr. Jarcho, 1980).

and noted that valvular regurgitation leads to ventricular dilatation because the cavities are "easily distended by the force of the blood that is regurgitated." (*Aneurysmatibus*, Proposition L, tr. Wright, 1952.) Lancisi noted that the cavity of the left ventricle does not dilate in severe aortic stenosis; this was seen at autopsy in a Canon of St. Peter's who died of "suffocative asthma":

> [O]f the valves of the aortic orifice one [was found to have] become ossified and two cartilaginous, and from this cause the path of the blood from the heart into that artery had become remarkably narrow . . . we observed, not without surprise, that the left cavities of the heart were quite sound and had not suffered at all from dilatation (*Aneurysmatibus*, Proposition LIII, tr. Wright, 1952).

Giovanni Battista Morgagni (1682–1771) (Fig. 1-12) published additional insights regarding the pathophysiology of cardiac hypertrophy in a series of letters entitled

Figure 1-12: Giovanni Battista Morgagni. Reprinted from Major RH (1954). *A History of Medicine.* Springfield IL, CC Thomas.

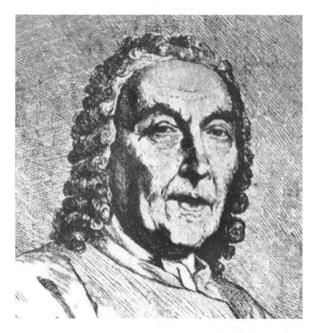

De sedibus et causes morborum. This text, published in 1761, describes 640 autopsies that include not only his own cases but also those of others, including Vieussens' patient with mitral stenosis described above. Morgagni recognized the adaptive nature of over-load-induced right ventricular hypertrophy in mitral stenosis, where increased pressure behind the narrowed mitral valve restricts right ventricular ejection; as a result:

> [B]oth the auricles, with their adjoining [veins] . . . and the trunk of the pulmonary artery, and the right ventricle, were much distended, and the columnae and fibers of the same ventricle, were become very thick; which might happen because . . . a greater thickness of the muscles is the consequence of their more frequent and stronger actions (*The Seats and Causes of Diseases*, Letter XVII, Article 13, tr. Alexander, 1769).

He described left ventricular hypertrophy with dilatation in a 33-year-old shoe-maker who had suffered from dyspnea for several years and whose aortic valve leaflets were "very lank, and contracted into themselves, somewhat rigid also, and a little hard." Morgagni noted:

> [B]y retaining the blood therein (which, as it was in greater quantity, would more irritate the fibres, and at the same time give more resistance to the increased efforts of the heart), could by degrees more and more distract, and dilate the heart (*The Seats and Causes of Diseases*, Letter XVIII, Article 4, tr. Alexander, 1769).

Jean-Baptiste de Sénac (1693–1770) distinguished between eccentric and concentric hypertrophy in 1749, when he wrote: "The volume of the heart can be contracted or it can dilate; this diminution and expansion present two illnesses that are not equally felt, but can be equally fearsome" (Sénac, 1749. *Treatise on the Structure of the Heart*, Book IV, Chapter VIII, I., tr. by the author).

Nicolas Corvisart (1755–1821) (Fig. 1-13), who was physician to Napoleon Bonaparte, is generally credited as having made the first clear clinical and pathological

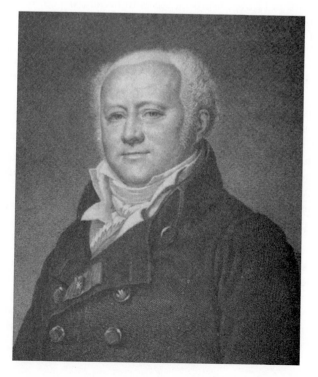

Figure 1-13: Jean Nicholas Corvisart. Reprinted from Major RH (1954). *A History of Medicine*. Springfield IL, CC Thomas.

distinctions between concentric and eccentric hypertrophy, which he called "active" and "passive" aneurism (enlargement) respectively. In his *Essai sur les maladies et les lésions organiques du coeur* (*Essai*), Corvisart stated:

> It is necessary to distinguish two species of aneurism of the heart [whose existence] is proved to the physician by symptoms different and appropriate to each; to the anatomist by constant and repeated observation of two very distinct states in which the heart is found when it has been the seat of the disease. . . . In the first species (active aneurism) the heart is [enlarged], its [walls] thickened, the energy of its action increased. . . . In the second (passive aneurism) there is likewise [enlargement], but an attenuation [thinning] of the [walls], and diminution of energy in the action of the organ (*Essai*, Second Class, Article I, Corvisart, 1812).

Corvisart equated *active aneurism,* in which the walls of the heart become thickened, to an "extraordinary evolution of the muscle of the body" that he viewed as adaptive:

> [The first effect is] to determine the extension and elongation of the fibres of the heart; the second to obtain a longer residence of blood in the cavities of this organ, and consequently a longer impression of its stimulus. In fine, the coronary arteries, as well as the capillaries of the heart, continuing in a permanent state of engorgement, will furnish more nutritive fluid to the fleshy substance of this organ. Hence the dilatation of the cavities, the elongation of the fibres, the thickening of their masses, the more vigorous the action of the organ (*Essai*. Second Class, Ch. I, Article II, Corvisart, 1812).

In describing differences between *passive aneurism* (dilatation) and *active aneurysm* (concentric hypertrophy), Corvisart wrote:

> [Passive aneurism] involves both thinning of its [walls], and debilitated action of the heart, [and] pursues in its formation, a course totally different from that of active aneurism. . . . The heart, in [active aneurism], seems to become the centre of a more active circulation, and nutrition. In that of [passive aneurism], this organ, on the contrary, is distended in the same manner as the bladder in cases of retention of urine. . . . The heart, which in [active aneurism] seems to employ . . . its own action to augment the organic lesion already existing, is, in [passive aneurism] an organ as passive as it appears to be active in the first (*Essai*, Second Class, Ch. II, Article I, Corvisart, 1812).

By recognizing that left ventricular dilatation seen in aortic and mitral regurgitation represents a response to increased diastolic stress, whereas concentric hypertrophy is the typical response to increased systolic stress, such as occurs in aortic stenosis, Corvisart anticipated by almost 200 years the current view that increased wall stress at different times during the cardiac cycle favors the appearance of specific phenotypes of cardiac hypertrophy (see Chapter 4).

Corvisart documented the terrible suffering once seen in end-stage heart failure when he defined three "periods" of cardiac aneurism:

In the *first period,* the patient "fears and suspects its evolution without being able to define the precise state." In this early phase, signs and symptoms are not specific. The latter include palpitation, dyspnea, and chest pain, while on physical examination the heart is not enlarged to percussion.

In the *second period,* cardiac enlargement is more obvious and the clinical manifestations are more troublesome: "A portion of the patient's apparent health is gone; there is swelling of the feet and ancles while standing, which commonly disappears during night. . . . Respiration has become extremely difficult. . . . He cannot breathe in a horizontal posture; to facilitate respiration, he is obliged to assume a sitting posture and to bend the body forward, resting as it were the thorax on his knees."

In the *third period*, the signs and symptoms of the disease "cannot be misunderstood." The patient is "attended by such inexpressible languor that he can scarcely move his limbs." All parts of the body are edematous, pleural effusions are evident as the chest is dull to percussion, and the extremities are cold. The cardiac impulse can no longer be felt: "The pulse is mostly small, frequent, unequal, intermittent . . . the veins are swoln, especially in the neck. . . . Suffocation is incessantly more threatening. . . . The integument of every part of the body, the muscles, cellular membrane &tc. are swoln, and dropsical. Ruptures are sometimes made on the extremities that discharge a vast quantity of water, which gives the patient momentary relief" (*Essai*, Second Class, Ch. III, Article I, Corvisart, 1812).

Corvisart observed that death, which "always intervenes to terminate the painful scene which this combination of symptoms presents," can occur in two ways: progressive heart failure, which "advances slowly, [until] life is insensibly extinguished," and sudden death, which can occur at any time in the natural history of this syndrome. Of the latter he wrote:

[T]he disease barely having reached its second period, when the patient dies (which sometimes occurs) the death is generally sudden and unexpected. On getting out of his bed, drinking &tc. he expires; and the attendants are often surprised to find him dead when he was left but a moment (*Essai*, Second Class, Ch. III, Article I, Corvisart, 1812).

John Bell (1763–1820), a contemporary of Corvisart who worked at the University of Edinburgh, also described the clinical implications of cardiac enlargement in the second edition of *The Anatomy of the Human Body*, published in 1802:

But the heart may be too big for its system, is a melancholy fact; for when it becomes relaxed, it enlarges, and as it grows in bulk loses its power. . . . While the heart gradually enlarges, the system changes, and accommodates itself to its powers. There is little distress; often we find a heart enlarged to a degree such as we never could have suspected before death. But slowly there is formed such an accumulation of ill oxydated blood as oppresses the vital powers, and chokes the motions of the heart, and draws after it those other disorders (Bell, 1802, 223).

Réné-Joseph-Hyacinthe Bertin (1767–1828), who served as a surgeon in Napoleon's army before becoming Professor of Hygiene at the Cochin Hospital in Paris, described the poor prognosis associated with eccentric hypertrophy (dilatation):

Now it is very evident, that, considered in the abstract, the dilatation of the heart has the effect to weaken the contractile power of the muscular substance of that organ, in consequence of the distention to which it is subjected. The muscular fibres lose in strength what they acquire in extent (Bertin, 1833, 380).

and the better prognosis is patients with concentric hypertrophy:

[T]he progress of [concentric] hypertrophy is, in general, slow, tardy and *chronic*; but that in some cases, however, it affects a more rapid, active and, as it were, *acute* form . . . frequently the hypertrophy does not merit on its own account any thing more than a secondary consideration (Bertin, 1833, 361–362).

Like most 19th century authorities, Bertin attributed overload-induced cardiac hypertrophy to an increase in the blood supply:

When from any cause the blood is obstructed in its course, it accumulates in the cavities of the heart and distends them: it enters in too great a quantity, and reverts upon the coronary arteries. The heart, irritated by the presence of this increased quantity of fluid, redoubles its energies, struggles, as it were, with all its powers against the resistance which it meets with: but these violent exertions themselves have the effect to solicit a new afflux of blood into the texture of the organ; so that the effect soon begins to take part with the cause. Stimulated beyond measure, the heart augments in bulk and thickness, and acquires an energy of contraction proportioned to the development of its hypertrophy (Bertin, 1833, 342).

Bertin is said by Vaquez (1924) to have believed that the valve abnormalities commonly found in patients with heart failure were largely irrelevant to the clinical disability, which he attributed to myocardial weakness. As described in the subsequent text, uncertainty regarding the relative importance of abnormalities in the heart's valves and changes in its muscular walls continued into the 20th century.

James Hope (1801–1841), who received his medical degree at Oxford and studied in Paris, described the hemodynamic consequences of a number of structural abnormalities in the heart. He was probably referring to myocarditis when he described the ability of inflammation to cause the heart to dilate:

Another class in whom debility of the heart exists as a cause of dilatation, comprises those who have had the organ softened or otherwise enfeebled by disease: an effect not uncommonly produced by typhoid fever, by inflammation of the heart (Hope, 1832, 296).

He also noted that dilatation is progressive:

When dilatation has progressed so far as to occasion *morbid* dyspnea, it has a constant tendency to increase unless the circulation be kept tranquil by a very quiet life and judicious medical treatment (Hope, 1832, 309).

To appreciate the natural history of heart failure before the modern era, one need only read Hope's description of the final stages of left heart failure (which he calls "cardiac asthma"); this paints a picture of this syndrome that, fortunately, is almost never seen today:

The respiration, always short, becomes hurried and laborious on the slightest exertion or mental emotion. The effort of ascending a staircase is particularly distressing. The patient stops abruptly, grasps at the first object that presents itself and fixing the upper extremities in order to afford a fulcrum for the muscles of respiration, gasps with an aspect of extreme distress.

Incapable of lying down, he is seen for weeks, and even for months together, either reclining in the semi-erect posture supported by pillows, or sitting with the trunk bent forward and the elbows or fore-arms resting on the drawn-up knees. The latter position he assumes when attacked by a paroxysms of dyspnea - sometimes, however, extending the arms against the bed on either side, to afford a firmer fulcrum for the muscles of respiration. With eyes widely expanded and starting, eye-brows raised, nostrils dilated, a ghastly and haggard countenance, and the head thrown back at every inspiration, he casts around a hurried, distracted look of horror, of anguish, of supplication: now imploring, in plaintive moans, or quick broken accents, and half-stifled voice, the assistance already often lavished in vain: now upbraiding the impotency of medicine; and now in an agony of despair, drooping his head on his chest, and muttering a fervent invocation for death to put a period to his sufferings. For a few hours–perhaps only for a few minutes - he tastes an interval of delicious respite, which cheers him with the hope that the worst is over, and that his recovery is at hand. Soon that hope vanishes. From a slumber fraught with the horrors of a hideous dream, he starts up with a wild exclamation that "it is returning." At length, after reiterated recurrences of the same attacks, the muscles of respiration, subdued by the efforts of which the instinct of self-preservation alone renders them capable, participate in the general exhaustion, and refuse to perform their function. The patient gasps, sinks, and expires (Hope, 1832, 381–382).

Hypertrophic Cardiomyopathy

Concentric left ventricular hypertrophy in patients without valvular disease was described by several 19th century physicians. Bell provided an early description of what may have been hypertrophic cardiomyopathy when he wrote:

The heart, which is so often dilated by weakness, is sometimes reduced in size by an increase in strength and action. It becomes dense, firm, thick in substance, but small in its cavity; it appears to be dilated without, but is, in fact, contracted within. This thickening of the wall of the ventricles is what I cannot understand, though I have cut many such hearts with the utmost care. There is no ossification of the valves, no straightening of the aorta, nor any other obstruction to excite the heart . . . I shall never forget the miseries I have seen such patients endure for having such a heart. They often have a full and bloated habit of body . . . a pulse weak at times, but trembling, and hardly sensible, when a fit of difficult circulation approaches; then the pulse vanishes, the patient sometimes faints; the anxieties, oppressed breathing, languid pulse, actual faintings, and all the intermediate conditions less than fainting, but like it, and infinitely more miserable, make their chief sufferings. After struggling long under this disease, the patients grow languid for a few days, often become dropsical, and then die (Bell, 1802, 231–232).

Another example of concentric left ventricular hypertrophy in the absence of valvular disease was provided by Austin Flint (1812–1886), who is now known largely for mid-diastolic murmur heard in severe aortic insufficiency that bears his name. Flint, who was educated at Amherst and Harvard and held positions in several cities in the United States, integrated physiology and clinical observation to explain heart disease in terms of pathophysiological abnormalities, rather than simply as diagnostic entities. He noted that hypertrophy is "almost always a secondary affection," but described the following patient who died suddenly and was found to have unexplained left ventricular hypertrophy:

I.S., age 23, residing in Brooklyn, breakfasted with his family and shortly after breakfast left for New York, apparently in good health to enter for the first time upon duties connected with a new mercantile arrangement. He had not proceeded far when he was noticed to stagger and fall heavily forward on the sidewalk. He was almost immediately taken to a police station-house near at hand but expired before reaching it. A post-mortem examination . . . was made eight hours after death. . . . [Aside from engorged blood vessels] there was no . . . morbid appearance within the skull. The heart . . . weighed 15 1/2 ounces [~450 gm]. . . . The aortic valves were competent. . . . The mitral orifice and valves were normal. . . . The left ventricular cavity . . . appeared to be diminished in size. The kidneys were of normal size and presented no appearance of disease. [The patient had] appeared to be always in excellent health. He was accustomed to take very active exercise without any inconvenience; and he complained of no ailments pointing to an affliction of the heart (Flint, 1870, 31–32).

However, as noted in the subsequent text, the unexplained hypertrophy described by Bell, Flint, and others could have resulted from systemic hypertension.

Hypertensive Heart Disease

Peter Mere Latham (1789–1875), an Oxford-trained physician who taught at the Middlesex Hospital in London, suggested that vascular disease might play a role in causing cardiac hypertrophy in the absence of valvular abnormalities:

> In truth the dropsies, the congestions, or the hemorrhages, or the diseases, functional or structural, of brain, lungs, or liver were not, as they seemed, the effects solely of the hypertrophied heart. But these and the hypertrophied heart were secondary to something, which preceded them all, and was the cause of them all, viz. disease pervading the whole arterial system (Latham, 1845, Vol II, 259).

A role for kidney disease as a cause for left ventricular hypertrophy had been suggested in 1836 by Richard Bright (1789–1858), the first of a group of outstanding physician-pathologists at Guy's Hospital in London. Bright noted that both cardiac hypertrophy and dropsy are common in patients with renal disease:

> The obvious structural changes in the heart [in patients with shrunken kidneys] have consisted chiefly of hypertrophy with or without valvular disease; and, what is most striking, out of 52 cases of hypertrophy, no valvular disease whatsoever could be detected in 34. . . . This naturally leads us to look for some less local cause for the unusual efforts to which the heart has been impelled; and the two most ready solutions appear to be either that the altered quality of the blood affords irregular and unwonted stimulus to the organ immediately, or that it so affects the minute and capillary circulation as to render greater action necessary to force the blood through distant subdivisions of the vascular system (Bright, 1836).

Twenty years later Traube, who found the heart to be hypertrophied in more than 90% of patients with shrunken kidneys, by then called Bright's disease, proposed that cardiac hypertrophy occurs when capillary obstruction in the atrophied kidneys elevates arterial blood pressure. However, according to Vaquez (1924), Traube wavered in this interpretation because he realized that obstruction to the renal circulation is not likely to increase arterial pressure enough to cause cardiac hypertrophy. After small peripheral arteries were observed to be thickened and narrowed in Bright's disease (Johnson, 1868), a process later called "arterio-capillary fibrosis" (Gull and Sutton, 1872), Traube returned to the view that left ventricular hypertrophy occurs when arteriolar narrowing increases aortic pressure (Traube, 1871). This hypothesis found critical support in 1863 when Marey, using an instrument that compresses the radial artery to provide an index of arterial pressure, found that systemic blood pressure is increased in patients with Bright's disease. Mahomed, using a modification of Marey's device to quantify arterial blood pressure, documented the correlation between hypertension, heart failure, and "chronic Bright's disease without albuminuria" (Mahomed, 1881). As a result, within ten years Osler was able to write that cardiac hypertrophy could be caused by

[A]ll states of increased arterial tension induced by the contraction of the smaller arteries under the influence of certain toxic substances, which act, as Bright suggested, by affecting the minute capillary circulation, to render greater action necessary to send the blood through distant subdivisions of the vascular system (Osler, 1892).

Riva-Rocci's introduction of the sphygmomanometer to measure brachial artery pressure at the end of the 19th century (Riva-Rocci, 1896) made it possible to define the pathophysiological correlations between arterial hypertension, pressure overload, left ventricular hypertrophy, and heart failure (Mancia, 1997).

Dilatation, Hypertrophy, and Valvular Disease in the Late 19th Century

Many classifications of cardiac enlargement were published in the 19th century; these included various combinations of dilatation, with and without thickening of the ventricular wall, and hypertrophy, with and without reduction in cavity volume. Viewed in the light of our current knowledge, most of these distinctions add little to an understanding of the hypertrophic response in patients with heart failure (see Chapter 4). However, the early clinical distinctions between what today would be called *concentric* and *eccentric hypertrophy* provide fascinating insights regarding prognosis. This distinction depended on meticulous physical examination, as evidenced by the following passage, published in 1855 by William Stokes, who trained in Ireland and provided a classical description of syncope in complete heart block:

The diagnosis of [simple uncomplicated dilatation of the heart] is one of extreme rarity ... I cannot produce any original observations of such a condition. ... The following should be the theoretical diagnostics of such an affection:

1. Increase in the area of dullness over the heart.
2. Feebleness of impulse.
3. Feebleness and smallness of pulse.
4. Feebleness of the sounds of the heart.
5. Absence of true valvular murmur.

Presuming that the contractile force of the heart is at least not below the normal state, the following signs will be observed [in dilatation with hypertrophy of the heart]:

1. Increase of dullness, generally commensurate with the extent of the organ.
2. Increase of the force of the impulse at the side, and of the extent of surface over which the impulse can be perceived.
3. The sounds are augmented (Stokes, 1855, 285–289).

A few years later, George Bacon Wood (1797–1879), an American physician-scientist who was educated at the University of Pennsylvania, wrote:

The physical signs of hypertrophy differ with the degree to which the heart is enlarged. In *simple hypertrophy*, the impulse is much stronger than in health, and may be felt over a somewhat larger extent of the chest. ... In *hypertrophy with dilatation*, the field of the impulse is extended in proportion to the expansion of the heart. There is a sensation of slow, heaving, and forcible movement imparted to the hand. ... The physical signs of *dilatation*, compared with those presented in health, are an impulse felt over a larger space, but soft, neither forcible nor heaving, and sometimes, in very feeble cases, quite wanting (Wood, 1858).

Similarly, William Orlando Markham (1818–1891), an English physician who edited the British Medical Journal, noted:

> Hypertrophy and dilatation of the heart increase the extent of praecordial dull percussion-sound, and in proportion to their degree. . . . When the dilatation exceeds the hypertrophy, the dullness increases chiefly on the transverse direction; and when the reverse of this occurs, it increases also in a direction from above downwards, - that is, in the long diameter of the heart (Markham, 1860, 150).

Sir Dominic John Corrigan (1802–1880), who trained in Dublin, suggested how regurgitation of blood through the leaky aortic valve can cause the left ventricle to dilate:

> In the perfect state of the valvular apparatus at the mouth of the aorta, the valves support by intervals the column of blood in the aorta, and the heart, with its ordinary complement of fibre and of muscular strength, is with this assistance competent to the office it has to perform. But when, in consequence of a deficiency in the valvular apparatus, the heart does not receive its due share of assistance from these valves, and is obliged to perform not only its own function of propelling the blood, but has in addition to support after each contraction a portion of that weight of blood which should then be wholly supported by the valves, it is no longer in its ordinary state equal to the task imposed upon it. In such circumstances, nature, to enable the heart to perform the additional labour thrown upon it, increases its strength by an addition of muscular fibre, and the heart thus becomes hypertrophied, in accordance with the general law, that muscular fibres become thickened and strengthened when there is additional power required from it (Corrigan, 1832).

After observing that when the heart "is at length incapable of sustaining the column of blood pressing upon it; it ceases to contract and is found after death largely distended with blood." Corrigan, described the terrible suffering that was once common in end-stage heart failure:

> For some days, or even weeks, before death, nature appears to be struggling against overwhelming exhaustion. The patient is constantly in the most heart-rending tone imploring to be relieved of the weight that is upon him; the countenance expresses the greatest sinking and distress; there are anxious calls for fresh air and continual restlessness, similar to what is seen in the patient sinking from hemorrhage; and when in this state the patient in some trifling motion dies exhausted (Corrigan, 1832).

Francois Aran (1817–1861), who trained in Paris, described the adaptive nature of cardiac hypertrophy when he wrote:

> Every time that a muscle takes on increased action, it receives an increased flow of blood; and consequently a proportional increase in nutrition results. What is seen in the arm of blacksmiths, in the legs of dancers, is also seen in the heart. . . . In proportion as the walls are thickened, its contractile power augments" (Aran, 1843, 100–101).

However, Aran was also aware that the hearts of patients with eccentric hypertrophy deteriorated prematurely:

> If the dilatation [has] reached a certain degree, and so far as to induce a morbid dyspnoea, the disease has a marked tendency to increase, unless the circulation be maintained in a state of complete repose. We may consider the tendency of dropsy to be reproduced immediately after its disappearance under proper treatment, as a fatal sign (Aran, 1843, 117).

The poor prognosis in dilatation was also noted in 1862 by Walter Hayle Walshe, who was born in Dublin and, after studying in Paris and Edinburgh, settled in London. Walshe wrote: "The more dilatation predominates over hypertrophy, the more serious becomes the prognosis" (Walshe, 1862). Markham, at about the same time, emphasized the compensatory nature of hypertrophy: "Hypertrophy of the heart must therefore be regarded as the result of an effort of nature, striving to compensate for the defective condition of other parts, than as a disease tending to the destruction of life" (Markham, 1860, 141–142). Austin Flint also highlighted the adaptive role of hypertrophy in *The Heart and Its Diseases*, published in 1879:

> [Overload] excites a more forcible ventricular action which for a time enables the ventricles to expel their contents. Meanwhile, hypernutrition follows, and hypertrophy is produced. The increased muscular growth for a certain period protects against the occurrence of dilatation. At length, the hypertrophy reaches a point beyond which it cannot advance; for the muscles of the heart, like other muscles, cannot increase indefinitely. There is a limit to the hypertrophic enlargement, and this limit varies in different persons just as the voluntary muscles in different persons attain, by the same efforts, to different degrees of development. The causes, however, persist and perhaps become more and more operative after the utmost degree of hypertrophy which is possible has taken place. These causes then can produce only dilatation, and from this period the progressive enlargement is due to augmentation of the cavities. This view is not only rational, but sustained by the facts derived from clinical experience. . . . According to this view, hypertrophy becomes an important conservative provision, first, against over-accumulation of blood, and second, against the more serious form of enlargement, viz., dilatation (Flint, 1870, 33).

The ability of excess wall stress imposed during systole and diastole to produce different types of hypertrophy was recognized by J. Milner Fothergill (1841–1888). Fothergill, who was trained in England, postulated that increased systolic stress (pressure overload, as seen in hypertension and aortic stenosis) causes concentric hypertrophy, and that increased diastolic stretch (volume overload, as seen in mitral and aortic insufficiency) leads to eccentric hypertrophy:

> [W]ith increase in the distending force [aortic insufficiency], hypertrophy is always combined with dilatation of the cardiac chambers; in obstruction . . . without any increase in the distending force, as in aortic stenosis, there is pure hypertrophy, usually without dilatation (Fothergill, 1879, 113).

He also observed that concentric hypertrophy, by "adding to the heart's power . . . tends to maintain itself, while dilatation tends downwards" (Fothergill, 1879, 133–134). In explaining the maladaptive effects of left ventricular dilatation caused by severe aortic regurgitation, he wrote:

> [Because of] escape of the blood backwards past the coronary orifices, the nutrition of the heart walls soon becomes impaired, and the hypertrophy, though massive, is not durable; muscular degeneration soon leads to further and uncontrollable dilatation, ending commonly by cessation of the action of the ventricle in diastole (Fothergill, 1879, 135).

The adverse effects of cardiac hypertrophy were emphasized in 1876 by Leopold Schroetter (1837–1908), an Austrian physician who was trained in Vienna:

Hypertrophy always occurs wherever a portion of the heart has been called upon to per-form work beyond its normal capacity, either to overcome mechanical obstacles or in consequence of increased innervation. . . . Hypertrophy may exist for many years, and the individual still continue to have relatively good health, but in the end it certainly leads to a so-called catastrophe through some of its sequels, at all events by fatty degen-eration and subsequent dilatation to disturbances of the circulation, which are of them-selves full of danger to the patient (Schroetter, 1876, in Ziemssen's *Practice of Medicine*, 191, 217).

Byrom Bramwell (1847–1931), who was trained in Medicine and Neurology at Edinburgh, observed in 1884 that hypertrophy is a "compensatory and beneficial condition, in fact, nature's effort to meet a difficulty," and observed that dilatation is an essential element of the heart's response to chronic volume overload:

In regurgitant valvular lesions dilatation of the cavity which is situated behind the affected orifice is beneficial, providing that it is just sufficient to accommodate the blood which is regurgitated at each systole [but is] usually bad [because it is] the direct opposite of hypertrophy, inasmuch as it impairs the efficiency of the cardiac pump" (Bramwell, 1884).

The same year, however, Constantin Paul (1833–1896) highlighted the adverse effects of hypertrophy and its ability to cause fibrosis:

It has frequently been said that the heart hypertrophies in order to establish a sort of compensation, and this process has been called providential. This view would be correct if the hypertrophy remained stationary; but experience has shown that the excess of work imposed upon the heart finally deteriorates its fibres, which become changed either by fatty degeneration or by the process of irritation of the connective tissue, which develops excessively and finally strangulates the muscular fibres (Paul, 1884, 319).

The fact that hypertrophy can be both adaptive and maladaptive was clearly described by William Osler (1849–1917) in the first edition of *The Principles and Practice of Medicine*, published in 1892. Osler, who was born and educated in Canada and became the first Professor of Medicine at Johns Hopkins, provided a remarkably modern view of the natural history of heart failure, noting that although enlargement of the overloaded heart is initially beneficial, maladaptive features of the hypertrophic response eventually cause the myocardium to deteriorate in a process that he divided into three stages (Table 1-3):

(a) The period of development, which varies with the nature of the primary lesion. For example, in rupture of an aortic valve . . . it may require months before the hyper-trophy becomes fully developed; or indeed, it may never do so and death may follow from an uncompensated dilatation. On the other hand, in sclerotic affections of the valves, with stenosis or incompetency, the hypertrophy develops step by step with the lesion, and may continue to counterbalance the progressive and increasing impair-ment of the valve.

(b) The period of full compensation - the latent stage - during which the heart's vigor meets the requirements of the circulation. This period has an indefinite time and the patient may never be made aware by any symptoms that he has a valvular lesion.

(c) The period of broken compensation, which may come on suddenly during very severe exertion. Death may result from acute dilatation [pulmonary edema]; but more commonly takes place slowly and results from degeneration and weakening of the heart muscle (Osler, 1892, 634).

TABLE 1-3

Three Stages in the Hypertrophic Response to Increased Afterload

Phase 1: Osler: *Development*; Meerson: *Transient breakdown*
Clinical: Symptomatic left ventricular dysfunction after mild overload; acute left ventricular failure and cardiogenic shock after severe overload
Pathophysiology: Left ventricular dilatation, pulmonary congestion, low cardiac output, early hypertrophy
Phase 2: Osler: *Full compensation;* Meerson: *Stable hyperfunction*
Clinical: Class I–II heart failure
Pathophysiology: Improved symptoms, resolved pulmonary congestion, increased cardiac output, established myocardial hypertrophy
Phase 3: Osler: *Broken compensation;* Meerson: *Progressive cardiosclerosis*
Clinical: Class III–IV heart failure
Pathophysiology: Worsening congestion, hemodynamic deterioration, continued hypertrophy with progressive ventricular dilatation, myocardial cell death, fibrosis

However, Osler followed the changing trends in medicine in the eighth edition of his textbook, which was published in 1918 after Starling had described his "law of the heart" (see subsequent text). This led Osler to replace his analysis of hypertrophy with a discussion of cardiac hemodynamics, a revision that attests to the shift in focus from pathology to hemodynamics that was stimulated by Starling's work (see subsequent text).

Hypertrophy and Hyperplasia

In the middle of the 19th century, refinements of the compound microscope led to a major conceptual advance in understanding the pathophysiology of heart failure. Rudolph Virchow (1821–1902), generally viewed as "the father of pathology," identified inflammation (myocarditis) as a potential cause of dilatation in some failing hearts. Most important was his distinction between hypertrophy (increased cell size) and hyperplasia (increased cell number)

> Hypertrophy, according to the meaning which I attach to the word, designates those cases in which the individual elements of structure take up a considerable amount of matter, and thereby become larger; and in which, in consequence of the simultaneous enlargement of a number of elements, at last the whole of the organ may become [enlarged]. When a muscle becomes thicker, all its primitive fasciculi become thicker . . . Essentially different from this process are the cases in which an enlargement takes place in consequence of an *increase in the number of the elements* (Virchow, 1860, 65).

This distinction between increased cell size and increased cell number in the heart's response to overload heralded a controversy that continues today, whether failing human cardiomyocytes undergo hyperplasia as well as the obvious hypertrophy (see Chapter 4).

The Early 20th Century

The controversy regarding the relative importance of valve abnormalities and myocardial dysfunction in causing clinical heart failure was revisited in 1908 by Sir James Mackenzie (1853–1925), who in the first edition of his *Diseases of the Heart,* highlighted the importance of myocardial abnormalities in causing this clinical syndrome. He noted that because "the heart muscle supplies the force which maintains the circulation," valve abnormalities produce no clinical manifestations of heart failure "so long as the heart can overcome the impediment" by means of normal adjustments. This reasoning led Mackenzie to state:

> [H]eart failure is simply inability of the heart muscle to maintain the circulation, and . . . this failure of the heart muscle is due to disturbance of the normal adjustment of the various factors concerned in the circulation (Mackenzie, 1908, 2).

The role of heart muscle, he wrote, is "of such prime importance in what we call heart failure, that a close and intimate study of its properties is essential." He sought to explain these properties using his concept of the "reserve force of the heart," stating:

> The more I study the symptoms of heart failure, and the more I reflect on the part played by the heart muscle, the more convinced am I that the explanation of heart failure can be summed up in the general statement that heart failure is due to the exhaustion of the reserve force of the heart muscle as a whole, or of one or more of its functions. This statement may seem so self-evident as scarcely to need amplification, but as a matter of fact, this, the essential principle on which diagnosis, prognosis and treatment should be based, is often practically ignored (Mackenzie, 1908, 2).

Mackenzie went so far in attributing heart failure to myocardial abnormalities that in 1923, after learning that Elliot C. Cutler, Chief of Surgery at the Peter Bent Brigham Hospital in Boston, had incised the narrowed mitral valve in a child with mitral stenosis, sent a letter to the child's physician, Samuel A. Levine, which stated:

> What a foolish thing you have done. It doesn't matter that the patient lived. You, of all physicians, should know that patients with mitral stenosis are in trouble primarily because of their sick myocardium and not because of the narrowed valve orifice (Cited by Shumacker, 1992, 39).

Mackenzie recognized the difficulty of defining the "reserve force of the heart," which he equated to the ability to increase output in response to an increase in the demands of the circulation. In the 1908 edition of *Diseases of the Heart*, Mackenzie listed five physiological mechanisms that lead to "exhaustion of the reserve force," which would now be called a decrease in myocardial contractility. These are tachycardia, dilatation, obstruction, imperfect nutrition, and degeneration; ten years later, in the 1918 edition of this text, he added a sixth: capillary obliteration. His view that heart failure is due largely to exhaustion of overloaded, damaged or energy-starved heart muscle provided the rationale for the recommendation, found in virtually all textbooks published until the end of the 20th century, that these patients should be treated with rest (see subsequent text).

Attempts to distinguish different forms of cardiac enlargement continued into the mid-1920s; for example, Henri Vaquez provided a classification that includes "essential hypertrophy" (the physiological hypertrophy associated with growth, exercise, and pregnancy), "symptomatic hypertrophy," and "dilatation" (Vaquez, 1924). However, efforts to understand the pathophysiology of heart failure shifted away from the architecture of failing hearts shortly after World War I, when Starling's description of the "law of the heart" returned the focus to hemodynamics.

Starling's Law of the Heart

The hemodynamic abnormalities in heart failure, while understood by a few highly trained physicians, came to the forefront in 1915, when Ernest Starling (Fig. 1-14) gave his Linacre Lecture on the "law of the heart," which was published 3 years later (Starling, 1918). Although physiologists in the late 19th century knew that increased diastolic volume leads to an increase in cardiac output (Katz, 2002), physicians had based their views of the effects of increased cavity size on the pathological evidence that dilatation is associated with a poor prognosis (see previous discussion). Starling's demonstration that increased end-diastolic volume increases the heart's ability to do work was confusing to physicians because it seemed to contradict the 19th century view that dilatation weakens the failing heart. This contradiction is highlighted in a Lumleian Lecture, delivered to the Royal College of Physicians of London by G.A. Sutherland (1917), which stated:

> Dilatation of the heart . . . has long been recognised amongst the changes associated with valvular disease. The view taken was that was a sign of weakness, a sign that the heart was yielding to some stress or strain more than it could effectively deal with. [However, the] whole subject of dilatation . . . is admittedly one of great difficulty. . . . On the physiological side Starling and his coworkers have recently promulgated some new views on this subject."

This contradiction was also noted by Sir James Mackenzie, whose first (1908) edition of *Diseases of the Heart* had emphasized the disadvantages of dilatation: "A certain size of the heart is also necessary for the perfect performance of contractions, and if the chambers be dilated the contractile force is placed at a disadvantage, and exhaustion results." However, 9 years later, in lectures given at the London Hospital, Mackenzie stated:

> *The real meaning of dilatation of the heart has, so far, eluded recognition.* . . . The latest researches by Starling show that a dilatation of any of the chambers of the heart is produced when there is an increase in the pressure during diastole - the increase of pressure being due to a larger influx of blood. Starling shows that, when the heart is stimulated to greater effort, it dilates slightly, because a slight increase in size gives the best condition of the heart for increased effort (Mackenzie, 1917).

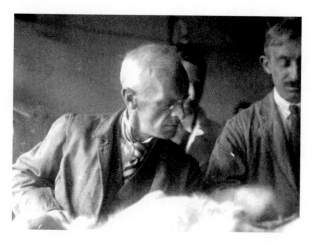

Figure 1-14: Ernest H. Starling in his laboratory. Photograph taken in 1925 by Louis N. Katz.

Cowan and Ritchie, in 1922, noted that Starling had found that increasing diastolic volume increases the work of the heart when "within physiological limits" (Cowan and Ritchie, 1922), and in 1925 Poulton distinguished between eccentric hypertrophy that "spells the onset of cardiac failure," and "compensatory dilatation," which occurs when a "particular chamber of the heart has to accommodate an extra quantity of blood." The latter wrote: "Starling's experiments suggest that [dilatation], too, may be a compensatory mechanism, enabling the heart to beat more forcibly...this is called Starling's 'Law of the Heart'" (Poulton, 1925). Vaquez (1924) addressed the question as to whether cavity enlargement is good or bad by first describing the late 19th century view that eccentric hypertrophy is "a reaction of distress testifying to the heart's inability to provide for an excess of work or even for the normal needs of the circulation." However, after noting that Starling described "the occasional providential or compensatory role of dilatation." Vaquez asked: "Is [dilatation] merely an exaggeration of that which normally follows exertion?.... Physiologists, notably Starling, have reached the conclusion that dilatation is one of the principal means of adaptation of the heart to the needs of the organism." In attempting to resolve these apparently contradictory effects, Vaquez distinguished between *physiological* dilatation, which is "essential for the heart's ability to respond to the various demands made upon it in normal existence," and *pathological* (or *passive*) dilatation, which "coincides with loss of energy of the cardiac systole," noting that the latter occurs in infectious, toxic, rheumatic and alcoholic myocarditis (Vaquez, 1924).

Rediscovery of the applicability of the law of Laplace to the heart (Burton, 1962, Burch et al. 1965), which led to measurement of wall stress in living human hearts, allowed three groups to demonstrate that hypertrophy normalizes wall stress in patients with compensated aortic stenosis (Sandler and Dodge, 1963; Hood et al., 1968; Grossman et al., 1975). Although these observations made it clear that overload-induced hypertrophy is initially adaptive, the importance of maladaptive hypertrophy did not come into focus until the last decade of the 20th century (see Chapter 5).

It is now apparent that Starling's law of the heart is a short-term *functional* response that operates on a beat-to-beat basis to allow increased end-diastolic volume to increase the work of the heart, whereas the much slower dilatation caused by eccentric hypertrophy, which was described by the great clinical pathologists of the 19th century, represents a long-term *architectural* response caused by abnormal proliferative (transcriptional) signaling (Table 1-4). That the latter is both adaptive

---

TABLE 1-4

Two Causes of Ventricular Dilatation

Hemodynamic (Acute)

An increase in venous return or a decrease in ejection increases end-diastolic volume, which stretches the myocytes in the walls of the ventricles. According to the length–tension relationship, the greater sarcomere length increases the ability of the ventricle to do work (Starling's law of the heart).

Architectural (Chronic)

Dilatation caused when hypertrophy increases cardiac myocyte length. By increasing wall stress, this growth response increases the energy demands of the heart and decreases cardiac efficiency, thereby initiating a vicious cycle that worsens heart failure. This form of dilatation occurs when abnormal transcriptional (proliferative) signaling causes eccentric hypertrophy (systolic dysfunction), and tends to progress (remodeling).

and maladaptive underscores one of today's key unanswered questions, which is how hypertrophy can be beneficial and deleterious, *and at the same time*. For some answers, keep reading this book!

Diuretics

From antiquity until the third decade of the 20th century, little progress had been made in the management of patients with heart failure. This is apparent in the following description of end-stage heart failure, published in 1916:

> A physician receives an emergency call, and knows, if it is not a patient who has hysteria, that it is his duty to see the patient immediately. The friends of the patient all anxiously await the physician's arrival; front doors are often wide open, and the servants and the whole household are in a great state of excitement and anxiety. The position in which the patient will be found is that which he has learned gives him the greatest comfort. If the physician knows his patient, he will know how he will find him. He may be sitting up in bed; he may be standing, leaning over a chair; he may be sitting in a chair leaning over a table or leaning over the back of another chair; but he is using every auxiliary muscle he possesses to respire. He is generally bathed in cold perspiration; the extremities are often icy cold; he calls for air, and to stop fanning all in one breath; he wishes the perspiration wiped off his brow, and nearly goes frantic while it is being done; there is agony depicted on his face; his eyes stare; his expirations are often groaning. Sometimes there is even incontinence of urine and feces, often hiccup or short coughs, perhaps vomiting, and possibly sharp pangs of pain in the cardiac region. A patient with these symptoms may die at any moment, and the wonder is that so many times one lives through these paroxysms.
>
> The patient can hardly be questioned, can certainly not be carefully examined; and herein lies the advantage of the family physician who knows the patient and his heart, and in whom the patient has confidence. In fact, this confidence which such a patient has in the physician who has more or less frequently aided him in weathering these terrible attacks is alone the greatest boon the patient can have.
>
> Two factors may normally, without treatment, stop these paroxysms, and the "bad heart turn" may be cured spontaneously. The first of these is self control. If the patient does not lose his head, by an effort of the will he saves himself from becoming nervous or frightened and therefore escapes the result of mental excitement; the increased peripheral blood pressure from fear does not occur, and in a shorter or longer time the heart quiets down. The physician recognizes this power, and gives his patient immediate assurance that he will be all right; the patient who knows his physician immediately feels this assurance and is quickly improved. The second factor in spontaneous cure of the heart attack is relaxation. The exhaustion from the respiratory muscular efforts, together with the drowsy condition caused by cerebral hyperemia and from the imperfectly aerated blood, causes finally a dulling of the mental activity, and the nervous excitement abates, which with the exhaustion, gives a relaxation of peripheral arterioles; the resistance to the flow of blood is removed, the surface of the body becomes warm, the heart quiets down by the equalization of the circulation, and the paroxysm is over (Osborne, 1916).

This horrible suffering, which hardly differed from that described during the previous 250 years (see previous discussion), changed dramatically less than a decade later when organic mercurial diuretics became available.

Fluid retention had been proposed as a cause of dropsy as early as the 16th century, but there had been no safe way to get rid of the excess fluid. Although the diuretic effect of inorganic mercurials was well known, their toxic/therapeutic ratio is so low that they usually did more harm than good. For this reason, discovery of the safety and predictable diuretic effect of organic mercurials had an enormous impact on the treatment of heart failure. This occurred shortly after World War I, when Saxl and Heilig (1920) injected an organic mercurial to kill the spirochetes in a patient with syphilitic heart disease and observed a massive diuresis that was subsequently demonstrated to be due to inhibition of sodium resorption by the renal tubules. However, organic mercurials have to be administered parentally, and, because they lose their efficacy when given more than two to three times each week, they are of little benefit in end-stage heart failure. This discovery, which came at a time when knowledge of renal physiology was increasing rapidly, shifted the focus of heart failure research to the development of more powerful diuretics that could be given orally. This effort ended successfully in the late 1950s and early 1960s with the discovery first of the thiazides and then of loop diuretics. One only need read descriptions such as those of Hope, Corrigan, and Osborne to appreciate the enormous impact that this research had on the management of heart failure.

Changing Etiologies of Heart Disease

The most common cause of heart failure throughout the period reviewed up to this point had been rheumatic valvular disease, one of the sequelae of rheumatic fever, an autoimmune process initiated by childhood streptococcal infections. In developed countries, improved public health and the antibiotics that became available in the 1940s have virtually eliminated acute rheumatic fever, for which there had been no treatment aside from aspirin, corticosteroids, and prolonged bed rest (Fig. 1-15). Today, in societies where this disease has become a rarity, it is difficult

Figure 1-15: Rheumatic fever ward of the Boston Children's Hospital in the 1930s, when the standard treatment for acute rheumatic fever was a year of bed rest. Reproduced courtesy of the Children's Hospital Archives, Boston, Massachusetts.

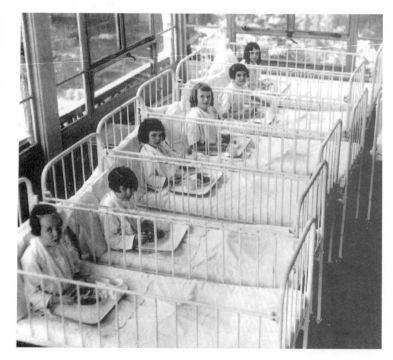

to appreciate the impact of rheumatic heart disease, which had been a scourge since antiquity.

In the early 20th century, Coombs (1926) reported that about three fourths of patients hospitalized for heart disease in England had structural abnormalities (51% rheumatic heart disease, 11% subacute bacterial endocarditis, 9% cardiovascular syphilis, and 2% congenital heart disease). Similarly, in the United States rheumatic heart disease was responsible for as many as 60%–80% of the adult heart disease seen in the 1920s (Cabot, 1914; Cohn, 1927; Paul, 1930; Wilson, 1940). Less common, though equally devastating, was congenital heart disease, which at the end of the first half of the 20th century affected about 0.1% of children (MacMahon et al., 1953). The high prevalence of structural heart disease highlighted the work of Starling, Carl J. Wiggers (Fig. 1-16), Louis N. Katz (Fig. 1-17), and other physiologists who studied the hemodynamics of valvular, congenital, and ischemic heart disease between World Wars I and II. Most investigations used animal models until the 1940s, when the introduction of cardiac catheterization by André Cournand and Dickinson W. Richards (Fig. 1-18) made it possible to incorporate the enormous body of basic hemodynamic physiology into clinical medicine.

Advances in the treatment of cardiac injury during World War II demonstrated the feasibility of operating on human hearts. This made it possible for Dwight Harkin and Charles Bailey in the United States, and Russell Brock in Great Britain, to develop operations that could open the narrowed valve in patients with rheumatic mitral stenosis. The development of open heart surgery and prosthetic valves, which began in the 1960s, allowed cardiac surgeons to palliate many other forms of structural heart disease, both rheumatic and congenital. However, the

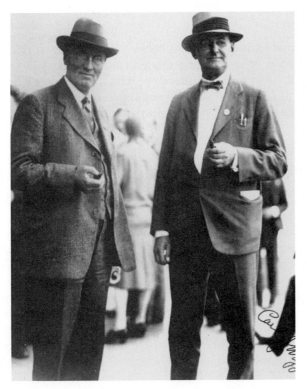

Figure 1-16: Carl J. Wiggers in the mid-1950s (*right*); at the **left** is Anton J. Carlson, whose position as intellectual leader in Gastrointestinal Physiology during the first half of the 20th century was similar to that held by Dr. Wiggers in Cardiovascular Physiology. Photograph by AMK in Atlantic City at a meeting of the American Physiological Society.

Figure 1-17: Louis N. Katz. Photograph in the possession of AMK.

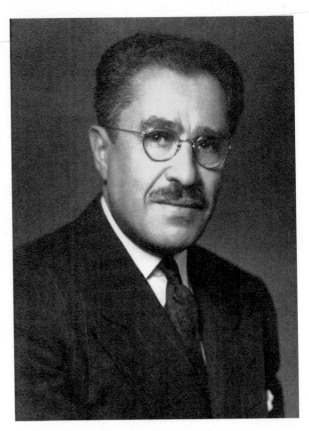

challenges posed by heart failure continued because new causes of this syndrome have emerged; ischemic heart disease and dilated cardiomyopathies are now the major causes of systolic heart failure in developed countries, while systemic arterial hypertension and the reduced aortic compliance that accompanies normal aging led to an epidemic of diastolic heart failure in today's aging population (see Chapter 2).

Abnormal Biochemistry

Energy Starvation

Most experimental studies of heart failure carried out between the 1930s and 1950s used animal models in which, although the hemodynamic abnormalities resemble those seen clinically, the pathophysiology is entirely different; these include deteriorating heart–lung preparations, where the heart fails largely because particulates in the perfusates occlude the coronary microcirculation, and acute right heart dilatation created by pulmonary artery constriction and tricuspid valve avulsion. It is not surprising that studies using these models reached the erroneous conclusion that cardiac energetics in the human heart failure are normal, a conclusion that was reinforced by data, which for technical reasons were inaccurate, suggesting that heart failure is caused by a change in the molecular weight of cardiac myosin (Olson and Piatnek, 1959).

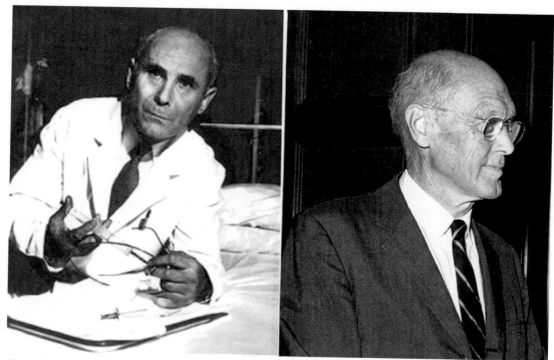

Figure 1-18: André Cournand (**left,** picture courtesy of the National Library of Medicine) and Dickenson W. Richards (**right,** photograph in the possession of AMK).

Myocardial Contractility

Between the 1920s and the 1960s, it was commonly taught that the failing heart operates on the descending limb of the Starling curve, where increasing chamber volume decreases the heart's ability to eject (Fig. 1-19). This was incorrect, and overlooked the fact that Starling, in his Linacre Lecture, had noted that when dilatation exceeds "the optimum length of the muscle fibre and the muscle has to contract at

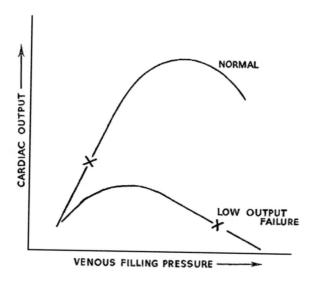

Figure 1-19: Diagram illustrating the view that the failing heart operates on the descending limb of the Starling curve. Modified from McMichael J (1950). *Pharmacology of the Failing Heart.* Springfield IL, CC Thomas.

such a mechanical disadvantage . . . the heart fails altogether" (Starling, 1918). However, it was not until 1965, when it was pointed out that a heart operating on the descending limb of the Starling curve cannot function at a steady state (Katz, 1965), that this erroneous view began to disappear from the literature. This fallacy, which until the 1980s was believed by a majority of medical students at a prominent United States medical school, was selected to illustrate "a pervasive and powerful misconception" in medical education (Feltovich et al., 1989).

Understanding of the causes for the obviously weak contraction of failing hearts began to emerge in 1955, when Stanley J. Sarnoff (1955) demonstrated that hearts can operate on different Starling curves (Fig. 1-20). A few earlier investigators had been aware of this possibility, but Sarnoff's introduction of the concept of a "family of Starling curves" shifted the focus in heart failure research from length-dependent regulation (Starling's law) to changes in what came to be called *myocardial contractility*. Application of this new knowledge to patients was hampered by difficulties in defining myocardial contractility and the fact that, although most investigators had some idea as to what contractility was, no one knew how to measure it (Harris, 1972). Much of the research on this subject during the 1960s and 1970s had been based on the work of A.V. Hill, whose classical studies of muscle mechanics in tetanized frog sartorius muscle, where curves relating muscle load to shortening velocity are hyperbolic, had dominated muscle physiology for almost a half century. However, efforts to measure maximal shortening velocity (V_{max}), which in the 1970s was viewed as the gold standard in quantifying contractility, in mammalian myocardium overlooked the fact that the heart pumps, rather than hops, and that accurate force–velocity curves cannot be measured because it is not possible to tetanize cardiac muscle (Abbott and Mommaerts, 1959). After almost two decades of heated controversy, it became clear that it is impossible to determine V_{max} in the heart and that myocardial contractility cannot be precisely quantified in patients (Katz, 2006). In spite of these theoretical limitations, however, it was possible to show convincingly that contractility is reduced in failing hearts (Spann et al., 1967).

This emphasis on myocardial contractility occurred at a time of rapid progress in muscle biochemistry, which by the mid-1960s had shown that calcium delivery to the cytosol and its binding to troponin, a regulatory protein in the myofilaments, are major determinants of myocardial contractility (Katz, 1967). These discoveries, which provided clues as to the mechanisms that depress contractility in failing hearts, stimulated efforts to develop inotropic drugs more powerful than digitalis, whose benefits in heart failure were then viewed as resulting from their ability to increase contractility.

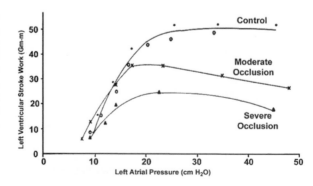

Figure 1-20: Effects of restricted coronary flow on left ventricular stroke work in an anesthetized dog showing a family of Starling curves. Modified from Case RB, Berglund E, Sarnoff SJ (1954). Ventricular function. II. Quantitative relationship between coronary flow and ventricular function with observations on unilateral failure. Circ Res 2:319–325.

The Neurohumoral Response

In a remarkable series of papers, Peter Harris (1983) provided a clear explanation for the adverse effects of the powerful neurohumoral responses to lowered cardiac output, notably vasoconstriction, salt and water retention, and adrenergic stimulation. Although these responses are essential to maintain cardiac output during exercise, and provide valuable support for the circulation during a transient fall in cardiac output such as after a hemorrhage, when sustained in chronic heart failure they become harmful and worsen prognosis (see Chapter 3). This is largely because fluid retention, cardiac stimulation, and vasoconstriction all have adverse long-term effects in heart failure (Francis et al., 1984).

Inotropic Agents

Efforts to develop powerful inotropic agents during the 1970s and 1980s were aided by clarification of the role of calcium in contraction, relaxation, and excitation–contraction coupling, and by the discovery that cyclic AMP mediates the positive inotropic response to sympathetic stimulation (see Chapter 3). The widely held belief that increasing contractility would benefit patients with heart failure was reinforced by observations that norepinephrine and other β-agonists, which increase cellular cyclic AMP levels, cause short-term hemodynamic improvement in patients with *acute* heart failure. However, evidence that the failing heart is energy starved led a minority to believe that the energy cost of the inotropic and chronotropic responses to cyclic AMP could harm patients with *chronic* heart failure (Katz, 1986). This provoked a sharp controversy that ended when several clinical trials showed that long-term inotropic therapy with β-agonists and phosphodiesterase inhibitors does more harm than good (see Chapter 7). In addition, a large clinical trial showed that cardiac glycosides, in spite of their inotropic effect, do not improve survival in heart failure patients with sinus rhythm (The Digitalis Investigation Group, 1997). However, the latter differed from Withering's patients, who were generally in atrial fibrillation and so benefited from the ability of digitalis to slow ventricular rate.

Vasodilators

Recognition of the adverse effects of the increased afterload commonly found in heart failure (Ross, 1976) provided the rationale for the use of vasodilators to treat these patients (Cohn and Franciosa, 1977). The short-term benefits of afterload reduction, which include an immediate increase in ejection, decreased ventricular end-diastolic pressure, and improved cardiac energetics, led Jay N. Cohn to organize VHeFT I (Veterans Administration Heart Failure Trial I), which examined the effects of several vasodilators on long-term prognosis (Cohn et al., 1986). This randomized double-blind trial showed a trend toward improved survival after administration of isosorbide dinitrate, a long-acting nitrate that is mainly a venodilator, and hydralazine, an arteriolar vasodilator that inhibits nitric oxide breakdown; however, the α_1-adrenergic blocker prazosin, another vasodilator, had no benefit (Fig. 1-21A). This study, which was the first of the large clinical trials that now represent the gold standard in evaluating therapy for heart failure, clearly documented the poor prognosis in heart failure and so led to additional trials that sought to document a survival benefit for other vasodilators. However, the majority of these trials were disappointing because, even though all

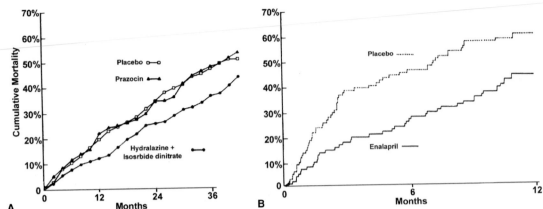

Figure 1-21: Clinical trials showing effects of vasodilators on mortality in patients with heart failure. **A:** Comparison of prazosin, the combination of isosorbide dinitrate and hydralazine, and placebo. Modified from Cohn JN, Archibald DG, Ziesche S, Franciosa JA, Harston WE, Tristani FE, Dunkman WB, Jacobs W, Francis GS, Cobb FR, Shah PM, Saunders R, Fletcher RD, Loeb HS, Hughes VC, Baker B (1986). Effect of vasodilator therapy on mortality in chronic congestive heart failure. Results of a Veterans Administration cooperative study (V-HeFT). N Engl J Med 314:1547–1552. **B:** Comparison of enalapril and placebo. Modified from CONSENSUS Trial Study Group (1987). Effects of enalapril on mortality in severe congestive heart failure. Results of the Cooperative North Scandinavian Enalapril Survival Study. N Engl J Med 316:1429–1434.

vasodilators are of short-term benefit, most worsen long-term prognosis. A major exception was CONSENSUS I (1987) which documented a significant benefit of angiotensin II–converting enzyme (ACE) inhibitors (Fig. 1-21B). The broad implications of this discovery became apparent when the results of CONSENSUS I were first presented in 1986 at a meeting in Oslo, Norway, where a member of the audience stood up and said that these results could not be true because, to paraphrase, "No other vasodilator has this marked effect on survival." This question overlooked the fact that, unbeknownst to most in the audience, investigators had already begun to explore the possibility that angiotensin II is not only a vasodilator but can also stimulate proliferative signaling (Katz, 1990a).

Molecular Abnormalities

Although the rapid advances in physiology and biochemistry during the 20th century had relegated studies of the architecture of the failing heart to the background, this earlier work had not been entirely forgotten. Felix Meerson, who in the 1950s was the first to use modern methods to study the hypertrophic response to overload in animal models (Meerson, 1961), observed the three phases of overload-induced myocardial degeneration that had been described by Osler in 1892 (Table 1-3). In the 1960s and 1970s, after cardiology rediscovered the law of Laplace (which although known to 19th century physiologists had been virtually forgotten since the 1920s), the initial hypertrophic response in patients with aortic stenosis and insufficiency was shown to be adaptive because it normalizes wall stress (see previous discussion). These findings made it clear that deterioration of hypertrophied hearts is not due simply to continued overload, but instead that maladaptive features of this growth response play an important role in causing the poor prognosis in patients

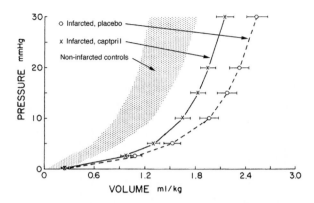

Figure 1-22: Effect of the ACE inhibitor captopril on left ventricular diastolic pressure–volume relationships following myocardial infarction. Diastolic volumes (abscissa) and pressures (ordinate) after 3 months are shown for noninfarcted control rats (*shaded area,* mean ± 2 SD), infarcted hearts of untreated rats (*o*), and infarcted hearts of rats treated with captopril (*x*). The difference between the latter is significant (p <0.05). Modified from Pfeffer JM, Pfeffer MA, Braunwald E (1985). Influence of chronic captopril therapy on the infarcted left ventricle of the rat. Circ Res 1985;57:84–95.

with heart failure (Katz, 1990b). The key to solving the puzzle as to how hypertrophy can be both adaptive and maladaptive emerged at a joint meeting of the International Society for Heart Research and American Heart Association, held in Boston in 1987, at which molecular biology moved to center stage in cardiology (Katz, 1988).

The mechanisms responsible for the survival benefits of ACE inhibitors had been presaged in 1985, when Janis Pfeffer, Mark Pfeffer, and Eugene Braunwald showed that these drugs slow the progressive cavity enlargement that follows experimental myocardial infarction (Pfeffer et al., 1985) (Fig. 1-22). Because these investigators viewed progressive dilatation as "compensatory remodeling [that allows] preservation of forward output at any filling pressure," they described the increase in cavity volume as *remodeling*, which highlights similarities to the beneficial short-term hemodynamic of increased end-diastolic volume described by Starling, rather than the deleterious long-term effects of eccentric hypertrophy noted in the 19th century (Table 1-4). Another early clue regarding the maladaptive effects of cardiac hypertrophy had been published in 1962, when Norman R. Alpert and Michael S. Gordon (1962) reported that ATPase activity is reduced in myofibrils isolated from failing human hearts. This study, by demonstrating that molecular composition can change in diseased hearts (see Chapter 5), heralded the importance of molecular biology in understanding the pathophysiology of heart failure.

CONCLUSIONS

The clinical impact of the advances in understanding the pathophysiology of heart failure are summarized in Figure 1-23, which shows the changes in therapy recommended by successive editions of two major cardiology textbooks. Most striking has been the addition of several major classes of drugs since the era of "dig, diuretics, and bed rest" ended in the late 1980s. Because there are many individual drugs in each class shown in Figure 1-23, and because devices, such as implantable defibrillators and cardiac resynchronization therapy, are not included, the changes that have taken place during the past 40 years are even more extensive than shown in this figure. The many new avenues for individualized treatment of this syndrome (see Chapter 7) means that optimal management of this syndrome now requires an understanding of both the pathophysiology that operates in the individual patient and the mechanisms of action of the drugs and devices that are available today.

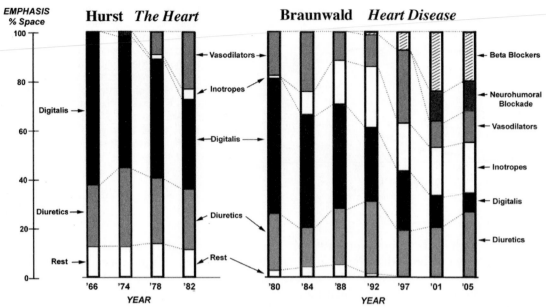

Figure 1-23: Changing emphasis on the management of heart failure over the past 40 years. A count of the approximate number of pages devoted to rest and drug treatment was used to estimate the overall patterns of therapy in four editions of Hurst's *The Heart* and seven editions of Braunwald's *Heart Disease*. Forty years ago, recommended treatment centered on rest, diuretics, and cardiac glycosides; the large amount of space devoted to the latter reflected the need to describe the toxicity of these drugs. Discussions of positive inotropic drugs that appeared in the late 1970s initially focused on β-adrenergic agonists and later on phosphodiesterase inhibitors. Sections on afterload reduction began to include neurohumoral blockade in the 1990s, when it became clear that the ability of some vasodilators to improve long-term prognosis are due in part to inhibition of maladaptive neurohumoral signaling. This shift continued during the late 1990s when it became clear that β-adrenergic blockers, in spite of short-term negative inotropic actions, prolong long-term survival. The amount of space devoted to the cardiac glycosides continued its decrease in 2005. The use of devices has been omitted.

REFERENCES

Abbott BC, Mommaerts WFHM (1959). A study of inotropic mechanisms in the papillary muscle preparation. J Gen Physiol 42:533–551.

Adams F (1856). *The Extant Works of Aretæus, The Cappadocian*. London, The Sydenham Soc.

Adelmann HB (1966). *Marcello Malpighi and the Evolution of Embryology*. Ithaca NY, Cornell University Press.

AHA Statistical Update (2006). Heart disease and stroke statistics—2006 update. Circulation 113:e85–e151.

Alpert NR, Gordon MS (1962). Myofibrillar adenosine triphosphatase activity in congestive heart failure. Am J Physiol 202:940–946.

Aran FA (1843) *Practical Manual of the Diseases of the Heart and Great Vessels*. tr Harris WA. Philadelphia, Barrington and Haswell.

Bell J (1802). *The Anatomy of the Human Body*. 2nd ed. London, Strahan.

Bertin RJ (1833). *Treatise on the Diseases of the Heart and Great Vessels*. Tr. Chauncy CW. Philadelphia, Carey, Lea and Blanchard.

Bramwell B (1884). *Diseases of the Heart and Thoracic Aorta*. New York. Appleton.

Bright R (1836). Cases and observations illustrative of renal disease accompanied with secretion of albuminous urine. Guy's Hosp Rep 1:339–379.

Buchan W (1774). *Domestic Medicine; or, The Family Physician*. London, Cruikshank.

Burch GE, DePasquale NP, Cronvich JA (1965). Influence of ventricular size on the relationship between contractile and manifest tension. Am Heart J 69:624–628.

Burton AC (1962). Physical principles of circulatory phenomena: the physical equilibria of the heart and blood vessels. In: *Handbook of Physiology*, Section 2: Circulation, Vol. 1. Hamilton WF, Dow P, eds. 85–106. Washington, DC, American Physiological Society.

Cabot RC (1914). The four common types of heart disease. An analysis of six hundred cases. JAMA 43:1461–1463.

Celsus (1938). *De Medicina*, Vol. I. Tr. Spencer WG. London, Heinemann.

Cohn AE (1927). Heart disease from the point of view of the public health. Am Heart J 2:275–301, 386–407.

Cohn JN, Franciosa JA (1977). Vasodilator therapy of cardiac failure, N Engl J Med 297:27–31, 254–258.

Cohn JN, Archibald DG, Ziesche S, et al. (1986). Effect of vasodilator therapy on mortality in chronic congestive heart failure. Results of a Veterans Administration cooperative study (V-HeFT). N Engl J Med 314:1547–1552.

CONSENSUS Trial Study Group (1987). Effects of enalapril on mortality in severe congestive heart failure. Results of the Cooperative North Scandinavian Enalapril Survival Study. N Engl J Med 316:1429–1434.

Coombs CF (1927). The aetiology of cardiac disease. Bristol Med-Chir J 43:1.

Corrigan DJ (1832). On permanent patency of the mouth of the aorta, or inadequacy of the aortic valves. Edinburgh Med Surg J37:225–245. (Reprinted in: Willius FA, Keyes TE. *Cardiac Classics*. St. Louis, MO, Mosby.)

Corvisart JN (1812). *An Essay on the Organic Diseases and Lesions of the Heart and Great Vessels*. Tr. Gates J. Boston, Bradford & Read.

Cowan J, Ritchie WT (1922). *Diseases of the Heart*. London, Arnold.

De Lacy P (1984). *Galen, on the Doctrines of Hippocrates and Plato*. Berlin, Akademie.

The Digitalis Investigation Group (1997). The effect of digoxin on mortality and morbidity in patients with heart failure. N Engl J Med 336:525–533.

East CT (1958). Failure of the circulation and its treatment. Lecture 4 in: *The Story of Heart Disease*. 127–145. London, Dawson and Sons.

Feltovich PJ, Spiro RJ, Coulson RL (1989). The nature of conceptual understanding in biomedicine: the deep structure of complex ideas and the development of misconceptions. Chapter 4 in: Evans DA, Patel VL. *Cognitive Science in Medicine*. 113–165. Cambridge, The MIT Press.

Flint A (1870). *Diseases of the Heart*. 2nd ed. Philadelphia, HC Lea.

Fothergill JM (1879). *The Heart and Its Diseases*. 2nd ed. Philadelphia, Lindsay & Blakiston.

Francis GS, Goldsmith SR, Levine TB, et al. (1984). The neurohumoral axis in congestive heart failure. Ann Int Med 101:370–377.

Grossman W, Jones D, McLaurin LP (1975). Wall stress and patterns of hypertrophy in the human left ventricle. J Clin Invest 56:56–64.

Gull WW, Sutton HG (1872). On the pathology of the morbid state commonly called "Bright's disease with contracted kidney" ("arterio-capillary fibrosis"). Med-Chir Tr (Lond) 55:273–329.

Gunther RT (1932). *Early Science in Oxford*, Vol IX: Lower R. *De Corde*. Tr. KJ Franklin. London, Dawsons.

Harris CRS (1973). *The Heart and Vascular System in Ancient Greek Medicine*. Oxford, Oxford University Press.

Harris P (1972). Contractility revealed. J Mol Cell Cardiol 4:179–184.

Harris P (1983). Evolution and the cardiac patient. Cardiovasc Res 17:313–319, 373–378, 437–445.

Harvey W (1957). *Movement of the Heart and Blood in Animals*. Tr. Franklin KJ. Oxford, Blackwell.

Hippocrates (1923–1931). Tr. Jones WHS. London, William Heinemann.

Hood WP Jr, Rackley CE, Rolett EL (1968). Wall stress in the normal and hypertrophied human left ventricle. Am J Cardiol 22:5550–5558.

Hope J (1842). *A Treatise on the Diseases of the Heart and Great Vessels*. Philadelphia, Haswell & Johnson.

Horace (1983). *The Complete Odes and Epodes*. Tr. Shepherd WG. London, Penguin.

Jarcho S (1980). *The Concept of Heart Failure. From Avicenna to Albertini*. Cambridge, Harvard University Press.

Johnson G (1868). I. On certain points in the anatomy and pathology of Bright's disease of the kidney. II. On the influence of the minute blood vessels upon the circulation. Med-Chir Tr (Lond) 51:57–78.

Katz AM (1965). The descending limb of the Starling curve and the failing heart. Circulation 32:871–875.

Katz AM (1967). Regulation of cardiac muscle contractility. J Gen Physiol 50:185–196.

Katz AM (1978). A new inotropic drug: its promise and a caution. N Engl J Med 299:1409–1410.

Katz AM (1986). Potential deleterious effects of inotropic agents in the therapy of heart failure. Circulation 73(Suppl III):184–190.

Katz AM. (1988). Molecular biology in cardiology, a paradigmatic shift. J Mol Cell Cardiol 20:355–366.

Katz AM (1990a). Angiotensin II: hemodynamic regulator or growth factor? J Mol Cell Cardiol 22:739–747.

Katz AM (1990b). Cardiomyopathy of overload. A major determinant of prognosis in congestive heart failure. N Engl J Med 322:100–110.

Katz AM (2002). Ernest Henry Starling, his predecessors, and the "law of the heart." Circulation 106:2986–2992.

Katz AM (2006). *Physiology of the Heart*. 4th ed. Philadelphia, Lippincott Williams & Wilkins.

Katz AM, Katz LA (1991). What is a paradigm and when does it shift? J Mol Cell Cardiol 23:403–408.

Katz AM, Katz PB (1962). Diseases of the heart in the works of Hippocrates. Br Heart J 24:257–264.

Katz AM, Katz PB (1995). Emergence of scientific explanations of nature in ancient Greece: the only scientific discovery? Circulation 92:637–645.

Kuhn TS (1970). *The Structure of Scientific Revolutions*. 2nd ed. Chicago, The University of Chicago Press.

Lathan PM (1845). *Lectures on Subjects Connected with Clinical Medicine Comprising Diseases of the Heart*. London, Longmans, Brown, Green and Longmans.

Littré E (1839–1861). *Oeuvres Complètes d'Hippocrate*. Paris, JB Baillière.

Mackenzie J (1908). *Diseases of the Heart*. London, Oxford University Press.

Mackenzie J (1917). *Principles of Diagnosis and Treatment in Heart Afflictions*. London, Oxford University Press.

MacMahon B, McKeown T, Record RG (1953). The incidence and life expectancy of children with congenital heart disease. Br Heart J 1953;15:121.

Mahomed FA (1881). Chronic Bright's disease without albuminuria. Guy's Hosp Rep (3rd series). 24:363.

Major RH (1945). *Classic Descriptions of Disease*. 3rd ed. Springfield IL, CC Thomas.

Major RH (1954). *A History of Medicine*. Springfield IL, CC Thomas.

Mancia G (1997). Scipione Riva-Rocci. Clin Cardiol 20:503–504.

Markham WO (1860). *Diseases of the Heart*. 2nd ed. London, Reed and Pardon.

Meerson FZ (1961). On the mechanism of compensatory hyperfunction and insufficiency of the heart. Cor et Vasa 3:161–177.

Morgagni JB (1769). *The Seats and Causes of Diseases Investigated by Anatomy, in Five Books*. Tr. Alexander B. London, Millar and Cadell.

Olson RE, Piatnek DA (1959). Conservation of energy in cardiac muscle. Ann N Y Acad Sci 72:466–478.

Osborne OT (1916). *Disturbances of the Heart*. Chicago, American Medical Association.

Osler W (1892). *The Principles and Practice of Medicine*. New York, Appleton.

Paul C (1884). *Diseases of the Heart*. New York, Wood.

Paul JR (1930). *The Epidemiology of Rheumatic Fever*. Printed by The Metropolitan Life Insurance Co.

Pfeffer JM, Pfeffer MA, Braunwald E (1985). Influence of chronic captopril therapy on the infarcted left ventricle of the rat. Circ Res 57:84–95.

Poulton EP (1925). *Taylor's Practice of Medicine*. 13th ed. London, Churchill.

Richards DW (1968). Hippocrates of Ostia. JAMA 206:377–378.

Riva-Rocci S (1896). Un nuovo sfigmomanometro. Gazz Med Torino 50-51:1001–1007.

Riva-Rocci S (1897). La tecnica sfigmomanometra. Gazz Med Torino 9-10:161–172.

Ross J Jr (1976). Afterload mismatch and preload reserve: a conceptual framework for the analysis of ventricular function. Prog CV Dis 18:255–264.

Saba MM, Ventura HO, Saleh M, et al. (2006). Ancient Egyptian medicine and the concept of heart failure. J Card Fail 12:416–421

Sandler H, Dodge HT (1963). Left ventricular tension and stress in man. Circ Res 13:91–104.

Sarnoff SJ (1955). Myocardial contractility as described by ventricular function curves. Physiol Rev 35:107–122.

Saxl P, Heilig R (1920). Über die diuretiche Wirkung von Novasurol und anderen Quecksilberinjektionen. Wien klin Wochenschr 33:943–944.

Schroetter L (1876). Diseases of the heart substance. In: Ziemssen H, ed. *Practice of Medicine*. Vol. VI: Diseases of the Circulatory System. New York, Wood.

Sénac J-B (1749). *Traité de la Structure du Coeur, de Son Action et de Ses Maladies*. Paris, Vincent.

Shumacker HB (1992). *The Evolution of Cardiac Surgery*. Bloomington, Indiana University Press.

Siegel RE (1968). *Galen's System of Physiology and Medicine*. Basel, Karger.

Singer C (1988). *The Fasciculus Medicinae of Johannes de Ketham*. Birmingham AL, Classics of Medicine.

Spann JF Jr, Buccino RA, Sonnenblick EH, et al. (1967). Contractile state of cardiac muscle obtained from cats with experimentally produced ventricular hypertrophy and heart failure. Circ Res 21:341–354.

Spencer WG (1938). *Celsus. De Medicina*, Vol. I. London, Heinemann.

Starling EH (1918). *The Linacre Lecture on the Law of the Heart*. London, Longmans Green & Co.

Stokes W (1855). *The Diseases of the Heart and the Aorta*. Philadelphia, Lindsay and Blakiston.

Sutherland GA (1917). The Lumleian lectures on modern aspects of heart disease. Lancet 1:401–406, 437–443, 477–482.

Traube L (1871). *Über den Zusammenhang von Herz und Nieren-Krankheiten Hirschwald. Gesammelte Beiträge zur Pathologie und Physiologie* Vol 2. Berlin pp 290–353.

Vaquez H (1924). *Diseases of the Heart*. Tr. Laidlaw GF. Philadelphia, WB Saunders.

Virchow R (1860). *Cellular Pathology*. Tr Chance F. London, Churchill.

Walshe WH (1862). *A Practical Treatise on the Diseases of the Heart and Great Vessels*. London, Walton & Maberly.

White PD (1942). Heart failure. Ann N Y Acad Med (2nd series). 18:18–35.

White PD (1957). The evolution of our knowledge about the heart and its diseases since 1628. Circulation 15:915–923.

Wilson MG (1940). *Rheumatic Fever*. New York, The Commonwealth Fund,.

Wood GB (1858). *A Treatise on the Practice of Medicine*. Philadelphia, Lippincott.

Woodward WA, Strom EA, Tucker SL, et al. (2003). Changes in the 2003 American Joint Committee on Cancer Staging for Breast Cancer dramatically affect stage-specific survival. J Clin Oncol 21:3244–3248.

Wright WC (1952). *Lancisi's Aneurysms*. New York, MacMillan.

CHAPTER 2

The Failing Heart as a Damaged Pump

Arnold M. Katz • Marvin A. Konstam

INTRODUCTION

The heart, which expends energy to "lift" blood from the low pressures in the veins to the higher pressures in the arteries, can be compared to a mechanical pump that moves water out of a leaky basement into a hose (Fig. 2-1). Failure of the latter causes the basement to flood and reduces flow out of the hose, which in heart failure is analogous to increasing venous pressure and decreasing cardiac output. However, heart failure is more complex because the heart is a reciprocating pump in which phases of filling alternate with phases of ejection. This means that impaired ejection increases the amount of blood remaining in the heart at the end of systole, which reduces filling during the next diastole; conversely, reduced filling provides less blood that can be ejected in the following systole. Stated simply, a heart that ejects poorly during systole cannot fill normally during diastole, and a heart that fills poorly during diastole cannot eject normally during systole. The heart is also two pumps—the right and left ventricles—that operate in series; for this reason, blood backing up behind one ventricle makes it more difficult for the other ventricle to eject, and when less blood is pumped out of one ventricle less returns to the other. Another complexity arises because the interventricular septum is shared by both ventricles, which allows failure of one ventricle to modify the function of the other by ventricular interaction. Finally, once the heart begins to fail, it deteriorates rapidly (see Chapter 1). The following discussions highlight left ventricular abnormalities because left heart failure is predominant in developed countries.

THE WORK OF THE HEART

The ability of the heart to pump blood is reduced in heart failure. This decreases *stroke work,* which is the product of the volume of blood ejected during each beat (stroke volume, abbreviated SV) and the pressure (P) at which the blood is ejected:

$$\text{Stroke work} = \text{SV} \times \text{P} \qquad \text{Eq. 2.1}$$

Peak aortic systolic pressure is often used to calculate stroke work. Because arterial pressure changes throughout ejection, stroke work is more accurately calculated as the integral $\int P dV$, where P is the pressure at which each increment ($\int dV$) of the stroke volume is ejected; this refinement, however, is cumbersome, adds little to a practical understanding of heart disease, and is rarely used clinically. Stroke work represents a form of mechanical work, so that it is not surprising that the product of volume (cm^3) and pressure ($dynes/cm^2$) has the correct units for work ($dynes\ cm$).

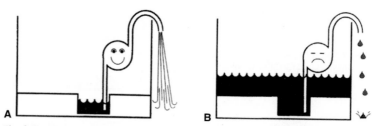

Figure 2-1: The failing heart as a defective pump. When a pump that moves water from a leaky basement into a hose (**A**) begins to fail, inadequate emptying of the basement can cause flooding (high venous pressure), reduced flow through the hose (low cardiac output), or both (**B**). From Katz AM (2006). *Physiology of the Heart.* 4th ed. Philadelphia, Lippincott Williams & Wilkins.

Stroke volume is end-diastolic volume (EDV) minus end-systolic volume (ESV, the residual volume remaining in the ventricle at the end of systole), so that the equation for stroke work can be expanded:

$$\text{Stroke work} = (\text{EDV} - \text{ESV}) \times \text{P} \qquad \textbf{Eq. 2.2}$$

Any or all of these three variables can be abnormal in a patient with heart failure (see subsequent text).

The external work of the heart is usually expressed as *minute work,* the work performed per minute, which in physics is a *power.* Minute work is simply stroke work (SV $\times$ P, see Eq. 2.1) multiplied by heart rate (HR):

$$\text{Minute work} = \text{HR} \times \text{SV} \times \text{P} \qquad \textbf{Eq. 2.3}$$

The product of HR $\times$ SV is the cardiac output (CO), so that:

$$\text{Minute work} = \text{CO} \times \text{P} \qquad \textbf{Eq. 2.4}$$

Because stroke volume = EDV $-$ ESV, there are actually four determinants of minute work:

$$\text{Minute work} = \text{HR} \times (\text{EDV} - \text{ESV}) \times \text{P} \qquad \textbf{Eq. 2.5}$$

As noted in the subsequent text, changes in each of these variables have different effects on the energy demands of the beating heart.

The heart performs a small amount of kinetic work to impart velocity to the blood as it leaves the ventricle. Kinetic work is normally only a small fraction of the stroke work and contributes to the "useful" work of the heart because most of the kinetic energy helps propel blood through the vascular system when flow velocity decreases.

In addition to the *external work* done to eject blood under pressure into the great vessels, the heart performs *internal work* to elongate viscous elements and stretch elasticities in the walls of the heart as pressure rises during systole. Because much of this internal work is degraded to heat when the heart relaxes, it contributes to the inefficiency of cardiac performance (see subsequent text).

LAW OF LAPLACE

Ventricular geometry plays an important role in determining the energy cost of ejection. This reflects the fact that cavity pressure is determined not only by the tension developed by the cardiac myocytes, but also by the size of the ventricular cavity. These effects are described by the law of Laplace, which states that *at any cavity*

Figure 2-2: The law of Laplace in a thin-walled cylinder relates wall tension (T) to the pressure within the cylinder (P) and the radius of curvature (R). From Katz AM (2006). *Physiology of the Heart.* 4th ed. Philadelphia, Lippincott Williams & Wilkins.

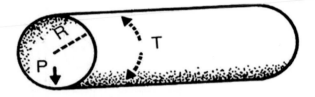

pressure, wall tension and wall stress are increased when the cavity becomes larger, and vice versa. The terms "wall tension" and "wall stress" are sometimes used interchangeably, but this is incorrect; *tension* describes a force exerted along a line, while *stress* is a force across an area.

In its simplest form, for a cylinder with an infinitely thin wall (Fig. 2-2), the law of Laplace states that wall tension is equal to the pressure within the cylinder times its radius:

$$T = P \times R \qquad \qquad \text{Eq. 2.6}$$

where T is wall tension (dynes/cm), P is pressure (dynes/cm^2), and R is radius (cm). The law of Laplace is more complex in the heart, where wall stress (σ) is inversely proportional to wall thickness (h). This is best understood in a thick-walled cylinder, where the stress across any area of the wall decreases when wall thickness is increased:

$$\sigma = \frac{P \times R}{h} \qquad \qquad \text{Eq. 2.7}$$

A greater wall stress is required to achieve a given cavity pressure when the heart dilates because, when diameter increases, a smaller proportion of the force developed by the cardiac myocytes is directed toward the center of the cavity (Fig. 2-3).

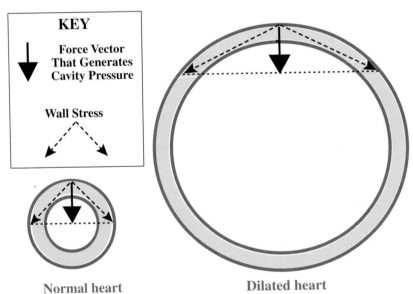

Normal heart   **Dilated heart**

Figure 2-3: Application of the law of Laplace to a dilated heart. The wall stress needed to achieve a given pressure is increased when the heart dilates because a smaller proportion of the force generated by the myocytes in the walls is directed toward the center of the cavity (downward arrow). As a result, to achieve the same cavity pressure, more stress must be developed in the walls of a dilated heart than a normal heart (dashed arrow). Modified from Katz AM (2006). *Physiology of the Heart.* 4th ed. Philadelphia, Lippincott Williams & Wilkins.

Two consequences of the law of Laplace contribute to the deleterious effects of cardiac dilatation: Wall stress at any cavity pressure is greater, and the decrease in wall stress during ejection is reduced (Fig. 2-4). The greater wall stress increases the internal work that must be done during systole to stretch elastic and viscous elements in the walls of the heart, whereas the smaller decrease in wall stress during ejection reduces the heart's ability to use energy stored in the stretched elasticities to perform external work. For these reasons, dilatation at any given wall thickness reduces cardiac efficiency (see subsequent text).

Stress is not distributed uniformly throughout the layers of the ventricular walls, but instead is greatest in the inner (endocardial) regions (Wong and Rauta-harju, 1968; Fenton et al., 1978). This might appear to contradict the law of Laplace, which states that wall stress increases as cavity diameter increases, but there is no contradiction because the *distribution* of stress among the layers of a thick-walled ventricle is not the same as the average *amount* of stress in the walls of ventricles that have different cavity sizes. The differences in wall stress in the various layers of the ventricle can be understood by viewing the ventricle as a series of concentric elastic spheres, where an increase in cavity volume causes the great-est increase in stress in the innermost layer. These differences are magnified when wall thickness increases, so that a marked increase in cavity pressure in a concen-trically hypertrophied heart can cause severe energy starvation, and even necrosis, of the subendocardium. The vulnerability of the inner layers of the ventricular wall to energy starvation is also due to compression of the muscular branches of the coronary arteries that penetrate the ventricular wall from their origins in epicardial coronary arteries.

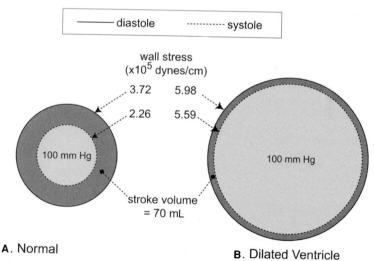

Figure 2-4: Effects of dilatation on the relationships between cavity pressure, wall stress, and the change in circumference during ejection. **A:** Normal ventricle. **B:** Dilated ventricle. Cavity outlines, which for ease in calculating wall stress are assumed to be spherical, are shown at end-diastole (*solid circles*) and at end-systole (*dashed circles*); the *shaded areas* between each pair of circles is the stroke volume, which is the same in both **A** and **B**. Because the dilated ventricle ejects its stroke volume with a smaller decrease in cir-cumference than the normal ventricle, dilatation has reduced the extent of the decrease in wall stress dur-ing ejection. Modified from Katz AM (2006). *Physiology of the Heart.* 4th ed. Philadelphia, Lippincott Williams & Wilkins.

PRELOAD AND AFTERLOAD

Two types of load play an important role in determining muscle performance: These are *preload* and *afterload*, which differ in the time at which they first interact with the contracting muscle. In a linear muscle, a preload stretches the relaxed muscle *before* it begins to contract, whereas the muscle does not encounter an afterload until *after* contraction has begun (Fig. 2-5). The beating heart also operates with a preload and an afterload, both of which are most accurately defined as the peak wall stress during diastole and during systole, respectively. Preload is therefore determined by ventricular cavity pressure and volume at the end of diastole, whereas afterload is determined by the cavity pressures and volumes after ventricular pressure exceeds aortic pressure.

Left ventricular afterload is often equated to systolic blood pressure, which approximates the pressure at which the ventricle ejects. Although it is more accurate to quantify afterload as systolic wall stress, this is not practical clinically because it is difficult to obtain simultaneous measurements of interventricular pressure, cavity size, and wall thickness, all of which influence wall stress according to the law of Laplace (Eq. 2.7). Furthermore, all of these variables change throughout ejection because ventricular pressure first rises and then falls, volume decreases, and wall thickness increases. In most ventricles, these changes cause wall stress to decrease as ejection proceeds.

Resistance and Impedance

Peripheral resistance and aortic impedance, along with stroke volume, determine systolic pressure in the aorta. Although related, resistance and impedance are not the same, nor are they determined in the same regions of the arterial system. Peripheral resistance, the major determinant of the rate at which blood flows out of the

Figure 2-5: Preload and afterload. A preload is supported by a resting muscle before it begins to contract (**left**), whereas an afterload, such as a weight resting on a support, is not encountered by the muscle until after it has begun to shorten and developed enough tension to lift the weight (**right**). From Katz AM (2006). *Physiology of the Heart*. 4th ed. Philadelphia, Lippincott Williams & Wilkins.

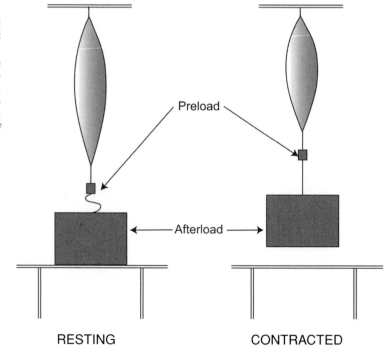

RESTING   CONTRACTED

arteries to perfuse the tissues, is determined largely by the diameter of small arterioles that are often called "resistance vessels." Aortic impedance, which determines the peak level of aortic pressure as blood is being ejected from the left ventricle, is influenced by the elasticities of the aorta and other large arteries as well as by peripheral resistance. Aortic impedance and systolic blood pressure become higher when the elasticity of the large arteries decreases during normal aging. This age-dependent increase in aortic impedance is accelerated by arteriosclerotic changes in the large arteries.

ENERGY COST OF THE WORK OF THE HEART, CARDIAC EFFICIENCY

The energy cost of cardiac work depends on the way in which the heart contracts. This was first shown by Evans and Matsuoka (1915), who found that cardiac oxygen consumption (which provides an excellent index of cardiac energy utilization because oxidative metabolism is the major source of the heart's energy) depends both on the *amount* of work performed and *how* it is performed. Not only do increases in pressure and stroke volume increase oxygen consumption, but more extra energy is expended when the heart contracts against an increased afterload than when it ejects a larger volume of blood. In other words, the energy cost of increasing pressure is greater than that of a similar increase in ejection.

It is now clear that the energy costs of the four determinants of minute work in Eq. 2.5 are not the same (see Katz, 2006). Most expensive are increases in P, HR, and EDV, while a decrease in ESV during ejection, even though it increases stroke volume, is energetically less costly. A major reason why stroke volume, while an important determinant of external work, makes only a small contribution to energy utilization is that some of the potential energy stored in stretched elasticities within the walls of the heart is converted to useful work during ejection, when the stretched elasticities shorten. The low energy cost of ejection explains why the product BP (blood pressure) × HR, called the *double product,* is a useful clinical index of left ventricular energy consumption.

Cardiac efficiency can be estimated by dividing the minute work of the heart by the energy equivalent of the oxygen consumed:

$$\text{Cardiac efficiency} = \frac{\text{minute work}}{\text{energy equivalent of oxygen consumption}} \qquad \textbf{Eq. 2.8}$$

Efficiencies between 5% and 20% have been documented in working hearts, the exact value depending on the amount and nature of the work performed (see previous discussion). Inefficiency is due largely to the energy expended in performing internal work during isovolumic contraction, which explains why efficiency is reduced by increases in HR, P, and EDV. A faster heart rate increases the frequency at which the heart expends energy to perform this internal work, while a rise in aortic pressure increases the amount of internal work done during each beat. Dilatation, like high aortic pressure, lowers cardiac efficiency by increasing systolic wall stress. Dilatation also reduces the amount of potential energy stored in the series elasticities that can be used to perform useful work because there is less wall shortening during ejection of a given stroke volume (Fig. 2-4).

The hemodynamic abnormalities in heart failure can be analyzed in three ways: Examination of the cardiac cycle, pressure–volume loops, and the interplay between venous return and cardiac output. Each highlights different features of the heart's activity, so that considered together they can provide a detailed understanding of the abnormal hemodynamics in the patient with heart failure.

THE CARDIAC CYCLE

Each cardiac cycle is initiated by a wave of electrical depolarization that is normally initiated by pacemaker cells in the SA (sinoatrial) node. Propagation of this electrical signal through the atria, AV (atrioventricular) junction, and His-Purkinje system initiates a series of mechanical events that ends with ventricular systole. These electrical and mechanical events can be depicted as a Wiggers diagram (Fig. 2-6). The following description of the cardiac cycle is modified from the 1949 edition of Carl J. Wiggers' classic text *Physiology in Health and Disease* (1949, 651–654).

The series of superimposed curves which are reproduced in Figure 2-6 unfold at a glance the story of cardiodynamic events in the left side of the heart which may be briefly summarized as follows:

Figure 2-6: The cardiac cycle (Wiggers diagram) showing seven phases of left ventricular systole. By convention, the cycle begins with ventricular systole. The top three curves represent aortic pressure (*upper dashed line*), left ventricular pressure (*solid line*) and left atrial pressure (*lower dashed line*). The *solid line* below these pressure curves is left ventricular volume, below which are the heart sounds: S_4, atrial (or fourth) sound; S_1, first heart sound; S_2, second heart sound; S_3, third heart sound. The bottom line shows the timing of the electrocardiogram (ECG) that records the electrical events during the cardiac cycle. Modified from Katz AM (2006). *Physiology of the Heart.* 4th ed. Philadelphia, Lippincott Williams & Wilkins.

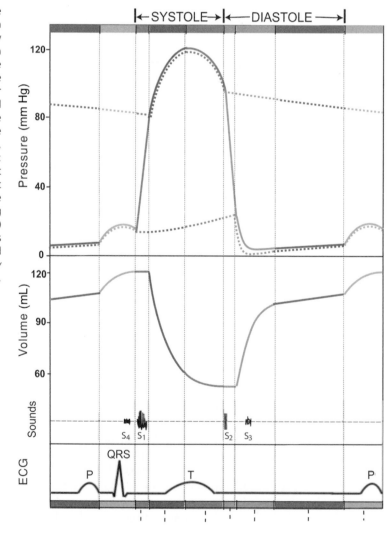

At the onset of ventricular systole the pressures are approximately equal in the atrium and ventricle, and the atrioventricular (AV) valves are in the act of floating into apposition. After the pressure has risen slightly within the ventricle, the AV valves close completely giving rise to the first heart sound [S_1]. Since the aortic valve is still closed, the ventricle contracts isovolumically, and the intraventricular pressure rises rapidly. The aortic valve opens when left ventricular pressure exceeds that in the aorta. As a result, aorta and ventricle become a common cavity, and the two pressure curves follow one another closely.

With the rapid expulsion of blood during the early moments of ejection - indicated by volume changes of the ventricles - the pressures in the left ventricle and aorta rise to a summit because the rate at which blood is expelled into the aorta exceeds that at which it flows from its branches through the arterioles. The rise is rounded chiefly because, with rather constant ejection rate, the runoff increases gradually with the progressive rise of aortic pressure. The rounded summit is reached when ejection and runoff become equal. Since the rate of ejection diminishes during the latter part of systole while flow out of the aortic branches continue to be high, aortic and ventricular pressures gradually decline. On the basis of pressure curves it is possible to separate the period of ejection into two phases, viz., maximum ejection and reduced ejection. Summarizing, the rise and fall of aortic and ventricular pressures always represent a balance between the rate at which blood is ejected into the aorta and the rate at which it leaves by its branches. However, the changes in rate of ventricular ejection normally dominate the shape of the curves during ejection.

At the onset of ventricular diastole, aorta and ventricle are still in communication. The first effect of relaxation consists in a sharp drop in pressure in the ventricle and aorta, the latter being quickly terminated by the closure of the semilunar valves, after which the aortic curve declines very gradually for the remainder of diastole. The closure of the semilunar valves is associated with the second heart sound [S_2]. The rate of aortic diastolic pressure decline is determined chiefly by the rate at which blood flows out of the aortic branches, but is affected to a variable extent by the increasing distensibility of arteries at different pressure levels.

Within the ventricle, the decline continues rapidly until the AV valves open, and the phase of isovolumic relaxation terminates. During this phase of ventricular relaxation the atrial pressure continues to rise slowly. As soon as intraventricular pressure has declined to a level lower than that in the atrium, the AV valves are opened again by the difference of pressure and a rapid inflow of blood into the ventricle begins. While this continues, pressures in the atrium and ventricle decline together, but the atrial pressure remains a trifle higher than the ventricular. In long cycles this is followed by a phase of slowed filling, or diastasis, during which ventricular inflow is exceedingly slow, and the pressure rises very gradually both in the atrium and ventricle. In young normal individuals, and in some pathological states, the rapid inflow of blood into the ventricle is associated with an audible sound, the third heart sound [S_3]. Occasionally, atrial systole also produces a sound sometimes called the fourth heart sound [S_4].

The Phases of the Cardiac Cycle: The succession of atrial and ventricular events constitutes the cardiac cycle. Since ventricular contraction is dynamically the most important it is fitting to start the cycle with this event. Accordingly, the cardiac cycle can be divided advantageously into ventricular systole and diastole, but each of these periods must be further subdivided. For the sake of clarity these subdivisions are designated as phases of systole and diastole. The vertical lines of Figure 2-6 serve to demarcate the successive periods and phases of systole and diastole. The first phase of systole is called isovolumic contraction, for the ventricle contracts essentially in this manner with all valves closed. The second phase is best referred to as ejection; it can be further subdivided by reference to the aortic pressure curve alone or with the aid of the ventricular volume curve into the phase of maximum ejection, and the phase of reduced ejection.

Diastole begins with closure of the semilunar valves. It is followed by isovolumic relaxation, which ends as soon as atrial pressure exceeds that in the ventricle. With *opening of the AV valves, rapid filling supervenes, and this is followed by a phase of slowed filling or diastasis, whose length depends on the heart rate. Finally, atrial systole terminates the period of ventricular diastole and the cycle begins again.*

PRESSURE–VOLUME LOOPS

Table 2-1 lists five major determinants of cardiac performance, of which three are properties of the heart and two are governed by the circulation. Among the former, heart rate is normally determined by pacemaker currents in the SA node, and inotropy and lusitropy by the biochemical and biophysical properties of the working cardiac myocytes. The key circulatory determinants of cardiac performance are venous return, which along with lusitropic properties, determines preload, and aortic pressure, which along with inotropy, determines afterload. A useful way to view the hemodynamic abnormalities in heart failure is to plot a pressure–volume loop, which describes changes in ventricular pressure as a function of cavity volume (Fig. 2-7). Pressure–volume loops do not describe the time dependence of these variables and so differ from the Wiggers diagram, where the variables are plotted as a function of time.

Each pressure–volume loop proceeds through four phases, beginning at the end of diastole. *Isovolumic contraction*, the first phase of systole, begins when myocyte contraction increases ventricular wall stress. The rising intraventricular pressure closes the mitral valve, after which pressure increases until it exceeds that in the aorta, which causes the aortic valve to open. Until this happens, blood can neither enter nor leave the ventricle, so that the increase of pressure at a constant volume inscribes an upward deflection (A in Fig. 2-7). The second phase, *ejection*, begins when ventricular pressure exceeds that in the aorta, after which blood is pumped into the aorta and the reduction in ventricular volume causes the pressure–volume loop to turn to the left (B in Fig. 2-7). Aortic pressure initially rises during ejection because blood is flowing into the aorta faster than it is running out into the tissues, and then falls as slowing of ejection allows blood to flow out of the aorta more rapidly than it enters from the ventricle. Even though aortic pressure rises and falls during ejection, wall stress falls throughout this phase of the cardiac cycle because of the decreasing cavity volume and thickening of the ventricular walls (the law of Laplace). Systole ends at a point along the *end-systolic pressure–volume relationship*, which describes the inotropic state of the ventricle.

Diastole begins with *isovolumic relaxation* (C in Fig. 2-7), which occurs after aortic valve closure; because the mitral valve is also closed, ventricular volume

---

TABLE 2-1
Major Determinants of the Work of the Heart
The Heart
Heart rate
Contractility (inotropy)
Relaxation (lusitropy)
The Circulation
Venous return (preload)
Arterial pressure (afterload)

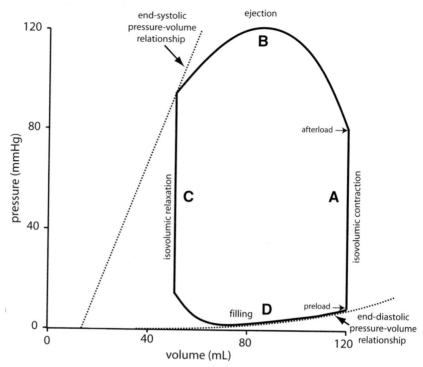

Figure 2-7: Pressure–volume loop generated by a normal left ventricle. The loop is constrained by the end-diastolic pressure–volume relationship, which is determined by the lusitropic state of the ventricle, and the end-systolic pressure–volume relationship, which is determined by the inotropic state. Systole begins at a point along the end-diastolic pressure–volume relationship that represents the preload, after which the mitral valve closes and pressure increases rapidly. Because both the aortic and mitral valves are closed, this phase is isovolumic (**A**). Ejection (**B**) begins when the aortic valve opens and the ventricle meets its afterload, the aortic pressure. Systole ends when ventricular pressure and volume reach the end-systolic pressure–volume relationship, which describes the inotropic state of the ventricle. After aortic valve closure separates the afterload (aortic pressure) and the ventricular cavity, blood can neither enter nor leave the ventricle; as a result, relaxation begins under isovolumic conditions (**C**). When left ventricular pressure falls below that in the left atrium, the mitral valve opens and blood flows from the atrium into the ventricle during the phase of filling (**D**). The cycle ends when ventricular pressure and volume reach the end-diastolic pressure–volume relationship. From Katz AM (2006). *Physiology of the Heart.* 4th ed. Philadelphia, Lippincott Williams & Wilkins.

cannot change. Diastole therefore proceeds at a constant ventricular volume until left ventricular pressure falls below that in the left atrium, which allows the mitral valve to open. This initiates the phase of *filling* (D in Fig. 2-7) during which blood flows across the mitral valve from the atrium into the relaxing ventricle. Left ventricular pressure and volume rise gradually during this phase as blood returning from the lungs generates the preload for the next contraction. Diastole ends at a point on the *end-diastolic pressure–volume relationship*, which describes the lusitropic state of the ventricle.

Two pressure–volume relationships constrain the pressure–volume loop: The end-systolic pressure–volume relationship, which is determined by the inotropic properties of the contracting ventricle, and the end-diastolic pressure–volume relationship, which is determined by the lusitropic properties of the relaxed ventricle. Ventricular end-diastolic volume, which must lie along the end-diastolic pressure–volume relationship, is determined by venous return, end-systolic volume (the residual volume left behind after the previous cardiac cycle), and the lusitropic properties of the ventricle (Table 2-2). End-systolic volume, which is determined by end-diastolic volume, aortic impedance, and contractility, lies along the end-systolic pressure–volume relationship, which characterizes the inotropic state. Changes in circulatory hemodynamics modify cardiac performance by shifting the end-diastolic and end-systolic points along the two pressure–volume relationships, but the limits imposed by the latter cannot be exceeded. Changes in inotropic and lusitropic state, on the other hand, alter these limits by shifting the end-systolic and end-diastolic pressure–volume relationships, respectively.

Inotropy and Lusitropy

The contractile state of a ventricle inotropy can be described as the relationship between end-diastolic volume, an index of preload, and the pressure developed during systole at each end-diastolic volume (Fig. 2-8). This relationship, commonly referred to as a Starling curve, can be plotted as the end-systolic pressure–volume relationship. The heart normally operates on the left-hand portion of the Starling curve, called the *ascending limb,* where increasing preload enhances the performance of the heart; this enables the heart to eject during systole what it receives during diastole. Because of the low compliance of cardiac muscle and the stiff pericardium, normal hearts cannot move onto the descending limb except at very high nonphysiological filling pressures. This is important because the heart cannot achieve a steady state on the descending limb where even a small increase in venous return would initiate a vicious cycle in which the additional filling, by increasing end-systolic volume, would further reduce ejection, which would cause more dilatation, which by decreasing the ability to eject would cause further dilatation, and so on. Unless preload or afterload are decreased, the heart has no way to recover from this vicious cycle, so that a ventricle that moves on to the descending limb of the Starling curve could burst like an overfilled balloon. However, ventricular rupture is prevented by the low compliance of the myocardium and the restraints exercised by the pericardium; instead, overdilatation can give rise to acute pulmonary edema (a clinical syndrome once referred to as "acute dilatation").

TABLE 2-2

Determinants of Ventricular Filling and Ejection

Filling
Venous return: Flow of blood toward the heart
End-systolic (residual) volume: Amount of blood left in the ventricle after the previous systole
Lusitropy: Ability of the heart to fill (end-diastolic pressure–volume relationship)

Ejection
Aortic impedance: Ability of the aorta to receive blood from the heart
End-diastolic volume: Amount of blood in the ventricle at the start of systole
Inotropy: Ability of the heart to eject (end-systolic pressure–volume relationship)

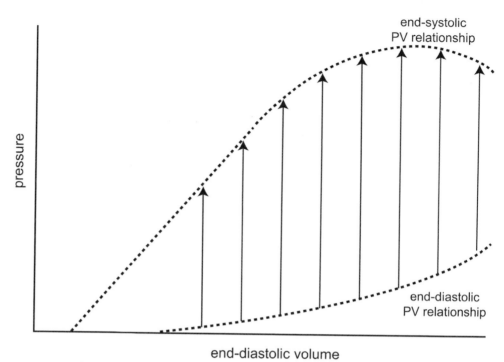

Figure 2-8: Effects of changing end-diastolic volume on the pressures developed in a series of isovolumic contractions (Starling's law of the heart). Developed pressure (*vertical arrows*) initially increases with increasing end-diastolic volume; at very high end-diastolic volumes, systolic pressure can decline with increasing volume. The *lower dashed line* is the end-diastolic pressure–volume relationship; the *upper dashed line* the end-systolic pressure–volume relationship. Modified from Katz AM (2006). *Physiology of the Heart*. 4th ed. Philadelphia, Lippincott Williams & Wilkins.

Starling curves, which describe the effect of changing cavity volume on the ability of a ventricle to develop pressure, are similar to end-systolic pressure–volume relationships. Because each curve describes a given level of contractility, a change in contractility generates a new curve; this allows the effects of changing inotropic state to be depicted as a family of Starling curves, each of which describes the end-systolic pressure–volume relationship at a given inotropic state (Fig. 2-9, CAB). A positive inotropic intervention, which by definition increases the ability of the heart to do work at any cavity volume (see Fig. 2-8), shifts the heart to a higher curve (Fig. 2-9, A → D), whereas a negative inotropic intervention causes a shift to a lower curve (Fig. 2-9, A → E). Figure 2-9 provides one way to view the interplay between regulation of cardiac performance by changing end-diastolic volume (Starling's law) and contractility.

Regulation of systolic function is traditionally attributed to the interplay between changing end-diastolic volume (Starling's law of the heart) and changing contractility. The former was viewed as the only determinant of myocardial performance until the mid-1950s, when description of the family of Starling curves clarified the interplay between regulation by end-diastolic volume and regulation by contractility. These two regulatory mechanisms were initially believed to reflect the operation of entirely different mechanisms, but it is now clear that both are brought about largely by variations in excitation-contraction coupling (see Chapter 5). However, the traditional distinction remains useful because the two mechanisms serve different physiological functions. Regulation by changing end-diastolic volume is a

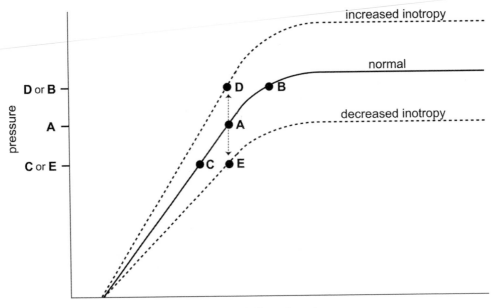

Figure 2-9: Family of Starling curves. The solid line (**CAB**) is an end-systolic pressure–volume relationship (Starling curve) that describes myocardial contractility; point **A** along this line represents the baseline state. The two *dashed lines* represent additional Starling curves recorded after contractility has changed. Changes in end-diastolic volume at a constant level of contractility shift the end-systolic point along each Starling curve, which allows a greater venous return to increase developed pressure (**A → B**), and a decrease in venous return to reduce pressure (**A → C**). The work of the heart can also be changed by interventions that modify myocardial contractility, which increase or decrease pressure at any end-diastolic volume; for this reason, positive and negative inotropic interventions shift the Starling curves. Starting from the baseline state at a given end-diastolic volume (point A), a positive inotropic intervention increases developed pressure (**A → D**) and a negative inotropic intervention decreases pressure from (**A → E**). Modified from Katz AM (2006). *Physiology of the Heart.* 4th ed. Philadelphia, Lippincott Williams & Wilkins.

"passive" hemodynamic mechanism that equalizes the outputs of the right and left ventricles and allows the heart to respond rapidly, often on a beat-to-beat basis, to changes in preload and afterload. Myocardial contractility, on the other hand, is modified more slowly by mediators of the neurohumoral response (see Chapter 3); drugs; changes in the environment of the myocardial cells such as occur in ischemia, hypoxia, and acidosis; and by disease.

Inotropy

Contractility is difficult to define. The simplest definition is *the ability of a cardiac myocyte to contract at a given preload (rest length) and afterload.* However this definition is of limited value because contractility is a manifestation of *all* of the biochemical and biophysical factors, except for preload and afterload, that influence the number and turnover rate of the interactions between the myosin cross-bridges and actin (see Chapter 5). A *change* in contractility, however, is easier to define; this is simply *any change in cardiac performance not caused by a change in preload (rest length) or afterload.*

In the 1960s and 1970s efforts were made to measure myocardial contractility using force–velocity curves to eliminate the effects of changing preload and afterload. This approach, which was based on A.V. Hill's classic analyses of tetanized frog skeletal muscle, where force–velocity curves are hyperbolic, was based on the premise that extrapolations of V_{max} could quantify myocardial contractility. In the heart, however, these curves are distorted by the slow onset and instability of the active state, the spiral arrangement of the fibers in the walls of the ventricles, the low compliance of heart muscle, and the influences of cavity size, inhomogeneities, and ventricular architecture. For these and other reasons, estimates of V_{max} in the heart are approximations that neither measure myocardial contractility nor distinguish the effects of changing fiber length from those of a change in inotropic state (Katz, 2006).

Lusitropy

Lusitropy defines the properties of the relaxed heart, so that changes in these properties generate a family of *filling curves*, which, like the Starling curves shown in Figure 2-9, regulate cardiac performance (Fig. 2-10); each filling curve (e.g., Fig. 2-10, VXW) represents an end-diastolic pressure–volume relationship. Changes in diastolic properties shift these filling curves by changing the end-diastolic volume at any filling pressure; increased lusitropy shifts the end-diastolic pressure–volume relationship downward and to the right (Fig. 2-10, X → Y), while a decrease in lusitropy shifts the curve upward and to the left (Fig. 2-10, X → Z).

Lusitropy is influenced by such variables as the rate and extent of calcium uptake into the sarcoplasmic reticulum, the calcium affinity of troponin, and the extent to

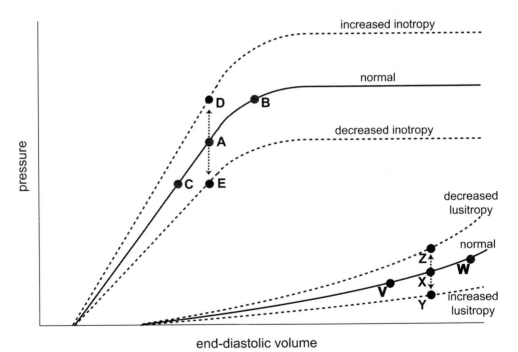

Figure 2-10: Family of filling curves. Three end-diastolic pressure–volume relationships have been added to the end-systolic pressure–volume relationships shown in Figure 2-9. The baseline end-diastolic pressure–volume relationship contains point **X**. A positive lusitropic intervention, which improves the ability of the ventricle to fill, shifts the end-diastolic pressure–volume relationship to the right and downward (curve containing point **Y**), while a negative lusitropic intervention, which reduces ventricular filling, shifts this relationship to the left and upward (curve containing point **Z**). From Katz AM (2006). *Physiology of the Heart.* 4th ed. Philadelphia, Lippincott Williams & Wilkins.

which the contractile proteins are dissociated after activator calcium has been removed from the troponin complex (see Chapter 5). Lusitropy is also influenced by changes in cytoskeletal proteins such as titin, ventricular interdependence, the pericardium, and the geometry and thickness of the ventricular walls.

INTERPLAY BETWEEN VENOUS RETURN AND CARDIAC OUTPUT

The fact that blood flows in a circle means that when the circulation is at a steady state, regulatory mechanisms are needed to ensure that venous return and cardiac output are the same. *Cardiac output is matched to venous return* by Starling's law of the heart, which increases stroke volume when more blood returning to the heart increases atrial and ventricular end-diastolic pressures, and decreases stroke volume when reduced venous return lowers atrial pressure (Fig. 2-11). *Atrial pressure also matches venous return to cardiac output* because increased atrial pressure reduces blood flow to the heart, and decreased atrial pressure increases venous return (Fig 2-11). Although ventricular diastolic pressure and volume are normally related to one another (the end-diastolic pressure–volume relationship [see previous discussion]), this relationship can be altered by disease; for example, pericardial effusion (tamponade) elevates diastolic pressure but lowers diastolic volume.

The effects of atrial pressure on venous return are not due to a physiological law, but instead result from a simple hydrostatic mechanism by which increased atrial pressure reduces blood flow from the venous system to the heart, and vice versa. This hydrostatic mechanism is depicted in Figure 2-12, which shows how changing

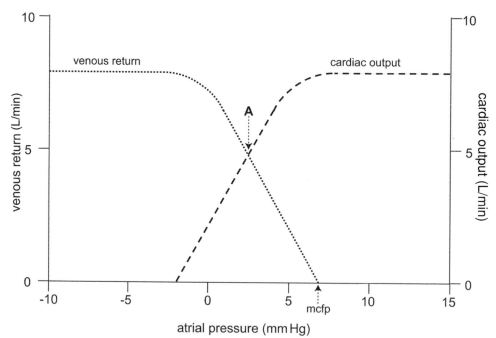

Figure 2-11: Guyton diagram showing how atrial pressure matches venous return (*dotted line*) and cardiac output (*dashed line*). Elevating atrial pressure increases cardiac output (Starling's law of the heart) but decreases venous return, whereas decreasing atrial pressure has the opposite effects. At any steady state, the two curves intersect at the atrial pressure at which flow into and out of the heart are the same (**A**). The mean circulatory filling pressure (mcfp) is the pressure recorded when the heart is stopped. From Katz AM (2006). *Physiology of the Heart.* 4th ed. Philadelphia, Lippincott Williams & Wilkins.

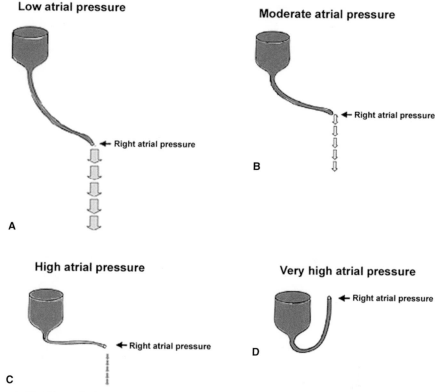

Figure 2-12: Effect of raising and lowering the outlet of a hose connected to a reservoir. Outflow from the reservoir depends on the pressure gradient between the outlet of the hose, which in the circulation is atrial pressure, and the pressure of the fluid in the reservoir, which is the mean circulatory filling pressure. When the outlet of the hose is at a low level (**A**), outflow from the reservoir is rapid. Outflow is reduced when the outlet of the hose is raised (**B** and **C**), and stops altogether when the height of the outlet is the same as that in the reservoir (**D**). From Katz AM (2006). *Physiology of the Heart.* 4th ed. Philadelphia, Lippincott Williams & Wilkins.

the height of a hose connected to a reservoir affects flow through the hose. Raising the outlet of the hose, like raising atrial pressure, slows outflow from the reservoir by reducing the pressure gradient between the reservoir and the tip of the hose. Flow stops completely when the level of the outlet and that in the reservoir are the same; this corresponds to the situation when the heart is stopped, blood flow ceases, and all pressures in the cardiovascular system come to equilibrium; the latter, called the *mean circulatory filling pressure,* is shown by the arrow labeled "mcfp" in Figure 2-11. Mean circulatory filling pressure in anaesthetized dogs is ~7 mm Hg, which is closer to the low pressure in the veins than the higher arterial pressures because there is much more blood in the venous circulation.

The curves in Figure 2-11, which is often called a "Guyton diagram" after Arthur Guyton who devised this plot, show that a rise in atrial pressure, when viewed from the circulation, reduces blood flow *toward* the heart but, when viewed from the heart, increases ejection of blood *from* the heart. Conversely, a fall in atrial pressure increases venous return and reduces ejection. The effects of changing atrial pressure on flow into and out of the heart are therefore opposite to one another; venous return falls with increasing atrial pressure, while cardiac output rises when atrial pressure increases. At any given steady state, the intersection of the two curves

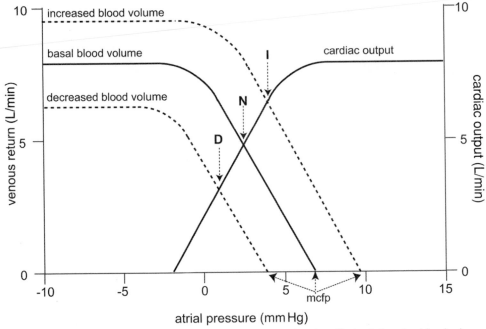

Figure 2-13: Curves relating venous return and cardiac output showing effects of changing blood volume. Increased blood volume increases venous return and mean circulatory filling pressure, whereas a decrease in blood volume reduces venous return and mean circulatory filling pressure. **D**, decreased blood volume; **I**, increased blood volume; **N**, normal. Modified from Katz AM (2006). *Physiology of the Heart.* 4th ed. Philadelphia, Lippincott Williams & Wilkins.

identifies the atrial pressure at which venous return and cardiac output are equal to one another.

Guyton diagrams help in understanding how changes in blood volume modify venous return and cardiac output. A decrease in blood volume, such as occurs after hemorrhage, lowers atrial pressure and reduces cardiac output (Fig. 2-13, N → D), whereas increased blood volume, as occurs after a blood transfusion, elevates atrial pressure and increases cardiac output (Fig. 2-13, N → I). Guyton diagrams also show how a positive inotropic intervention, which increases ejection and so lowers atrial pressure, increases venous return (Fig. 2-14, N → I), and how a negative inotropic intervention, which reduces ejection and increases atrial pressure, lowers venous return (Fig. 2-14, N → D). In all of these examples, shifts of the intersection between the curves relating atrial pressure to venous return and cardiac output establish new steady states at which venous return and cardiac output are equal.

HEMODYNAMIC ABNORMALITIES IN HEART FAILURE

There are many ways to classify the hemodynamic abnormalities in a patient with heart failure. Some are descriptive, while others imply the operation of distinct pathophysiological mechanisms. Unfortunately, none is entirely satisfactory because of the many mechanisms that can cause the heart to fail. Furthermore, efforts to link causal mechanisms to abnormal hemodynamics are complicated by effects of changing preload and afterload, the interplay between filling and ejection, and the fact

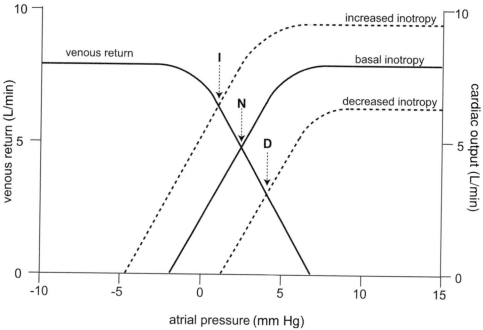

Figure 2-14: Curves relating venous return and cardiac output showing effects of changing contractility. Increased inotropy increases cardiac output and reduces atrial pressure, which allows venous return to increase. Conversely, decreased inotropy decreases cardiac output and increases atrial pressure, which causes venous return to decrease. **D**, decreased contractility; **I**, increased contractility; **N**, normal. Modified from Katz AM (2006). *Physiology of the Heart*. 4th ed. Philadelphia, Lippincott Williams & Wilkins.

that failure of one ventricle generally modifies the function of the other because blood flows in a circle and because of direct ventricular interdependence effects. For these reasons, pathophysiological classifications tend to be ambiguous and are often confusing.

A simple way to classify the hemodynamic abnormalities in heart failure is to define the reduced ejection of blood into the aorta and pulmonary artery as *forward failure,* and the increased pressure in the veins returning blood to the heart as *backward failure* (see Fig. 2-1). Heart failure can also be characterized according to whether the primary abnormality involves the left or right ventricle, so that there can be four distinct manifestations of this syndrome (Table 2-3). However, this is an oversimplification

TABLE 2-3

Hemodynamic Manifestations of Heart Failure

Site of failure	Type of failure	Major hemodynamic consequence
Right heart	Forward	Reduced ejection into pulmonary artery—low cardiac output
Right heart	Backward	Increased systemic venous pressure
Left heart	Forward	Reduced ejection into aorta—low cardiac output
Left heart	Backward	Increased pulmonary venous pressure

because filling is a major determinant of ejection, ejection is a major determinant of filling, and the two sides of the heart operate in series. Attempts to classify the hemodynamics of heart failure in terms of forward and backward failure are further complicated by the neurohumoral response, which alters hemodynamics by increasing myocardial contractility, accelerating relaxation, constricting arteries and veins, and causing fluid retention by the kidneys (see Chapter 3). Local factors, notably autoregulation, also affect these hemodynamics, for example when reduced blood flow increases the accumulation of tissue metabolites that cause arteriolar dilatation.

Although most components of the neurohumoral response initially alleviate the hemodynamic abnormalities in patients with heart failure, they also have adverse long-term effects. The latter include myocardial energy starvation (see Chapter 5), and activation of proliferative responses that adversely modify the size, shape, and composition of the failing heart. As noted in Chapter 3, the influence of the neurohumoral response is often so great that it can dominate the clinical picture in these patients.

The hemodynamic consequences of changing vascular tone differ in the arterial and venous circulations. Constriction of the arterioles, which contribute most of the *resistance* to flow but contain relatively little blood, increases arterial pressure but has no direct effect on venous pressures, whereas constriction of the veins, which are large vessels that contain most of the blood in the vascular system, increases venous return to the heart by reducing venous *capacitance,* but has little effect on arterial pressure. Fluid retention by the kidneys, a devastating consequence of the neurohumoral response (see Chapter 3), plays a key role in heart failure by worsening both pulmonary and systemic venous congestion.

Backward and Forward Failure

Heart failure can reduce ejection of blood under pressure into the aorta and pulmonary artery (*forward failure*) and cause inadequate emptying of the venous reservoirs (*backward failure*) (see Fig. 2-1). Although forward failure is sometimes equated with depressed myocardial contractility (decreased inotropy), and backward failure with impaired relaxation (decreased lusitropy), the link between these abnormalities of pump function and altered hemodynamics is tenuous. As already noted, a heart that fills poorly cannot empty normally, and vice versa; furthermore, the clinical manifestations of forward and backward failure are influenced when extracardiac responses to neurohumoral activation modify the interactions between the peripheral circulation and the heart. Increased afterload caused by reflex arteriolar vasoconstriction reduces cardiac output and so worsens forward failure, whereas the increased preload caused by venoconstriction and fluid retention by the kidneys increases venous pressure and so worsens backward failure. The pathophysiological value of the distinction between forward and backward failure is further diminished because these hemodynamic abnormalities are modified by the effects of therapy on the blood vessels and kidneys (Chapter 7). Vasodilator drugs, by reducing afterload, increase stroke volume and alleviate the low cardiac output that characterizes forward failure, while diuretics reduce blood volume and decrease venous pressures, which alleviates the major manifestations of backward failure. For these reasons, the severity of forward and backward failure, defined as reduced cardiac output and increased venous pressure, respectively, provides little information regarding the extent to which depressed contractility or impaired relaxation has caused the abnormal pump function.

Right and Left Heart Failure

In developed countries, where the major etiologies of heart failure are coronary and hypertensive heart disease (Table 2-4), the clinical picture is generally dominated by the signs and symptoms of impaired left ventricular function. Symptoms of left heart failure also dominate the clinical picture in most patients with dilated, hypertrophic, and infiltrative cardiomyopathies. Tachycardia-induced cardiomyopathy, which usually causes left heart failure, is rare but important because it is among the curable forms of heart failure. Primary right heart failure, which is less common, occurs in cor pulmonale, which can be caused by chronic lung disease, multiple pulmonary emboli, or primary pulmonary hypertension. Right heart failure secondary to left heart failure is also common (see subsequent text). Valvular heart disease can cause either left or right heart failure, depending on the valve abnormalities, while congenital heart disease often causes right heart failure, for example when pulmonic stenosis or pulmonary hypertension associated with an intracardiac shunt overloads the right heart.

Right heart failure often comes to dominate the clinical picture in patients in whom the primary abnormality involves the left heart. This sequence of events, which is elegantly described by Paul Wood in one of the outstanding clinical papers of the 20th century (Wood, 1957), occurs when chronic elevation of left atrial pressure causes vasoconstriction and proliferative changes in the pulmonary arterioles that increase pulmonary vascular resistance. The resulting pulmonary arterial hypertension, by reducing blood through the lungs, alleviates pulmonary congestion, but this response replaces left heart failure with right heart failure.

TABLE 2-4

Some Causes of Heart Failure and Their Most Common Clinical Manifestations

Etiology	Right/Left heart failure	Systolic/Diastolic heart failure	Global/Regional ventricular wall abnormality
Myocardial infarction	Left	Systolic	Regional loss of function
Dilated cardiomyopathy/ myocarditis	Left	Systolic	Global loss of function
Hypertensive heart disease/ aortic stenosis	Left	Diastolic	Global hypertrophy
Hypertrophic cardiomyopathy	Left	Diastolic	Hypertrophy, often regional
Incessant tachycardia	Left	Systolic	Global loss of function
Infiltrative diseases	Both	Diastolic	Wall thickening, usually global
Cor pulmonale	Right	Both	Global abnormalities
Pericardial effusion/tamponade	Right	Diastolic	Global restriction of filling
Valvular/congenital	Depends on structural abnormality		Varies

Systolic and Diastolic Dysfunction

Systolic and diastolic *dysfunction,* which describe different pathophysiological mechanisms, are not the same as systolic and diastolic *heart failure,* which refer to different subsets of patients (see subsequent text). Systolic dysfunction describes abnormalities of ventricular ejection that slow the rate of pressure rise during isovolumic contraction (+dP/dt) and the rate and extent of ejection (Fig. 2-15), whereas diastolic dysfunction, which impairs ventricular filling, slows the rate of pressure fall during isovolumic relaxation (−dP/dt) and, when diastolic stiffness is increased, decreases the rate and extent of filling (Fig. 2-16).

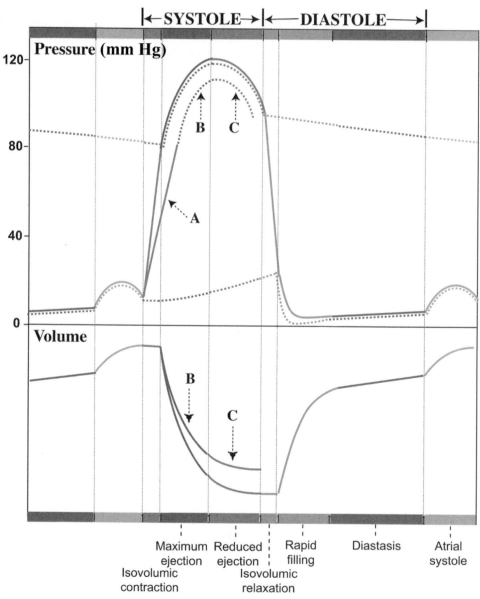

Figure 2-15: Pathophysiological mechanisms that can impair systolic function. **A:** Slowed rate of pressure rise during isovolumic contraction (+dP/dt). **B:** Slowed ejection. **C:** Reduced systolic wall stress, which reduces stroke volume.

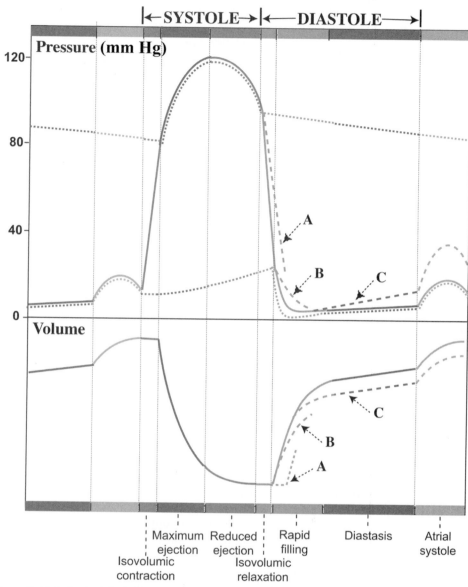

Figure 2-16: Pathophysiological mechanisms that can impair diastolic function. **A:** Slowed rate of pressure fall during isovolumic relaxation (−dP/dt). **B:** Slowed filling during early diastole. **C:** Reduced diastolic compliance, which slows filling throughout diastole. Modified from Katz AM (2006). *Physiology of the Heart*. 4th ed. Philadelphia, Lippincott Williams & Wilkins.

Systolic dysfunction can be initiated by damage to the ventricular wall such as occurs after a myocardial infarction, cardiac myocyte elongation (eccentric hypertrophy) in patients with dilated cardiomyopathies, and biochemical abnormalities that impair cardiac myocyte shortening. Systolic dysfunction impairs ejection in patients with viral myocarditis, or with toxic and metabolic abnormalities.

Causes of diastolic dysfunction include reduced cavity volume caused by cardiac myocyte thickening (concentric hypertrophy) in patients with hypertension or hypertrophic cardiomyopathies; reduced ventricular compliance associated with aging; restrictive diseases like amyloidosis, fibroelastosis, and pericardial diseases that impede filling; and cellular abnormalities that impair cardiac myocyte relaxation. Diastolic dysfunction caused by energy starvation impairs ventricular filling in hypertrophied hearts and when coronary flow is reduced.

Neither hemodynamic measurements, such as stroke volume or venous and arterial pressures, nor the clinical manifestations of forward or backward failure can distinguish between systolic and diastolic dysfunction in chronic heart failure. In both, aortic pressure and cardiac output usually decrease and ventricular diastolic pressures increase, so that additional data regarding ventricular function are needed to make this distinction. Systolic dysfunction is suggested by marked reductions in +dP/dt, ejection rate, or systolic compliance, whereas diastolic dysfunction is suggested by low −dP/dt, slowed ventricular filling, or reduced diastolic compliance. However, systolic and diastolic dysfunction commonly occur together, which makes it difficult for any single pathophysiological measurement to identify which of these mechanisms is responsible for impaired pump function.

Systolic and Diastolic Heart Failure

Definitions of systolic and diastolic heart failure are among the most controversial topics in cardiology today. Disputes arise largely because of the many etiologies of both of these pathophysiological entities and a lack of accepted gold standards for diagnosis. For these reasons, the following discussion should be viewed as a progress report rather than a definitive essay.

Criteria for the definition of *systolic heart failure* are elusive. Although the usual patient with this diagnosis presents with heart failure and a dilated left ventricle, definitions based solely on these criteria are oversimplified because of the many conditions that can give rise to these findings. In volume overload of the left ventricle caused by valvular regurgitation, either aortic or mitral, the primary problem is the abnormal valve and not the myocardium (see Chapter 1); other less common causes of volume overload include systemic arteriovenous fistula and vascular tumors. (More than 35 years ago, one of the authors cared for a lady with an inoperable melon-sized giant cell tumor of the jaw and heart failure that had been attributed to "ischemic heart disease"; it was not until the tumor was noted to be very warm and no other evidence for coronary disease could be found that it became clear that she had high output failure caused by the huge flow of blood through the tumor.) Other causes of heart failure and dilated left ventricle include acute myocardial infarction, where other clinical features point to the underlying abnormality in the coronary arteries; toxic causes such as severe alcohol intoxication, carbon tetrachloride, or cobalt poisoning; acute viral myocarditis; and noncardiac conditions such as severe anemia and thyrotoxicosis. The remaining causes—"old" (as opposed to acute) myocardial infarction, often called "ischemic cardiomyopathy", and a diverse group of diseases called "dilated cardiomyopathies" (see Chapter 5)—give rise to the syndrome called "systolic heart failure." Criteria for the diagnosis of diastolic heart failure, which are even more difficult, are detailed in the subsequent text.

In patients with systolic heart failure, the ventricle is dilated, whereas in diastolic heart failure ventricular cavity volume can be normal, minimally reduced, or slightly increased (Table 2-5). Systolic and diastolic heart failure are usually distinguished on the basis of the ejection fraction (EF), which is the ratio between stroke volume (SV) and end-diastolic volume (EDV):

$$EF = \frac{SV}{EDV}$$

Eq. 2.9

> **TABLE 2-5**
>
> ## Systolic and Diastolic Heart Failure
>
> **Systolic Heart Failure (Heart Failure With Low Ejection Fraction [EF]):**
> *Eccentric hypertrophy* (increased cavity volume)
>   Regional: Myocardial infarction
>   Global: Dilated cardiomyopathies, viral or toxic myocarditis
> **Diastolic Heart Failure (Heart Failure With Preserved EF):**
> *Concentric hypertrophy* (normal or reduced cavity volume)
>   Hypertrophic cardiomyopathies, hypertensive heart disease
> *Restrictive cardiomyopathies*

Because EF is significantly reduced in systolic heart failure, but not in diastolic heart failure, it is becoming common for these syndromes to be called *heart failure with low EF* and *heart failure with preserved (or normal) EF*, respectively.

The major cause of the decreased EF in systolic heart failure is ventricular dilatation, which increases the denominator (EDV), rather than a fall in cardiac output, which would reduce the numerator (SV). In fact, the ability of EF to distinguish between systolic and diastolic heart failure is due largely to differences in the denominator (EDV), which is increased when ejection is impaired and usually reduced when impaired filling is the underlying abnormality. Abnormalities in SV are much less important in making this distinction because cardiac output is low in most patients with both types of heart failure; exceptions such as high output failure, where EF is preserved by increased SV, are uncommon.

Because ejection fraction is the ratio between stroke volume, a *physiological* measurement, and end diastolic volume, an *architectural* measurement, EF cannot be used to quantify either ventricular function or ventricular architecture. Another reason that EF is of little value as an index of myocardial contractility is that it is influenced by heart rate, preload, afterload, and ventricular architecture. Because left ventricular volume is a useful predictor of survival in patients with systolic heart failure, patients with low EF generally have a poor long-term outcome; on the other hand, EF provides surprisingly little information about exercise intolerance or the extent of clinical disability (Benge et al., 1980; Franciosa et al., 1981; Lipkin and Poole-Wilson, 1986; Volterrani et al., 1994).

Systolic heart failure, which is characterized by left ventricular dilatation (eccentric hypertrophy), is usually caused by diseases that destroy, damage, or weaken the myocardium. The left ventricular wall motion abnormalities in systolic heart failure can be either regional or diffuse (global). *Regional* wall motion abnormalities are seen most often when occlusion of a major coronary artery has destroyed part of the left ventricle (myocardial infarction), whereas *global* wall motion abnormalities result from conditions like idiopathic dilated cardiomyopathy and myocarditis, in which function throughout the ventricle is impaired. As many as half of patients with dilated cardiomyopathies appear to have familial diseases (see Chapter 5), but the importance of viral infection as a cause of this syndrome is not clear (Kuethe et al., 2007). Patients with acute myocarditis, which is generally attributed to viral infection, can recover; surprisingly, among patients with active lymphocyte infiltration, those with fulminant myocarditis have been found to have a better long-term prognosis than those with less severe myocarditis, possibly because the latter has an autoimmune etiology (McCarthy et al., 2000).

Diastolic heart failure is characteristically seen in patients with concentric left ventricular hypertrophy. Underlying etiologies include hypertension and the decreased aortic impedance that accompanies aging, which is a major reason that diastolic heart failure is commonly diagnosed in the elderly. Episodes of acute pulmonary edema in patients whose hearts seem to be normal under basal conditions are common in diastolic heart failure where, because of the reduced compliance of these ventricles, even a small increase in preload or afterload can cause a sharp rise in end-diastolic pressure that "tips" the patient onto the descending limb of the Starling curve (see subsequent text). It is for this reason that these patients frequently develop acute pulmonary edema following a rapid increase in preload, such as occurs after a large salt-rich holiday meal, or when exercise or an emotional upset reduces left ventricular ejection by causing a sudden rise in arterial blood pressure. Less common causes of heart failure with normal ejection fraction include familial hypertrophic cardiomyopathies (see Chapter 5) and restrictive cardiomyopathies. The latter can be caused by fibrosis or infiltrative processes that stiffen the walls of the heart; etiologies include amyloid, sarcoidosis, hemochromatosis, and endocardial processes such as endomyocardial fibroelastosis and eosinophilic (tropical) endomyocardial fibrosis (Hancock, 2001). The hemodynamic abnormalities in restrictive cardiomyopathies resemble those caused by constrictive pericarditis, which can make it difficult to diagnose these diseases (Kabbani and LeWinter, 2000).

SIGNS AND SYMPTOMS OF HEART FAILURE

The clinical abnormalities in heart failure include *signs,* which are objective manifestations of depressed cardiac performance, and *symptoms,* which are perceived by the patient. The consequences of increased diastolic pressure are readily understood because transmission of this pressure upstream into the venous system behind a failing ventricle elevates capillary pressure and so increases fluid transudation across the capillary endothelium into the tissues. In left heart failure, the resulting edema appears in the lungs, whereas right heart failure causes peripheral edema, ascites (fluid in the peritoneal cavity), and pleural and pericardial effusions. Fatigue, the major symptom associated with decreased cardiac output, occurs in virtually all patients with heart failure.

The previously described signs and symptoms are not specific for heart failure. *Circulatory failure,* which can be defined as a disorder in which hemodynamic abnormalities resembling those caused by heart failure occur in patients with increased blood volume but normal hearts, can occur when renal or hepatic disease, or infusion of large amounts of blood or saline, elevate systemic and pulmonary venous pressures to levels that produce signs and symptoms similar to those of backward heart failure. Conversely, reduced blood volume, which can be caused by hemorrhage, extensive burns, or toxic shock syndrome, can mimic forward failure. In *heart failure,* similar hemodynamic abnormalities are caused by abnormalities that involve the heart, such as valvular stenosis and regurgitation, septal defects, pulmonary emboli, and, pericardial effusion. The same clinical findings are seen in *myocardial failure,* where the underlying abnormality is impaired cardiac myocyte function. However, distinctions between heart failure and myocardial failure are blurred because both chronic hemodynamic overloading and the neurohumoral response cause deleterious effects on the myocardium (see Chapters 3 and 5).

Backward Failure of the Left Heart

Backward failure of the left heart causes shortness of breath (dyspnea) largely by increasing the work required to ventilate the congested lungs. In contrast to normal breathing, which is rarely perceived, the increased respiratory effort seen when elevated pulmonary venous pressure causes the lungs to become stiff and inelastic, like a water-logged sponge, cannot be ignored (Mancini et al., 1992). Cardiac dyspnea is exacerbated by pulmonary interstitial edema and weakness of the respiratory muscles (see subsequent text). Arterial hypoxia occurs when pulmonary interstitial edema impairs oxygen exchange; ventilation–perfusion mismatch can also contribute to cardiac dyspnea (Sullivan et al., 1988; Poole-Wilson and Ferrari, 1996; Wasserman et al., 1997). As noted previously, reactive pulmonary vasoconstriction and obliteration of small pulmonary arteries, which occur in many patients with chronic backward failure of the left heart, can protect the lungs from overfilling but exchanges one problem (left heart failure) for another (right heart failure) (Wood, 1954).

Dyspnea is worsened by exertion in patients with both left heart failure and pulmonary disease, but cardiac dyspnea generally becomes more severe when the patient lies down (*orthopnea*) because elevation of the lower extremities drains blood from the leg veins, which increases central blood volume. *Paroxysmal nocturnal dyspnea,* the sudden onset of severe shortness of breath in a patient who has been recumbent for several hours, occurs when slow resorption of interstitial fluid from the edematous legs increases blood volume.

High pulmonary venous pressure causes fluid transudation across the pulmonary capillaries; this fluid appears first in the interstitium, from which it is carried to the systemic veins via lymphatic vessels. If the rate of transudation exceeds the rate at which the fluid can be removed by the lymphatics, the interstitium becomes edematous. Interstitial edema can be seen on an ordinary chest x-ray film as thin horizontal lines, called *Kerley B lines* that, due to the effects of gravity, initially appear in the lower lung fields. Because of gravity, this interstitial fluid compresses the veins that drain the lower lobes and blurs the borders of the lower lobe vessels, which results in a radiological pattern called "cephalization," in which the pulmonary veins draining the upper lobes appear larger than those that drain the lower lobes. In contrast to right-sided filling pressure, which is readily measured by examination of the jugular veins (see subsequent text), clinical estimation of left ventricular diastolic pressure is difficult; several noninvasive indices correlate with left atrial pressure, but precise measurements may require catheter measurement.

Accumulation of large amounts of interstitial fluid interferes with gas exchange between the pulmonary capillaries and the alveoli; most prominent is arterial hypoxia because oxygen is much less soluble in water than carbon dioxide. When backward failure of the left heart becomes severe, fluid entering the small bronchi causes rales, which are crackling sounds described by Hippocrates as like the "seething of vinegar" (see Chapter 1). Because of gravity, rales appear initially at the lung bases. In severe left heart failure, when pulmonary capillary pressure—which drives fluid into the interstitium—greatly exceeds plasma protein oncotic pressure—which causes fluid resorption—flooding of the airspaces leads to pulmonary edema that can literally drown a patient.

Backward Failure of the Right Heart

Backward failure of the right heart elevates jugular venous pressure, which provides an accurate bedside measurement of right atrial pressure. In addition to quantifying the severity of backward failure of the right heart, examination of the neck veins can provide valuable information regarding the state of the tricuspid valve and the stiffness of the right ventricle.

Right heart failure also causes fluid to be transudated into the soft tissues (edema) and the pleural, pericardial, and abdominal spaces (anasarca). Massive fluid accumulation, once called dropsy, caused horrible suffering in patients before the development of effective therapy to rid the body of the excess fluid (see Chapter 1). Fortunately, this misery can generally be avoided by modern diuretics, which along with salt (sodium) restriction have changed the clinical manifestations of this syndrome by making fatigue, rather than fluid retention, the most common cause of disability in these patients. For this reason, the term *congestive heart failure* (CHF) is being replaced by the more general *heart failure*.

Forward Failure

Fatigue, which has emerged as one of the most common and troublesome problems in patients with heart failure, has several causes. In addition to reduced skeletal muscle perfusion caused by low cardiac output, a major cause of fatigue in these patients is a skeletal muscle myopathy whose underlying mechanisms include disuse, malnutrition, inflammation, apoptosis, and molecular abnormalities in the skeletal myocytes that include changes in myosin isoforms and mitochondrial dysfunction (Mettauer et al., 2006). The latter, by impairing oxidative ATP regeneration, increases anaerobic lactate production that reduces skeletal muscle performance by accelerating the appearance of systemic acidosis during exercise. Cytokines and other inflammatory mediators, along with activation of the receptors that bind these peptides, also appear to play an important causal role in this myopathy (Niebauer et al., 2005). The ability of exercise training to alleviate the symptoms associated with this myopathy, and possibly to improve prognosis (van Tol et al., 2006; Ventura-Clapier et al., 2007) argues strongly against the once widely held view that heart failure should be treated with prolonged rest (see Chapter 1).

Low cardiac output, by increasing anaerobic metabolism in exercising skeletal muscle, can also contribute to exertional dyspnea.

PATHOPHYSIOLOGICAL MECHANISMS IN HEART FAILURE

The Descending Limb of the Starling Curve

During the mid-20th century it was commonly taught that chronically failing hearts operate on the descending limb of the Starling curve (McMichael, 1950; Wiggers, 1952; Guyton, 1961), even though Starling himself had made it clear that the heart cannot achieve a steady state when increasing chamber volume decreases its ability to eject (see previous discussion). It is now clear, however, that extremely high diastolic pressures are required to force the heart onto the descending limb (Spiro and Sonnenblick, 1962; Elzinga, 1992), and that the heart cannot achieve a steady state when it operates on the descending limb (Katz, 1965) (see Chapter 1).

There remains some controversy regarding the extent to which increased end-diastolic volume can enhance performance in failing hearts (Schwinger et al., 1994; Holubarsch et al., 1996; Weil et al, 1998; Brixius et al., 2003, 2005; Gill et al., 2006). Starling curves appear to become flatter in systolic heart failure, which, by reducing the heart's ability to eject an increased preload, contributes to progressive left ventricular dilatation by increasing diastolic stress. In diastolic heart failure, blunting of the ability of increased end-diastolic volume to increase stroke volume is one reason why these patients are prone to developing severe acute pulmonary edema (see previous discussion).

Impaired Ejection and Filling

Although both ejection and filling are impaired in patients with heart failure, attention has traditionally been directed to the abnormal systolic function. Historically, this reflects the relative ease with which the latter could be estimated during cardiac catheterization by measurements of the rate of pressure rise during isovolumic contraction ($+dP/dt$). In contrast, changes in the rate of pressure fall during isovolumic relaxation ($-dP/dt$), an index of the heart's ability to relax, are difficult to interpret because this variable is highly dependent on aortic pressure. For this reason, little attention was paid to relaxation abnormalities until technological advances in echocardiography and nuclear cardiology provided accurate noninvasive measurements of wall motion and ventricular volume that could quantify the rate and extent of ventricular filling. As already noted, impaired ejection (systolic dysfunction) and impaired filling (diastolic dysfunction) cannot be equated to abnormalities in contraction (negative inotropy) and relaxation (negative lusitropy) by cardiac myocytes because both have many other causes.

Left ventricular ejection can be reduced by hemodynamic abnormalities such as aortic stenosis and the high afterload caused by hypertension (Table 2-6). Other causes of impaired ejection include ventricular dilatation, which according to the law of Laplace lowers cavity pressure at any systolic wall stress; concentric hypertrophy, which reduces ventricular volume, cardiac myocyte death such as occurs in patients following a myocardial infarction; and fibrosis of the walls of the heart. Cardiac myocyte abnormalities that impair ejection include reduced calcium influx via L-type calcium channels, impaired calcium release from the sarcoplasmic reticulum, and reduced calcium binding to troponin that occurs when the calcium affinity of this regulatory protein is decreased (see Chapter 5).

TABLE 2-6

Some Mechanisms That Impair Ejection by Failing Hearts

1. Hemodynamic abnormalities
  Valvular disease (aortic stenosis)
  Increased afterload (hypertension)
  Impaired filling (decreased end-diastolic volume)
2. Architectural and structural abnormalities
  Dilatation (eccentric hypertrophy)
  Loss of cardiac myocytes
  Increased connective tissue, fibrosis
3. Cardiac myocyte abnormalities
  Decreased calcium influx via L-type calcium channels
  Decreased calcium release from the sarcoplasmic reticulum
  Decreased calcium affinity of the contractile proteins

> **TABLE 2-7**
>
> ## Some Mechanisms That Impair Filling by Failing Hearts
>
> **1. Hemodynamic abnormalities**
>   Valvular diseases (mitral stenosis)
>   Constrictive pericarditis, pericardial effusion
>   Abbreviation of systole (tachycardia)
>   Impaired ejection (increased end-systolic volume)
> **2. Architectural and structural abnormalities**
>   Concentric hypertrophy
>   Increased connective tissue, fibrosis
>   Loss of cardiac myocytes
> **3. Cardiac myocyte abnormalities**
>   Decreased calcium uptake by the sarcoplasmic reticulum
>   Increased calcium affinity of the contractile proteins
>   Energy starvation
>   Cytoskeletal abnormalities

Pathophysiological mechanisms that impair filling include hemodynamic abnormalities like the once-common mechanical obstruction to ventricular filling caused by mitral stenosis (see Chapter 1), pericardial disease, and reduced filling time in patients with rapid tachycardias (Table 2-7). Filling is also decreased when impaired ejection increases ventricular volume. Architectural and structural abnormalities that impair filling include reduced cavity volume in patients with concentric hypertrophy; decreased compliance caused by fibrosis, glycogen storage diseases, amyloid, and other restrictive diseases; and loss of cardiac myocytes. Cardiac myocyte abnormalities that impair filling include changes in the biochemical systems that relax the myocardium, notably reduced content of the calcium pump ATPase protein (SERCA2a) and decreased calcium affinity of this pump caused by abnormalities in phospholamban, both of which decrease calcium uptake into the sarcoplasmic reticulum (see Chapter 5). Relaxation is also impaired by abnormalities of the proteins of the thin filament that increase the calcium affinity of troponin C, isoform shifts involving cytoskeletal proteins such as titin, and energy starvation, which increases the persistence of rigor bonds linking the thick and thin filaments and impairs calcium removal from the cytosol (see Chapter 5).

INTERPLAY BETWEEN THE FAILING HEART AND THE PERIPHERAL CIRCULATION

The immediate consequences of heart failure are reduced blood flow into the arteries and accumulation of blood in the veins behind the failing ventricle (Fig. 2-1), but the actual clinical syndrome is much more complex because of responses involving both the heart and the peripheral circulation. Starling's law, which increases cardiac output when diastolic pressures are elevated, helps compensate for the initial fall in stroke volume, while the neurohumoral response can both alleviate and exacerbate the hemodynamic abnormalities (see Chapter 3). Cardiac performance is improved by increased inotropy, but the accompanying increase in cardiac energy demands can damage the myocardium. Other elements of the neurohumoral response include

Fluid retention

The kidneys

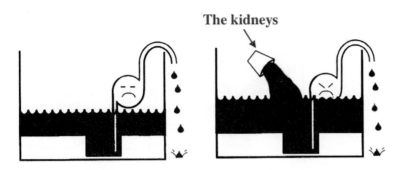

Figure 2-17: Effect of fluid retention. When the failing heart is viewed as a defective pump in a leaky basement (Fig. 2-1), fluid retention by the kidneys worsens flooding of the basement. Modified from Katz AM (2006). *Physiology of the Heart*. 4th ed. Philadelphia, Lippincott Williams & Wilkins.

venoconstriction and fluid retention by the kidneys, which worsen backward failure (Fig. 2-17), and peripheral arteriolar vasoconstriction, which worsens forward failure (Fig. 2-18). Therapy also modifies hemodynamics in heart failure; for example, diuretics improve backward failure by reducing blood volume (Fig. 2-19) and vasodilators, which increase cardiac output by reducing afterload, alleviate both forward and backward failure (Fig. 2-20). Understanding of these and other hemodynamic responses is facilitated by examining pressure–volume loops (Fig. 2-7) and Guyton diagrams (Fig. 2-11) that can clarify the interplay between arterial pressure, cardiac output, and inotropic state during systole; and between blood volume, venous return, ventricular diastolic pressure, and the lusitropic state of the heart during diastole.

Effects of Heart Failure on Pressure–Volume Loops

Pressure–volume loops depict the interplay between *lusitropy*, which determines the end-diastolic pressure–volume relationship; *inotropy*, which determines the end-systolic pressure–volume relationship; and *preload* and *afterload*, which determine the positions of the end-diastolic and end-systolic points along the corresponding pressure–volume relationships (see Fig. 2-7). The following discussion describes the events that occur when a decrease in contractility impairs the heart's ability to eject, and when increased diastolic stiffness impairs the ability of the heart to fill.

Impaired Ejection

A sudden decrease in contractility, such as occurs after complete occlusion of a coronary artery, shifts the end-systolic pressure-volume relationship (the Starling curve) to

Vasoconstriction

Arteriolar resistance vessels

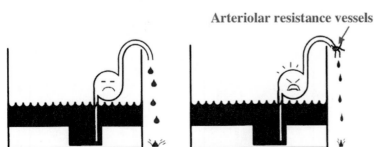

Figure 2-18: Effect of vasoconstriction. When the failing heart is viewed as a defective pump in a leaky basement (Fig. 2-1), arteriolar vasoconstriction reduces forward flow. Modified from Katz AM (2006). *Physiology of the Heart*. 4th ed. Philadelphia, Lippincott Williams & Wilkins.

Figure 2-19: Diuretics, which inhibit fluid retention, improve backward failure.

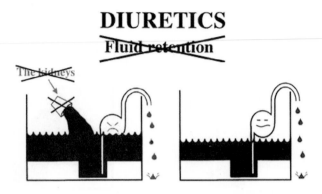

the right and downward (Fig. 2-21A). Because ejection is reduced, end-systolic (residual) volume increases; as a result, addition of a normal venous return to the greater end-systolic volume increases end-diastolic volume in the next cardiac cycle (Fig. 2-21B). This hemodynamic adjustment increases preload by moving the end-diastolic point upward and to the right along the end-diastolic pressure–volume relationship, which, according to Starling's law of the heart, increases stroke volume. Additional hemodynamic changes are initiated by the neurohumoral response; these include arteriolar vasoconstriction, which increases afterload, and venoconstriction and fluid retention by the kidneys, which increase preload. The higher afterload increases aortic pressure but worsens forward failure by reducing stroke volume (Fig. 2-21C), while the increased preload increases stroke volume, but at the expense of a further increase in filling pressure that worsens backward failure (Fig. 2-21D). β-Adrenergic stimulation of the heart, another element of the neurohumoral response, increases inotropy and lusitropy; the positive inotropic response increases the ability of the failing heart to eject (Fig. 2-21E), while the positive lusitropic response reduces end-diastolic pressure, which, by increasing end-diastolic volume, increases ejection (Fig. 2-21F).

Impaired Filling

A decrease in the ability of the heart to fill, such as occurs when the heart becomes energy-starved (see Chapter 5), shifts the end-diastolic pressure-volume relationship to the left and upward (Fig. 2-22A). Because ejection is reduced, end-systolic

Figure 2-20: Vasodilators, which reduce afterload, improve forward failure.

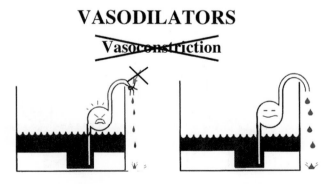

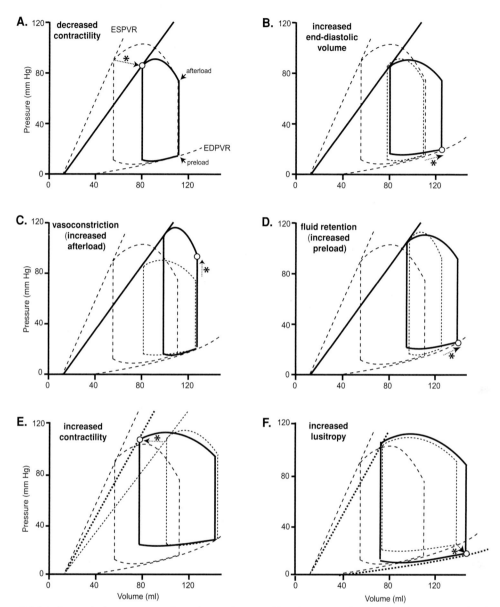

Figure 2-21: Left ventricular pressure–volume loops after a sudden decease in the heart's ability to eject; for clarity, the responses to the fall in the end-systolic pressure–volume relationship are shown sequentially. Hemodynamic and other changes are identified by *dotted arrows* (indicated by *asterisks*) that point to *open circles* that represent the new condition. In all six panels the heart operating under baseline conditions is depicted using *dashed lines*; in panels **B–F** the pressure–volume loop in the preceding panel is shown as a *dotted line*. **A:** Impaired ejection shifts the end-systolic pressure–volume relationship to the right and downward (*solid curve*), which, if afterload remains constant, reduces stroke volume by shifting the end-systolic point (*open circle*) to a lower volume. **B:** Reduced ejection increases end-diastolic pressure and volume (*open circle*), which according to Starling's law increases stroke volume; this is apparent when the solid curves in **A** and **B** are compared. **C:** Vasoconstriction increases afterload (*open circle*), which moves the end-systolic point upward, thereby increasing ejection pressure but reducing stroke volume; this is apparent when the solid loops in **B** and **C** are compared. **D:** Fluid retention increases preload (*open circle*), which increases stroke volume but at the expense of increasing end-diastolic pressure and volume; this is apparent when the solid loops in **C** and **D** are compared. **E:** Increased contractility (*dotted line*) increases stroke volume, which is apparent when the solid loops in **D** and **E** are compared. **F:** Increased lusitropy (*dotted line*) increases stroke volume, which is apparent when the solid loops in **E** and **F** are compared. EDPVR, end-diastolic pressure–volume relationship; ESPVR, end-systolic pressure–volume relationship. Modified from Katz AM (2006). *Physiology of the Heart*, 4th ed. Philadelphia, Lippincott Williams & Wilkins.

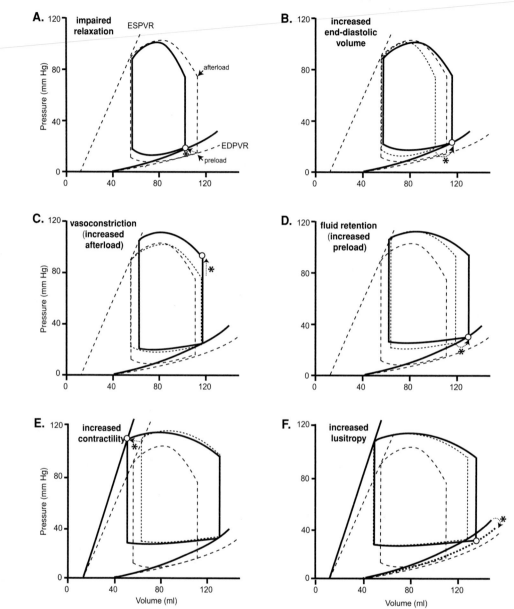

Figure 2-22: Left ventricular pressure–volume loops after a sudden decease in the heart's ability to fill; for clarity, the responses to the upward shift in the end-diastolic pressure–volume relationship are shown sequentially. Hemodynamic and other changes are identified by *dotted arrows* (indicated by *asterisks*) that point to *open circles* that represent the new condition. In all six panels the heart operating under baseline conditions is depicted using *dashed lines*; in panels **B–F** the pressure–volume loop in the preceding panel is shown as a *dotted line*. **A:** Impaired relaxation shifts the end-diastolic pressure–volume relationship to the left and upward (*solid curve*), which causes the end-diastolic point (*open circle*) to move to a lower volume at a higher pressure; if afterload remains constant stroke volume will be reduced. **B:** Reduced ejection increases end-diastolic pressure and volume (*open circle*), which according to Starling's law increases stroke volume; this is apparent when the solid loops in **A** and **B** are compared. **C:** Vasoconstriction increases afterload (*open circle*), which moves the end-systolic point upward, thereby increasing ejection pressure but reducing stroke volume; this is apparent when the solid loops in **B** and **C** are compared. **D:** Fluid retention increases preload (*open circle*), which increases stroke volume but at the expense of increased end-diastolic pressure and volume; this is apparent when the solid loops in **C** and **D** are compared. **E:** Increased contractility (*solid line*) increases stroke volume, which is apparent when the solid loops in **D** and **E** are compared. **F:** Increased lusitropy (*dotted line*) increases stroke volume, which is apparent when the solid loops in **E** and **F** are compared. EDPVR, end-diastolic pressure-volume relationship; ESPVR, end-systolic pressure-volume relationship.

(residual) volume increases so that addition of the venous return to the greater end-systolic volume increases end-diastolic volume in the next beat which, according to Starling's law of the heart, increases stroke volume (Fig. 2-22B). Vasoconstriction and fluid retention, which are initiated by the neurohumoral response, increase both preload and afterload. The higher afterload caused by arteriolar constriction increases aortic pressure but reduces stroke volume (Fig. 2-22C), while the higher end-diastolic volume caused by venoconstriction and fluid retention increases stroke volume, but at the expense of a further increase in diastolic pressure (Fig. 2-22D). β-Adrenergic stimulation of the heart increases contractility, which increases ejection (Fig. 2-22E) and, by stimulating the biochemical mechanisms that relax the heart, reduces end-diastolic pressure and increases ejection (Fig. 2-22F).

In diastolic heart failure, the steeper end-diastolic pressure–volume relationship caused by decreased lusitropy has two important hemodynamic consequences (Fig. 2-23). The first is an increase in venous pressure, which because of the reduced diastolic compliance in diastolic heart failure rises more steeply than in systolic heart failure (Fig. 2-23C). The second, which magnifies the adverse effect of the high venous pressure, is blunting of the ability of Starling's law to increase stroke volume; this occurs because the steep end-diastolic pressure–volume relationship in diastolic heart failure impairs the ability of the ventricle to dilate (Fig. 2-23E). Together, the high venous pressure and impaired ability of Starling's law to increase cardiac performance can explain the rapid onset of severe pulmonary congestion (often called "flash pulmonary edema") that is commonly seen in diastolic heart failure.

Combination of Impaired Ejection and Impaired Filling

Impairment of both ejection and filling "compresses" the pressure volume loop (Fig. 2-24). The smaller area within the pressure-volume loop reduces the ability of the failing heart to perform external work, which decreases both stroke volume and the ability of the ventricle to develop pressure.

Ventricular Architecture

The effects of architectural changes on ventricular performance are often more important than those caused by changes in inotropy and lusitropy. This is shown in Figure 2-25, which shows how concentric and eccentric hypertrophy shift the pressure–volume loops to lower and higher volumes, respectively. Concentric hypertrophy impairs both filling and ejection by reducing cavity volume; in addition, thickening and fibrosis of the ventricular walls increases the steepness of the end-diastolic pressure–volume relationship. Eccentric hypertrophy impairs filling in part because dilatation increases wall stress at any diastolic pressure (see Eq. 2.7 and Fig. 2-4); the steepness of the end-diastolic pressure–volume relationship can also be increased by the fibrosis that generally accompanies ventricular hypertrophy.

INTERPLAY BETWEEN VENOUS RETURN AND CARDIAC OUTPUT

The interplay between venous return and cardiac output depicted in Figs. 2-11 to 2-14 provides an additional way to view the effects of heart failure on cardiac performance and circulatory hemodynamics. Figure 2-26 shows the sequence of events that begins when impaired ejection increases atrial pressure and reduces cardiac output (Fig. 2-26B), which shifts the intercept between these curves to the right and downward. The decreased stroke volume causes atrial pressure to rise, which moves

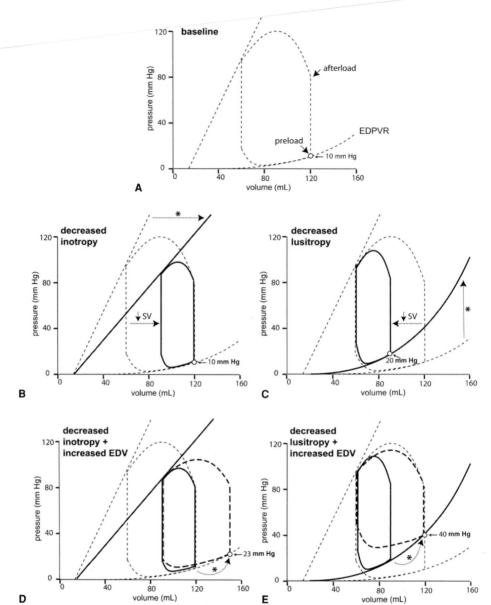

Figure 2-23: Differences in the hemodynamic effects of systolic and diastolic heart failure. In all five panels the heart operating under baseline conditions is depicted by dashed lines. Pressure–volume loops under baseline conditions (**A**), after a decrease in inotropy that causes systolic heart failure (**B, D**), and after a decrease in lusitropy that causes diastolic heart failure (**C, E**). **B:** The first beat after a reduction in inotropy that reduces stroke volume by 50% (*arrow* labeled ↓SV); note that end-diastolic pressure and volume are unchanged. **C:** The first beat after a reduction in lusitropy that reduces stroke volume by 50% (*arrow* labeled ↓SV); because the decrease in diastolic compliance shifts the end-diastolic pressure–volume relationship upward and to the left, end-diastolic pressure increases from 10–20 mm Hg. **D:** The decrease in stroke volume shown in **B** increases end-systolic volume, which, when added to the venous return, causes end-diastolic volume to increase in subsequent beats (heavy dashed line). If venous return remained unchanged, the increased end-diastolic volume would restore stroke volume to normal by increasing end-diastolic pressure to ~23 mm Hg (*dotted arrow* marked by an *asterisk*). **E:** The increased end-diastolic pressure shown in **C** causes end-diastolic volume to increase, which, if the venous return in the next beat restored stroke volume to normal, would increase end-diastolic pressure to ~40 mm Hg (*dotted arrow* marked by an *asterisk*). The higher diastolic pressures in diastolic heart failure (**C** and **E**) than in systolic heart failure (**B** and **D**) can be seen to result from the shift of the end-diastolic pressure–volume relationship upward and to the right.

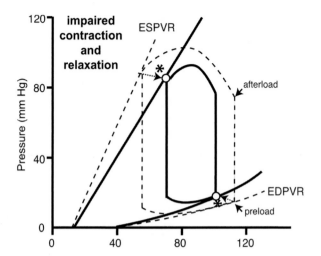

Figure 2-24: Left ventricular pressure–volume loop after sudden deceases in the heart's ability both to eject and to fill (*solid lines*). Hemodynamic and other changes are identified using *dotted arrows* (indicated by *asterisks*) that point to *open circles* that represent the new condition. The pressure–volume loop for the heart operating under baseline conditions is depicted using *dashed lines*.

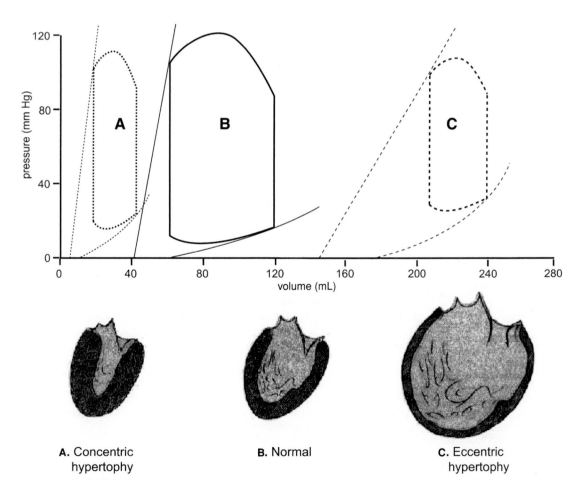

A. Concentric hypertophy

B. Normal

C. Eccentric hypertophy

Figure 2-25: Effects of different phenotypes of ventricular hypertrophy (**below**) on pressure–volume loops (**above**). **A:** Concentric hypertrophy. **B:** Normal. **C:** Eccentric hypertrophy. Major causes of the reduced stroke volume in both types of hypertrophy are changes in ventricular architecture. Based on data of Kass (1988). From Katz AM (2006). *Physiology of the Heart*, 4th ed. Philadelphia, Lippincott Williams & Wilkins.

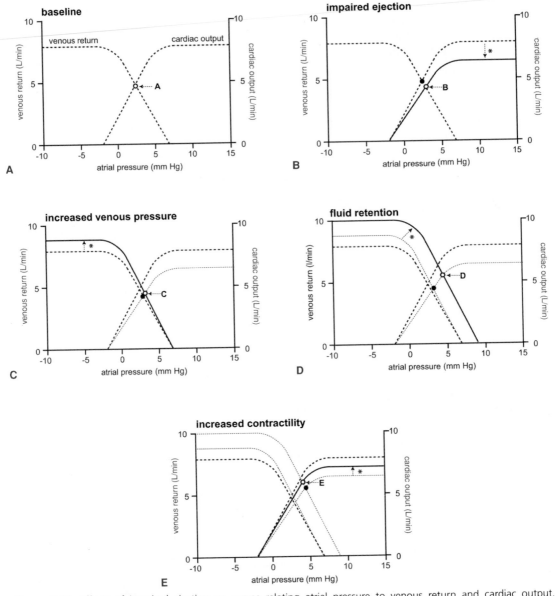

Figure 2-26: Effects of impaired ejection on curves relating atrial pressure to venous return and cardiac output. **A:** Control curves showing the intercept (*open circle A*) that defines the steady state where blood flow into and out of the heart are equal. In **B–E**, hemodynamic changes are identified by *dotted arrows* (indicated by *asterisks*), new steady states by *open circles*, and previous steady states by *closed circles*. **B:** Reduced ejection caused by a decrease in contractility decreases cardiac output and so shifts the intercept to a lower cardiac output and a higher atrial pressure (*open circle B*); the shift to a lower Starling curve is apparent when the solid curve is compared to that under baseline conditions. **C:** Atrial pressure becomes higher because impaired ejection increases end-systolic and end-diastolic volumes; according to Starling's law, the latter increases ejection by moving the intercept upward and to the right (*open circle C*). **D:** Fluid retention shifts the curve relating atrial pressure upward and to the right; the increased mean circulatory filling pressure is seen as an increase in the atrial pressure where venous return and cardiac output are zero. The resulting increase in preload increases cardiac output (*open circle D*). **E:** Increased contractility (*solid line*) shifts the intercept upward and to the left, which increases cardiac output and reduces atrial pressure (*open circle E*).

the intercept upward along the depressed curve relating atrial pressure to cardiac output. These changes do not initially affect blood volume, so that mean circulatory filling pressure (the atrial pressure at which venous return and cardiac output are zero) does not change.

Two components of the neurohumoral response (see Chapter 3) modify these curves. The first, an increase in blood volume caused when the kidneys retain fluid, shifts the curve relating venous return to atrial pressure upward and to the right (Fig. 2-26D); this response increases cardiac output (according to Starling's law of the heart), but leads to a further rise in venous pressure because mean circulatory filling pressure is increased. The second component of the neurohumoral response, an increase in myocardial contractility (Fig. 2-26E), causes an upward shift of the curve relating atrial pressure to cardiac output, which by shifting the intercept upward and to the left, increases cardiac output and lowers atrial pressure. At the same time, however, this inotropic effect increases cardiac energy demands.

CONCLUSION

The hemodynamic abnormalities described in this Chapter are responsible for many of the clinical signs and symptoms in most patients with heart failure. These abnormalities are modified by the neurohumoral response, which, although its adaptive effects alleviate some of the hemodynamic abnormalities, also has maladaptive consequences that cause more problems than it solves. The latter include vasoconstriction, fluid retention (see Chapter 3), and changes in proliferative signaling that worsen long-term prognosis by accelerating progressive deterioration of the failing heart (see Chapters 3 and 4).

REFERENCES

Benge W, Litchfield RL, Marcus ML (1980). Exercise capacity in patients with severe heart failure. Circulation 61:955–959.

Brixius K, Reuter H, Bloch W, et al. (2003). Reduced length-dependent cross-bridge recruitment in skinned fiber preparations of human failing myocardium. Eur J Appl Physiol 89:249–256.

Brixius K, Reuter H, Bloch W, et al. (2005). Altered hetero- and homeometric autoregulation in the terminally failing human heart. Eur J Heart Fail. 7:29–35.

Elzinga G (1992). Starling's law and the rise and fall of the descending limb. News Physiol Sci 7:134–137.

Evans CL, Matsuoka Y (1915). The effect of various mechanical conditions on the gaseous metabolism and efficiency of the mammalian heart. J Physiol (Lond) 49:378–405.

Fenton TR, Cherry JM, Klassen GA (1978). Transmural myocardial deformation in the canine left ventricular wall. Am J Physiol 235:H523–H530.

Franciosa JA, Park M, Levine TB (1981). Lack of correlation between exercise capacity and indexes of resting left ventricular performance in heart failure. Am J Cardiol 47:33–39.

Gill RM, Jones BD, Corbly AK, et al. (2006). Exhaustion of the Frank-Starling mechanism in conscious dogs with heart failure induced by chronic coronary microembolization. Life Sci 79:536–544.

Guyton A. (1961). Cardiac Failure. Chapter 36 in: *Textbook of Medical Physiology*. Philadelphia, Saunders.

Hancock EW (2001). Cardiomyopathy: differential diagnosis of restrictive cardiomyopathy and constrictive pericarditis. Heart 86:343–349.

Holubarsch C, Ruf T, Goldstein D, et al. (1996). Existence of the Frank-Starling mechanism in the failing human heart. Investigations on the organ, tissue and sarcomere levels. Circulation 94:683–689.

Kabbani SS, LeWinter MM (2000). Diastolic heart failure. Constrictive, restrictive, and pericardial. Cardiol Clin 18:501–509.

Kass DA (1988). Evaluation of left-ventricular systolic function. Heart Failure 4:198–205.

Katz AM (1965). The descending limb of the Starling curve and the failing heart. Circulation 32:871–875.

Katz AM (2006). *Physiology of the Heart*. 4th ed. Philadelphia, Lippincott Williams & Wilkins.

Kuethe F, Sigusch HH, Hilbig K, et al. (2007). Detection of viral genome in the myocardium: lack of prognostic and functional relevance in patients with acute dilated cardiomyopathy. Am Heart J 153:850–858.

Lipkin DP, Poole-Wilson PA (1986). Symptoms limiting exercise capacity in chronic heart failure. Br Med J 292:653–655.

Mancini DM, LaManca J, Henson D (1992). The relation of respiratory muscle function to dyspnea in patient with heart failure. Heart Failure 8:183–189.

McCarthy RE III, Boehmer JP, Hruban RH, et al. (2000). Long-term outcome of fulminant myocarditis as compared with acute (nonfulminant) myocarditis. N Engl J Med 342:690–695.

McMichael J (1950). *Pharmacology of the Failing Heart*. London, Blackwell.

Mettauer B, Zoll J, Garnier A, et al. (2006). Heart failure: a model of cardiac and skeletal muscle energetic failure. Pflugers Arch 452:653–666,

Niebauer J, Clark AJ, Webb-Peploe KM, et al. (2005). Exercise training in chronic heart failure: effects on proinflammatory markers. Eur J Heart Failure 7:189–193.

Poole-Wilson P, Ferrari R (1996). Role of skeletal muscle in the syndrome of chronic heart failure. J Mol Cell Cardiol 28:2275–2285.

Schwinger RHG, Böhm M, Koch A, et al. (1994). The failing human heart is unable to use the Frank-Starling mechanism. Circulation 74:959–969.

Spiro D, Sonnenblick EH (1962). Comparison of the ultrastructural basis of the contractile process in heart and skeletal muscle. Circulation Res 14(Suppl II):II-14–II-36.

Sullivan M, Higgenbotham M, Cobb F (1988). Increased exercise ventilation in patients with chronic heart failure: intact ventilatory control despite hemodynamic and pulmonary abnormalities. Circulation 77:552–559.

van Tol BA, Huijsmans RJ, Kroon DW, et al. (2006). Effects of exercise training on cardiac performance, exercise capacity and quality of life in patients with heart failure: a meta-analysis. Eur J Heart Failure 8:841–850.

Ventura-Clapier R, Mettauer B, Bigard X (2007). Beneficial effects of endurance training on cardiac and skeletal muscle energy metabolism in heart failure. Cardiovasc Res 73:10–18.

Volterrani M, Clark AJ, Ludman PF, et al. (1994). Predictors of exercise capacity in chronic heart failure. Eur Heart J 15:801–809.

Wasserman K, Zhang Y-Y, Gitt A, et al. (1997). Lung function and gas exchange in chronic heart failure. Circulation 96:2221–2227.

Weil J, Eschenhagen T, Hirt S, et al. (1998). Preserved Frank-Starling mechanism in end stage heart failure. Cardiovasc Res 37:541–548.

Wiggers CJ (1952). *Circulatory Dynamics*. New York, Grune & Stratton.

Wong AY, Rautaharju PM (1968). Stress distribution within the left ventricular wall approximated as a thick ellipsoidal shell. Am Heart J 1968;75:649–662.

Wood P (1954). An appreciation of mitral stenosis. Br Med J 1:1051–1063, 1113–1124.

CHAPTER 3

The Neurohumoral Response in Heart Failure: Functional Signaling

Andrew M. Katz • Marvin A. Konstam

Underfilling of the arteries, and to a lesser extent venous congestion, initiate a *neurohumoral response* that attempts to correct the hemodynamic abnormalities. This compensatory mechanism, which can both alleviate and exacerbate the abnormalities caused by reduced cardiac output and accumulation of blood behind the failing ventricle, plays a major role in heart failure.

Claude Bernard (1878) noted that a constant environment within our bodies, which he called the *milieu intérieur,* is essential for independent life. He observed that living organisms enclose themselves "in a kind of a hot-house [where the] perpetual changes of external conditions cannot reach it; it is not subject to them, but is free and independent." Constancy of the milieu intérieur, which Walter Cannon (1932) called *homeostasis,* is made possible by regulatory systems that compensate for changes in the ever-changing, often hazardous, external environment; the same responses help to alleviate problems created by malfunction of one or more of the body's components. In heart failure, the neurohumoral response minimizes the hemodynamic consequences caused by failure of the cardiac pump (see Chapter 2). However, this response is not well suited to deal with the long-term problems caused by heart failure, but instead provides mechanisms that adapt to short-term challenges, such as exercise and hemorrhage. This is why, when sustained in chronic heart failure, this response can fail to improve the situation and generally adds to the long-term problems in these patients.

Circulatory regulation requires effective communication between the heart, the rest of the body, and the external environment. Mechanisms are needed to generate signals that inform a structure, such as the heart or a blood vessel, that its function must be modified, and then to initiate appropriate responses. To ensure that these responses are turned on when needed, operate at an appropriate intensity, and end when no longer useful, biological signaling systems collect and integrate information from many sources. Appropriate safeguards are provided by interlocking control mechanisms that recognize challenges, amplify signals, and adjust and integrate the responses that compensate for changing hemodynamics.

MAJOR FEATURES OF THE NEUROHUMORAL RESPONSE

Underfilling of the arterial system, a major hemodynamic abnormality in heart failure, evokes a neurohumoral response that is similar to that evoked by exercise and hemorrhage. Even though they pose different challenges, exercise, hemorrhage, and heart failure initiate similar short-term *functional* signals (Fig. 3-1) that increase cardiac performance, constrict blood vessels, and inhibit salt and water excretion by the

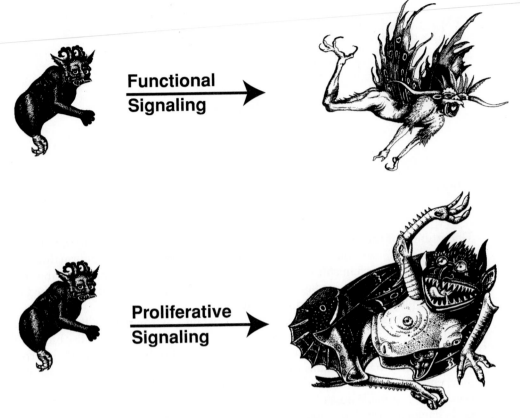

Functional Signaling

Proliferative Signaling

Figure 3-1: Functional and proliferative responses. Functional responses, which alter the properties of pre-existing structures by posttranslational mechanisms, aid survival by evoking responses like fight and flight. Proliferative responses, which take longer to evolve, allow organism to grow out of trouble. From Katz AM (2006). *Physiology of the Heart.* 4th ed. Philadelphia, Lippincott Williams and Wilkins.

kidneys (Table 3-1). When the challenge is exercise, cardiac stimulation and selective vasoconstriction appear rapidly, over a few seconds or minutes, and generally last until the exercise ends, usually a few minutes or hours. Urine output also decreases during exercise, but fluid retention becomes important only after activity has lasted several hours, as in a marathon runner (Table 3-2). More prolonged responses are initiated when blood volume is decreased by hemorrhage, severe diarrhea, endo-toxin, or an extensive burn; in these conditions the challenge lasts hours, at most a few days, after which the patient either dies or recovers (Table 3-2). In heart failure, which is usually progressive (see Chapter 2), the neurohumoral response persists and fluid retention commonly becomes a major clinical problem (see Chapter 1).

A very different feature of the neurohumoral response is mediated by *proliferative (transcriptional)* signaling (Fig. 3-1, Table 3-1). The resulting long-term responses, which are mediated by changes in gene expression that alter the com-position of myocardial cells and the structure of the heart, evolve over weeks, months, and often years. A third type of response, referred to in this text as *proinflammatory* (Table 3-1), evolved from mechanisms that combat infection. Like proliferative responses, proinflammatory responses develop slowly; if there is an infectious cause they can be turned off when the infectious agent is eliminated, but in heart failure they generally persist until the patient dies (see Chapter 4).

TABLE 3-1

Major Elements of the Neurohumoral Response

Signaling mechanism	Short-term adaptive	Long-term maladaptive
Functional	**Adaptive Responses**	**Maladaptive Consequences**
Cardiac β-adrenergic drive	↑ Contractility	↑ Cytosolic calcium
	↑ Relaxation	(arrhythmias, sudden death)
	↑ Heart Rate (increase cardiac output)	↑ Cardiac energy demand (cardiac myocyte necrosis)
Vasoconstriction	↑ Afterload (maintain blood pressure)	↓ Cardiac output
		↑ Cardiac energy demand (cardiac myocyte necrosis)
Salt and Water Retention	↑ Preload (maintain cardiac output)	Edema, anasarca, pulmonary congestion
Proliferative	**Adaptive Hypertrophy**	**Maladaptive Hypertrophy**
Transcriptional activation More sarcomeres	Cell thickening (normalize wall stress, maintain cardiac output)	Cell elongation (dilation, remodeling, increased wall stress)
		↑Cardiac energy demand (cardiac myocyte necrosis)
		↓ Cardiac energy supply (cardiac myocyte necrosis)
Apoptotic signaling		Apoptosis
Proinflammatory	**"Anti-Other"**	**"Anti-Self"**
	Antimicrobial, antihelminthic	Cachexia
	Adaptive hypertrophy	? Skeletal muscle myopathy

TABLE 3-2

Three Conditions That Evoke the Neurohumoral Response

Challenge	Duration	Stimulus	Functional response
Exercise	Minutes/hours	Increased blood flow to exercising muscles	Cardiac stimulation Selective vasoconstriction (fluid retention)
Shock	Hours/days	Decreased intravascular volume (e.g. hemorrhage, fluid loss)	Cardiac stimulation Vasoconstriction Fluid retention
Heart failure	Usually for life (progressive)	Impaired cardiac pumping	Cardiac stimulation Vasoconstriction Fluid retention Activation of proliferative and proinflammatory signaling

FUNCTIONAL COMPONENTS OF THE NEUROHUMORAL RESPONSE

Cardiac stimulation, vasoconstriction, and salt and water retention, the three major functional components of the neurohumoral response in heart failure (Tables 3-1 and 3-2), provide short-term support for the circulation during a brief challenge, but become maladaptive when called on in chronic heart failure; the consequences are vividly summarized in a brilliant essay by Peter Harris (1983):

> Success and survival in the animal kingdom have overwhelmingly depended on physical mobility and strength. To ensure this the body makes use of the neuro-endocrine defense reaction which is also life-saving in injury... When the output of the [failing] heart decreases, the body reacts in the way nature has programmed it. It cannot distinguish. But now the neuro-endocrine response persists. Over weeks or months or years the retention of saline threatens the cardiac patient with drowning in his own juice. And every hour of every day he is running for his life.

Exercise

The neurohumoral response evoked by *exercise*, the briefest of the challenges listed in Table 3-2, is initiated by several mechanisms that are integrated by autonomic centers in the brain stem. Most important is the baroreceptor reflex, which increases sympathetic activity and reduces parasympathetic tone in response to the fall in arterial blood pressure caused by vasodilatation in the exercising muscles. Chemoreceptor stimulation also increases sympathetic activity in response to CO_2 and lactic acid released by the exercising muscles. These responses are supplemented by nerve impulses that arise in the exercising muscles and the cerebral cortex; the latter explains the appearance of sympathetic stimulation before the start of exercise, for example when a sprinter hears the starter's gun.

The most important features of the response to exercise are brought about by changes in the heart and blood vessels. Cardiac output is increased when activation of the sympathetic nervous system causes an inotropic response that increases ejection, a lusitropic effect that augments filling, and a chronotropic effect that accelerates heart rate. Sympathetic stimulation also causes vasoconstriction, which helps maintain blood pressure by increasing resistance in arterial beds not dilated during exercise, and by constricting large veins, which increases the return of blood to the heart. Fluid retention, as previously noted, becomes important only during prolonged exercise.

Shock

The second challenge that activates the neurohumoral response is a clinical syndrome, called *shock*, whose most obvious abnormalities are low blood pressure and inadequate tissue perfusion. This syndrome, which usually lasts no more than several hours, can occur when hemorrhage, severe diarrhea, leaky capillary endothelium, or extensive vasodilatation decrease circulating blood volume. Cardiogenic shock, caused when cardiac output is reduced by severe left ventricular dysfunction, can follow a large myocardial infarction, valve rupture, pulmonary embolus, pericardial tamponade, acute myocarditis, and some arrhythmias. If the underlying cause is reversible and appropriate therapy started promptly, patients usually recover, but if treatment is delayed this syndrome becomes irreversible because, even after blood pressure is restored, severe tissue damage initiated by low blood flow causes the patient to die.

The neurohumoral response in shock differs from that evoked by exercise because the challenge is more intense and, more important, lasts longer. When prolonged, underfilling of the arteries causes the kidneys to retain salt and water, which by reducing fluid loss facilitates restoration of blood volume and, by increasing preload, helps maintain cardiac output.

Heart Failure

In *heart failure,* where underfilling of the arterial system can last for a lifetime, most of the functional responses listed in Table 3-1 become maladaptive. Tachycardia and increased contractility, while helping to maintain cardiac output, also increase cardiac energy utilization, which, because most failing hearts are energy starved, contributes to myocardial cell death. Arteriolar vasoconstriction increases afterload and so helps to maintain blood pressure, but at the same time reduces cardiac output and increases myocardial energy demand. The increased preload caused by venoconstriction and fluid retention do little to increase cardiac output because Starling curves are often flattened in heart failure (see Chapter 2); instead, these responses become deleterious because the increased preload adds to the problems caused by the already elevated systemic and pulmonary venous pressures.

REGULATORY AND COUNTERREGULATORY RESPONSES

Underfilling of the arterial system activates two opposing types of functional response (Table 3-3). The first, which include cardiac stimulation, vasoconstriction, and fluid retention (see previous discussion), are *regulatory* in that they help maintain blood pressure and cardiac output. At the same time, however, *counterregulatory* responses that oppose the dominant regulatory responses are also evoked; these include a negative inotropic effect on the heart, vasodilatation, and diuresis. (A similar dichotomy in proliferative signaling is described in Chapter 4.) The apparent paradox seen when a single stimulus activates opposing responses illustrates one

---

TABLE 3-3

Regulatory and Counterregulatory Neurohumoral Responses

Regulatory Responses
Functional responses
  Increased myocardial contractility, accelerated relaxation, faster heart rate
  Vasoconstriction
  Fluid retention by the kidneys
Proliferative responses
  Stimulate cell growth and proliferation, proapoptotic
Counterregulatory Responses
Functional responses
  Decreased myocardial contractility, slowed relaxation, slower heart rate
  Vasodilatation
  Diuresis
Proliferative responses
  Inhibit cell growth and proliferation, antiapoptotic

mechanism that avoids runaway signaling (see subsequent text). The functional responses to some neurohumoral mediators are predominantly regulatory, whereas others are mainly counterregulatory; most of the former also have proliferative effects that promote cardiac hypertrophy, while counterregulatory mediators generally inhibit cell growth and proliferation (Table 3-4). However there are many exceptions to this generalization and most neurohumoral mediators evoke *both* regulatory and counterregulatory responses.

Cardiac Stimulation

Increased inotropy, lusitropy, and chronotropy modify all of the three variables that determine cardiac output (CO):

$$CO = (EDV - ESV) \times HR \qquad \text{Eq. 3.1}$$

Increased contractility reduces end-systolic volume (ESV) by increasing ejection; the lusitropic response increases end-diastolic volume (EDV) by facilitating relaxation, and tachycardia increases heart rate (HR) by accelerating pacemaker activity in the SA node.

The most important mediator of the cardiac stimulation caused by underfilling of the arterial system is the baroreceptor response, which causes sympathetic activation and decreases parasympathetic tone. The major regulatory mediator is

---

TABLE 3-4

Regulatory and Counterregulatory Signaling Molecules

Signaling Molecules Whose Major Role is Regulatory

Mediators
  Catecholamines—peripheral effects
  Angiotensin II
  Arginine vasopressin
  Endothelin
Responses
  Fluid retention by the kidneys
  Vasoconstriction
  Increased cardiac contractility, relaxation, heart rate
  Stimulation of cell growth and proliferation

Signaling Molecules Whose Major Role is Counterregulatory

Mediators
  Catecholamines—central effects
  Dopamine
  Atrial natriuretic peptide
  Nitric oxide (NO)
  Bradykinin
Effects
  Reduce fluid retention by the kidneys
  Vasodilatation
  Decrease cardiac contractility, relaxation, heart rate
  Inhibition of cell growth and proliferation

norepinephrine, which stimulates the heart when it binds to β_1-adrenergic receptors; other regulatory mediators include angiotensin II, vasopressin, and endothelin, all of which have minor effects that increase contractility. Unfortunately, the benefits of cardiac stimulation in failing hearts are accompanied by proarrhythmic effects and an increase in energy expenditure that can cause myocardial cell death (see Chapter 5).

Vasoconstriction

Increased peripheral vascular resistance, the second major regulatory component of the neurohumoral response, helps maintain blood pressure. However, like cardiac stimulation, arteriolar vasoconstriction has deleterious effects in chronic heart failure; for example, the increased afterload reduces cardiac output (see Chapter 2) and increases cardiac energy expenditure (see Chapter 5). Other maladaptive effects of vasoconstriction contribute to the clinical deterioration of patients with end-stage heart failure by reducing perfusion of skeletal muscle, the kidneys, the liver, and other organs.

The most important stimulus for vasoconstriction occurs when sympathetic activation releases norepinephrine that binds to α_1-adrenergic receptors on arteriolar smooth muscle; other mediators include angiotensin II, endothelin, and vasopressin, whose levels become elevated in chronic heart failure. Some mediators of the neurohumoral response have counterregulatory effects that relax arteriolar smooth muscle; these include the natriuretic peptides, bradykinin, nitric oxide, and some prostaglandins, notably PGI_2 (prostacyclin). Furthermore, many regulatory mediators bind to receptors that relax vascular smooth muscle; for example, norepinephrine binding to central preganglionic α_2-receptors inhibits regulatory neural vasoconstrictor pathways, and adrenergic, angiotensin II, vasopressin, and endothelin receptors can activate vasodilator pathways (see subsequent text). In patients with heart failure, however, these counterregulatory effects are overwhelmed by the regulatory vasoconstrictor responses.

Fluid Retention

Edema, dropsy, anasarca, and dyspnea, once the most devastating clinical manifestations of heart failure (see Chapter 1), occur when fluid accumulates in the tissues. The most important causes of edema are salt and water retention by the kidneys, rather than the high venous pressure caused by impaired pumping of blood out of the venous system. This was noted more than 50 years ago, when Warren and Stead (1944) found that weight gain and the appearance of symptoms in early heart failure generally precede a significant increase in venous pressure. The enormous amount of salt and water that can be retained by patients with severe heart failure is apparent in the ability of diuretics to eliminate enough fluid to cause weight loss in excess of 20 kilograms within a few days. Harris (1983) observed that fluid accumulation in heart failure can be so dramatic that a visiting Martian could easily conclude that the primary problem in these patients involves the kidneys!

The major cause of the expanded extracellular fluid volume in heart failure is retention of sodium, rather than water. Although the excess water is more evident clinically, water retention is largely due to sodium retention, rather than the other way around. Stated simply, water follows salt. In some patients, however, water retention can become a serious problem, for example, when increased vasopressin levels or overly vigorous use of natriuretic diuretics leads to a fall in serum sodium concentration called "dilutional hyponatremia."

The potential causes of sodium retention by the kidneys are conceptually simple. Because most of the sodium eliminated in the urine is filtered by the glomeruli, inappropriate sodium retention could occur if too little sodium is filtered into the renal tubules, if too much of the filtered sodium is reabsorbed, or both. In patients with severe heart failure, the first mechanism operates when low cardiac output reduces glomerular filtration rate (GFR); more commonly, however, sodium reabsorption is increased when too much filtered sodium is transported from the tubules into the plasma by the renal tubular epithelial cells.

Selective constriction of the renal efferent arterioles, increased renal vein pressure, increased sodium reabsorption by the renal tubules, and increased water reabsorption by the collecting ducts can all cause fluid retention in heart failure. Selective constriction of the efferent arterioles that carry blood out of the glomeruli increases GFR by elevating glomerular pressure (Fig. 3-2). Because the glomerular membranes are impermeable to the proteins that maintain plasma oncotic pressure,

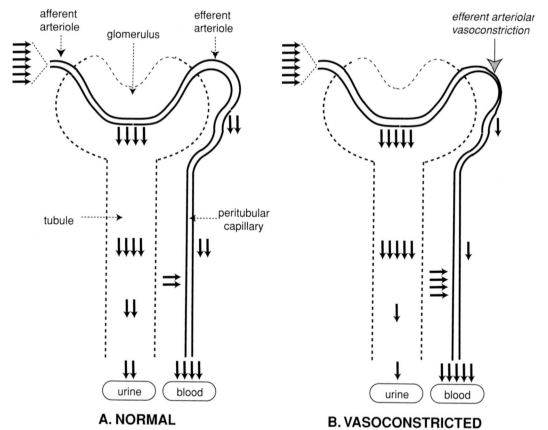

A. NORMAL   **B. VASOCONSTRICTED**

Figure 3-2: Effect of renal efferent artery constriction on sodium excretion. **A:** Under normal conditions, much of the sodium (*heavy arrows*) that enters the afferent arterioles supplying the glomeruli is filtered into the glomerulus. Some of this sodium is reabsorbed by the tubules; the remainder is excreted in the urine. **B:** Vasoconstriction of the efferent arterioles leading out of the glomeruli increases the amount of sodium and water that enters the tubules. However, because the increased glomerular filtration also reduces oncotic pressure within the tubules and increases oncotic pressure in the peritubular capillaries, a greater fraction of the tubular fluid is reabsorbed. Fluid resorption from the tubules is increased further by the higher hydrostatic pressure within the tubular lumen and lower hydrostatic pressure in the peritubular capillaries. Together, these changes in oncotic and hydrostatic pressures increase sodium retention. From Katz AM (2006). *Physiology of the Heart.* 4th ed. Philadelphia, Lippincott Williams and Wilkins.

increased GFR promotes fluid reabsorption from the tubules into the peritubular capillaries by reducing the oncotic pressure of the fluid that enters the renal tubules and increasing the oncotic pressure of the blood leaving the glomeruli to perfuse the tubules. Constriction of the efferent arterioles also increases renal tubular fluid resorption by lowering hydrostatic pressure in the peritubular capillaries downstream from the efferent arterioles and by raising the hydrostatic pressure within the tubules. Neurohumoral mediators that selectively constrict glomerular efferent arterioles include norepinephrine, angiotensin II, vasopressin, and endothelin. These constrictor effects are augmented by reduced sensitivity of the renal vasculature to the normal vasodilator effects of nitric oxide but partially offset by vasodilator effects of atrial natriuretic peptides and prostaglandins. Aldosterone and vasopressin, which also contribute to fluid retention, directly increase sodium and water reabsorption by the tubular epithelium and collecting ducts, respectively.

SIGNAL TRANSDUCTION CASCADES

Most components of the neurohumoral response are initiated when binding of extracellular signaling molecules to receptors on the heart, blood vessels, and kidneys activates multistep signaling cascades like that shown in Figure 3-3. The analogy in this figure, which illustrates how norepinephrine increases ventricular ejection, resembles an old-fashioned bucket brigade, but unlike the latter, where a single substance (water) is passed from fireman to fireman, biological signaling cascades utilize many different signaling molecules and chemical reactions.

It is reasonable to ask why so many steps are required for a signal to evoke a physiological response. The answer is that biological signaling cascades, whose complexity might seem almost perverse, use these steps to amplify, inhibit, and fine-tune responses; to integrate signal transduction cascades with one another; and to allow signals to turn themselves off automatically so as to prevent responses from going out of control ("runaway signaling"). In fact, the depiction of the signal cascade in Figure 3-3 is oversimplified because cellular responses are not linear cascades, where each step is coupled to a single downstream reaction; instead, biological pathways often branch, loop forward and backward, interconnect with other pathways, and generate multiple signals at a single step. These intricacies provide options for amplification, fine-tuning, and negative feedback by integrating each response with other parts of the cascade and with additional signaling systems, which would not be possible if each step simply evoked an "all-or-none" response. For these reasons, cascades similar to that shown in Figure 3-3 but different in detail mediate virtually every signal that modifies cardiovascular function.

EXTRACELLULAR SIGNALING MOLECULES

The role of chemical mediators in regulating cardiovascular function was discovered by Oliver and Schäfer (1895), who found that injection of adrenal extracts increases heart rate in anaesthetized cats. A decade later, Elliott (1905) suggested that sympathetic nerve stimulation, whose effects resemble those of adrenal extracts, might also be mediated by a chemical messenger. However, it was not until 1921 that Otto Loewi (1921) carried out a simple but inspired experiment that proved conclusively that a chemical can mediate a neurohumoral response, in this case to vagal stimulation. Early efforts to isolate the chemical mediator had proven fruitless because the neurotransmitter is inactivated very rapidly, but Loewi overcame this problem by

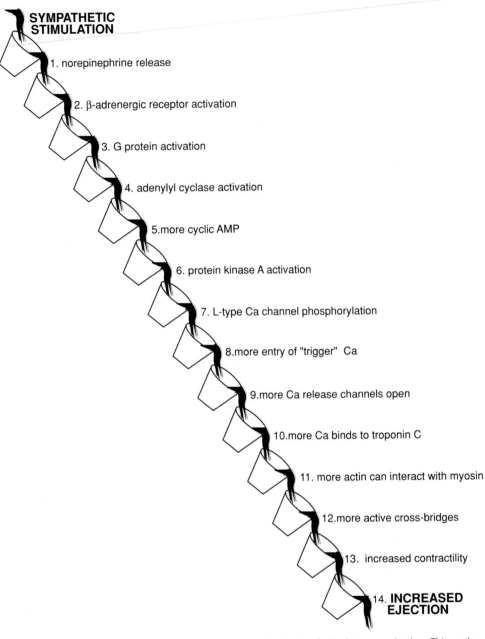

SYMPATHETIC STIMULATION

1. norepinephrine release

2. β-adrenergic receptor activation

3. G protein activation

4. adenylyl cyclase activation

5. more cyclic AMP

6. protein kinase A activation

7. L-type Ca channel phosphorylation

8. more entry of "trigger" Ca

9. more Ca release channels open

10. more Ca binds to troponin C

11. more actin can interact with myosin

12. more active cross-bridges

13. increased contractility

14. **INCREASED EJECTION**

Figure 3-3: Depiction of a signal cascade by which sympathetic stimulation increases ejection. This analogy shows 14 steps as a series of buckets where, in each step, the upstream signal causes the bucket to pour its contents into the next bucket, thereby transmitting the signal down the cascade. The response begins when sympathetic stimulation releases norepinephrine from nerve endings at the surface of cardiac myocytes (step 1), after which this neurotransmitter binds to and activates β-adrenergic receptors (step 2). The remaining steps, which all take place within myocardial cells, include activation of a G protein (step 3), activation of adenylyl cyclase activity (step 4), increased production of cAMP (step 5), activation of a cAMP-dependent protein kinase (step 6), phosphorylation of plasma membrane L-type calcium channels (step 7), increased calcium entry into the cell (step 8), increased opening of calcium release channels (step 9), increased calcium binding to troponin C (step 10), increased availability of actin in the thin filaments for interaction with myosin (step 11), participation of more cross-bridges in contraction (step 12), increased contractility (step 13), and a greater extent of ejection (step 14). From Katz AM (2006). *Physiology of the Heart*. 4th ed. Philadelphia, Lippincott Williams and Wilkins.

placing two frog hearts a short distance apart in a slowly moving stream of Ringer's solution. When he stimulated the vagus nerve supplying the upstream heart, not only did this heart slow, but the rate of beating also decreased in the unstimulated downstream heart; in contrast, stimulation of the vagus nerve supplying the downstream heart had no effect on the upstream heart. This elegant experiment proved that vagal stimulation releases a chemical that slows the heart; a few years later Loewi, who initially called this chemical *vagusstoff,* identified the mediator as acetylcholine. Sympathetic stimulation was subsequently shown to release norepinephrine, a catecholamine that—except for the absence of a methyl group—is the same as epinephrine (adrenaline), which had previously been isolated from the adrenal medulla. The list of signaling molecules that regulate cardiovascular function continues to grow (Table 3-4) and now includes *catecholamines* (e.g., epinephrine, norepinephrine, dopamine), *quaternary amines* (e.g., acetylcholine), and other small organic molecules (e.g., thyroxin, purines), *peptides* (e.g., angiotensin II, vasopressin, natriuretic peptides, endothelin, cytokines, growth factors), *steroid hormones* (e.g., aldosterone), *fatty acid derivatives* (e.g., prostaglandins), and even a *free radical gas* (nitric oxide).

Interactions between Extracellular Signaling Molecules (Ligands) and Their Receptors

Extracellular messengers are frequently called *ligands* because they bind with high affinity and specificity to *receptors* that recognize their presence as a signal to modify cell function. Most physiological ligands, as well as the majority of clinically useful drugs, are amphipathic molecules that contain hydrophilic moieties that prevent their crossing the lipid barrier in biological membranes. For this reason, their cellular actions depend on interactions with receptors on the extracellular surface of the plasma membrane. Exceptions include steroid and thyroid hormones, which are hydrophobic molecules that enter the cytosol where they interact with intracellular receptors.

The concept of specific receptors originated when Ahlquist (1948) found that epinephrine is a vasodilator at low concentrations and a vasoconstrictor at high concentrations, whereas norepinephrine is almost always a powerful vasoconstrictor; these and other observations led him to postulate that the response to an extracellular messenger is determined when it binds to a specific receptor. To explain why low concentrations of epinephrine relax blood vessels and high concentrations cause vasoconstriction, Ahlquist suggested that the catecholamine could bind to two types of receptor: one, which he called the *α-receptor,* mediates the constrictor action seen at high epinephrine concentrations; the other, which he called the *β-receptor,* was postulated to have a higher affinity for epinephrine and to be responsible for the vasodilator response at low concentrations of this catecholamine. Elucidation of the structures of these and other receptor molecules, along with the demonstration that different signal transduction pathways are activated when an extracellular messenger interacts with various receptors, have proven Ahlquist's hypothesis to be correct.

Routes by Which Ligands Gain Access to Their Receptors

Endocrine signaling (Table 3-5) was discovered by WM Bayliss and EH Starling (1902), who observed that instilling acid into the duodenum stimulates pancreatic secretion, even after both tissues are denervated. After finding that intravenous

TABLE 3-5
Routes By Which Extracellular Messengers Reach Cells
Endocrine (hormonal) signaling: An extracellular messenger is generated by a distant cell and delivered via the bloodstream to the tissue whose function is altered.
Neurotransmitter signaling: An extracellular messenger is generated by a nerve that releases the ligand at the surface of the cells whose function is altered.
Paracrine signaling: An extracellular messenger generated by a cell diffuses through the extracellular fluid to alter function in a nearby cell.
Autocrine signaling: An extracellular messenger is released into the extracellular fluid by the cell whose function is altered.
Cytoskeletal signaling: Mechanical stresses deform cytoskeletal structures to generate a signal that modifies cell function.

injection of a jejunal mucosa extract also stimulates pancreatic secretion, they proposed that a substance, which they called *secretin,* travels through the bloodstream from the jejunum, where it is produced, to the pancreas, where it exerts its effect. Less than 20 years after this discovery of *endocrine (hormonal signaling),* Loewi described *neurotransmitter signaling,* where the chemical messenger is released by the nervous system (see previous discussion). More recently, signaling molecules were found to reach their receptors by shorter routes; in *paracrine signaling* an extracellular messenger released by one cell diffuses to a receptor on a nearby cell, and by *autocrine signaling,* where a cell modifies its own function by releasing a ligand that binds to a receptor on its surface. *Cytoskeletal signaling* plays an important role in determining the size and shape of the heart by allowing mechanical interactions between neighboring cells and the surrounding extracellular matrix to modify gene expression. This type of signaling is initiated when cell deformation modifies cytoskeleton-bound proteins that are homologous to the ligands, receptors, and other molecules that participate in cell signaling (see Chapter 4).

Ligand Binding to Receptors: Receptor Number and Binding Affinity

The interactions between a ligand and its receptor can be characterized in terms of the *number* of receptors that can bind to the ligand and the binding *affinity* of the receptors for the ligand. Receptor number is often quantified by measuring B_{max}, the maximal amount of ligand that binds specifically to the receptor. A commonly used index of the affinity of a receptor for its ligand is the *dissociation constant* (k_d), which is the ligand concentration at which 50% of receptors are bound to the ligand; this means that the greater the affinity of the receptor for the ligand, the lower will be the k_d. Affinity can also be expressed as an *association (binding) constant* (k_b), which is the reciprocal of the dissociation constant. Ligands have a wide range of receptor-binding affinities; some peptides bind to their receptors at concentrations below 10^{-12} M, while most neurohumoral transmitters and drugs occupy their receptors at concentrations between 10^{-8} and 10^{-6} M. A few compounds, like ethanol, interact with a variety of membrane proteins at much higher concentrations (Table 3-6).

Binding affinity is an important determinant of the specificity of the biological response to a ligand. A ligand that binds to its receptor with high affinity usually evokes a specific response that is accompanied by few side effects because even low concen-

TABLE 3-6

Ligand-Binding Affinities of Some Cardiac Plasma Membrane Receptors

Ligand	Receptor	Approximate K_d[a]
Tetrodotoxin[b]	Sodium channel	10^{-12} M
Nitrendipine[c]	L-type calcium channel	10^{-10} M
Epinephrine	β-Adrenergic receptor	10^{-8} M
Ouabain[d]	Sodium pump (Na-K ATPase)	10^{-6} M
Ethanol	Nonspecific	10^{-3} M

[a] K_d, the dissociation constant, is the ligand concentration at which half of the receptors are occupied, so that a lower K_d means that the ligand binds more tightly to its receptor.
[b] A peptide toxin from puffer fish.
[c] A dihydropyridine calcium channel blocker.
[d] A cardiac glycoside.

trations of the ligand can be recognized by the receptor, which minimizes interactions of the ligand with other cell components. Ligands that bind to their receptors with low affinity, and so evoke responses only at high concentrations, often have additional nonspecific actions. The toxic effects of clinically useful drugs occur at concentrations higher than those that produce the desired therapeutic effects; exceptions include allergic or sensitivity reactions, which generally depend little on the concentration of the ligand. Specificity can be described as the ratio of the ligand concentrations that cause toxic and therapeutic effects; a higher toxic/therapeutic ratio means that a drug is less likely to cause unwanted side effects at doses that yield desirable therapeutic effects.

Receptor Blockade

Identification and characterization of plasma membrane receptors made it possible to design drugs that inhibit the binding of receptors to their ligands (see also Chapters 6 and 7. The inhibitory effects of these drugs, called *blockers* or *antagonists*, generally exhibit competitive kinetics and can be reversed by high concentrations of the physiological ligand (called an *agonist*). A few drugs inactivate receptors noncompetitively; aspirin, for example, irreversibly acetylates *cyclooxygenase*, an enzyme that generates a thrombogenic prostaglandin (see subsequent text).

The difference between most receptor blockers and physiological ligands is not *where* these molecules bind, but instead what happens *after* binding has occurred. Unlike an agonist, which activates the subsequent steps in a signal transduction cascade (e.g., after step 1 in Fig. 3-3), antagonists occupy the receptor but do not generate an intracellular signal. The clinical value of an antagonist (e.g., a *β-blocker)* therefore reflects the fact that the receptor-bound antagonist inhibits the ability of the receptor to bind to, and thus become activated by, the physiological agonist (e.g., norepinephrine).

Not all molecules that interact with receptors can be classified simply as agonists and antagonists. Some drugs, called *partial agonists,* bind to a receptor and cause weak activation of its signal transduction cascade but inhibit the ability of the receptor to interact with the more potent physiological agonists. By blocking binding of norepinephrine, for example, partial β-adrenergic agonists inhibit the response to surges of sympathetic activity while, at the same time, providing sustained but weak adrenergic stimulation called *intrinsic sympathomimetic activity (ISA).*

Types of Receptor

Cardiovascular function can be regulated by ligand binding to many types of receptor (Table 3-7). Most functional signals are mediated by *G protein–coupled receptors,* which are named for the heterotrimeric GTP-binding proteins that mediate their cellular actions (see subsequent text). *Enzyme-linked receptors,* most of which contain an intracellular protein kinase or other enzyme that is activated when the receptor binds to its ligand, were initially thought to mediate only proliferative responses, but are now known to participate in functional signaling. *Cytokine receptors,* whose major role is in inflammation, resemble enzyme-linked receptors except that instead of having intrinsic enzyme activity, the ligand-bound receptors form aggregates that modify the catalytic activity of other enzymes. *Ion channel–linked receptors* contain channels that are opened when the receptor binds its ligand, while *nuclear receptors* regulate gene expression when they bind to hormones, like aldosterone and thyroxin, whose hydrophobic structure allows them to cross the plasma and nuclear membranes. Cellular responses to nitric oxide, a gas that readily crosses the plasma membrane, are not mediated by a receptor; instead, this signaling molecule binds directly to *guanylyl cyclase,* its target enzyme within cells.

The following discussion highlights the G protein–coupled receptors, which are the most important mediators of functional signals in the heart and blood vessels. The other classes of receptor, which participate mainly in proliferative signaling, are described in Chapter 4.

TABLE 3-7

Some Receptors and Extracellular Messengers That Modify Cardiac Function

G protein–coupled receptors	**Enzyme-linked receptors**
Catecholamine	*Tyrosine kinase receptors*
Epinephrine and norepinephrine	Fibroblast growth factor (FGF)
Dopamine	Platelet-derived growth factor (PDGF)
Peptide	Insulin-like growth factor (IGF)
Angiotensin II	Vascular endothelial growth factor (VEGF)
Bradykinin	*Serine/threonine kinase receptors*
Arginine vasopressin (ADH)	Transforming growth factor-β (TGF-β)
Endothelin	Receptor guanyl cyclases
Neuropeptide Y	Natriuretic peptides
Adrenomedullin	*Cytokine receptors*
Ghrelin	Tumor necrosis factor α (TNF-α)
Other	Interleukins
Acetylcholine (muscarinic)	Growth hormone
Adenosine and other purines	Leptin
Prostaglandins	
	Nuclear receptors
Ion channel-linked receptors	Aldosterone
Acetylcholine (nicotinic)	Thyroxin

Direct binding to an intracellular target
Nitric oxide (NO)

TABLE 3-8

Some Important G Protein–Coupled Receptors in the Cardiovascular System

Ligand	Receptor	Target	G_α isoform	Second messenger/ effector
α-Agonists	α_1-Adrenergic	Phospholipase C	$G_{\alpha q}$	Diacylglycerol, InsP$_3$ ($\uparrow$)
β-Agonists	β_1-Adrenergic	Adenylyl cyclase	$G_{\alpha s}$	cAMP ($\uparrow$)
Acetylcholine	Muscarinic	K channel	$G_{\alpha o}$	Outward K current ($\uparrow$)
Acetylcholine	Muscarinic	Adenylyl cyclase	$G_{\alpha i}$	cAMP ($\downarrow$)
Adenosine	Purinergic (P$_1$)	K channel	$G_{\alpha o}$	Outward K current ($\uparrow$)
Adenosine	Purinergic (P$_1$)	Adenylyl cyclase	$G_{\alpha i}$	cAMP ($\downarrow$)
Angiotensin II	Angiotensin (AT$_1$)	Phospholipase C	$G_{\alpha q}$	Diacylglycerol, InsP$_3$ ($\uparrow$)
Endothelin	Endothelin	Phospholipase C	$G_{\alpha q}$	Diacylglycerol, InsP$_3$ ($\uparrow$)

InsP$_3$, inositol 1,4,5-trisphosphate; $\uparrow$, increased; $\downarrow$, decreased.

G Protein–Coupled Receptors

The most important regulators of cardiovascular function are *G protein–coupled receptors* (*GPCR*) (Table 3-8) that interact with the *guanyl nucleotide-binding proteins* (*G proteins*) described in the subsequent text. This family, which is among the largest in biology, includes more than 800 different proteins; in humans, ~1 in 80 genes encode members of this class of receptors (Clapham and Neer, 1997; Luttrell, 2006). G protein–coupled receptors contain seven membrane-spanning α-helices (Fig. 3-4) and so are sometimes called *heptahelical* or *seven-membrane–spanning* receptors. The ligand-binding sites, which interact with extracellular messengers, often include hydrophobic regions of the membrane-spanning α-helices. The

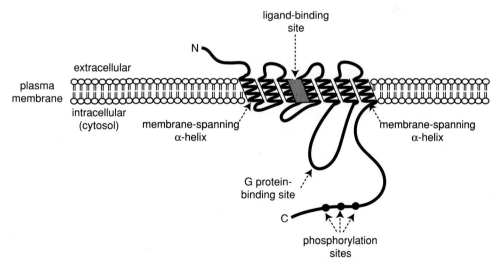

Figure 3-4: A G protein–coupled membrane receptor showing seven membrane spanning α-helices, portions of which contribute to the ligand-binding site. Sites that bind the heterotrimeric G proteins are located on the intracellular peptide chain that links the fifth and sixth membrane-spanning helices. Phosphorylation of the C-terminal intracellular peptide chain participates in receptor desensitization. Modified from Katz AM (2006). *Physiology of the Heart.* 4th ed. Philadelphia, Lippincott Williams and Wilkins.

G protein–binding sites lie within the cytosol and include a large intracellular C-terminal loop and portions of the membrane-spanning α-helices.

Enzyme-Linked Receptors

Binding of a ligand to an *enzyme-linked receptor* activates an intracellular enzyme, usually a protein kinase, that is part of the receptor molecule. This family includes *tyrosine kinase receptors* that contain catalytic sites that phosphorylate tyrosine moieties, *serine/threonine kinase receptors* whose catalytic site phosphorylates serine or threonine, *receptor guanyl cyclases* that synthesize cGMP, and *phosphatases* that catalyze dephosphorylations. *Cytokine receptors* lack enzymatic activity, but instead form aggregates with other membrane proteins that contain a latent tyrosine kinase that is activated when the receptor binds to a cytokine.

Ion Channel–Linked Receptors

Ion channel–linked (ionotropic) receptors contain channels that open when the receptor binds to its ligand. These include the nicotinic receptors, found at skeletal neuromuscular junctions, that generate a depolarizing sodium current that activates the motor end-plate when they are bound to acetylcholine. (Nicotinic receptors differ from the G protein–coupled muscarinic receptors that mediate the parasympathetic effects on the heart and vasculature described in the subsequent text.) Ion channel–linked receptors also mediate central responses to a variety of small molecules including agmatine, glutamine, serotonin, and γ-amino butyric acid.

Nuclear Receptors

Some lipophilic ligands, notably thyroxin and aldosterone, modify cardiovascular function when they bind to receptors within cells. When bound to their ligands, these receptors are transported to the nucleus where they participate in proliferative signaling.

G PROTEIN–COUPLED RECEPTORS AND HETEROTRIMERIC GTP-BINDING PROTEINS (G PROTEINS)

G protein–coupled receptors activate pathways whose cellular targets in the heart and blood vessels include phospholipase C, enzymes that synthesize intracellular second messengers, and voltage-gated potassium channels (Table 3-8). The responses initiated when these receptors bind to their ligands are mediated by heterotrimeric GTP-binding proteins that include one member of each of three protein families: G_α, G_β, and G_γ. G proteins can generate two signals; one carried by the GTP-binding protein G_α, the other by the $G_{\beta\gamma}$ dimer. The rich signaling diversity made possible by this coupling system reflects the fact that the large superfamily of G protein–coupled receptors interacts with at least 20 G_α subunits, 5 G_β subunits, and 12 G_γ subunits (Luttrell, 2006). Monomeric G proteins, like *ras*, also bind to GTP and participate in proliferative signaling (see Chapter 4).

G_α subunits, which are associated with the intracellular surface of the plasma membrane, bind GTP and contain a GTPase site. Four types of G_α subunit are important in cardiovascular regulation: $G_{\alpha s}$, which participates in the activation of adenylyl cyclase by norepinephrine; $G_{\alpha i}$ which mediates the inhibition of cAMP production by muscarinic and purinergic agonists; $G_{\alpha o}$, which activates (opens) potassium channels and inhibits cAMP production in response to muscarinic and purinergic agonists; and $G_{\alpha q}$, which participates in signaling cascades that activate phospholipase C (Table 3-8). $G_{\alpha i}$ and $G_{\alpha q}$ are generally regulatory, $G_{\alpha s}$ and $G_{\alpha o}$ are generally counterregulatory, while the heterodimers formed by G_{β} and G_{γ} can be both regulatory and counterregulatory. Some $G_{\beta\gamma}$ dimers activate phospholipase C and phospholipase A2, and a $G_{\beta\gamma}$ dimer activates $I_{K.Ach}$, an inward rectifying potassium channel that mediates vagal slowing of heart rate (see Chapter 5).

Ligand-bound G protein-coupled receptors generally interact with a single G_{α} to activate a single signaling pathway, but some can interact with more than one G_{α} subtype and/or $G_{\beta\gamma}$ dimer so as to activate several signal transduction cascades. In some cases ligand binding to a single receptor can activate up to 10 different G_{α} subunits, including members of all four families (Laugwitz et al., 1996).

Interactions between G Protein–Coupled Receptors and Heterotrimeric G Proteins

The interactions between a G protein–coupled receptor, its ligand, and the heterotrimeric G proteins can be described by the five-step sequence depicted schematically in Fig. 3-5.

STEP 1: Binding of the ligand to its receptor and activation of Gα: Inactive receptors, whose ligand-binding sites are unoccupied (Fig. 3-5A), are bound to the G protein trimer ($G_{\alpha\beta\gamma}$), which increases the affinity of the unoccupied receptor (R) for its ligand (L). Binding of the ligand to the receptor initiates the first step in the activation sequence (Fig. 3-5B):

$$\text{R-}G_{\alpha}\text{-GDP-}G_{\beta\gamma} + \text{L} \rightarrow \text{R-L-}G_{\alpha}\text{-GDP-}G_{\beta\gamma} \qquad \textbf{Eq. 3.2}$$

STEP 2: Formation of Gα-GTP and dissociation of Gβγ: Ligand binding to the receptor-G protein complex causes the GDP bound to G_{α} to be exchanged for GTP, which forms an activated G_{α}-GTP complex and releases activated $G_{\beta\gamma}$ (Fig. 3-5C) that can interact with its targets ($T_{\beta\gamma}$).

$$\text{R-L-}G_{\alpha}\text{-GDP-}G_{\beta\gamma} + \text{GTP} \rightarrow \text{R-L-}G_{\alpha}\text{-GTP} + \text{GDP} + G_{\beta\gamma} \rightarrow T_{\beta\gamma} \qquad \textbf{Eq. 3.3}$$

STEP 3: Dissociation of Gα-GTP from the receptor: G_{α}-GTP dissociates from the R-L-G_{α}-GTP complex (Fig. 3-5D), which allows free G_{α}-GTP to activate its own targets (T_{α}). Dissociation of G_{α}-GTP also reduces the ligand-binding affinity of the receptor, which releases the ligand.

$$\text{R-L-}G_{\alpha}\text{-GTP} \rightarrow \text{R} + \text{L} + G_{\alpha}\text{-GTP} \rightarrow T_{\alpha} \qquad \textbf{Eq. 3.4}$$

STEP 4: Dephosphorylation of Gα-bound GTP: Dissociation of the G_{α}-GTP complex from the receptor stimulates the intrinsic GTPase activity of G_{α}, which dephosphorylates the G_{α}-bound GTP to form G_{α}-GDP (Fig. 3-5E). This returns G_{α} to its basal state (G_{α}-GDP), which can no longer participate in signal transduction. G_{α}-GDP then rebinds and inactivates $G_{\beta\gamma}$ released in step 2, which ends signal transduction by $G_{\beta\gamma}$.

$$G_{\alpha}\text{-GTP} + G_{\beta\gamma} \rightarrow G_{\alpha}\text{-GDP-}G_{\beta\gamma} + P_i \qquad \textbf{Eq. 3.5}$$

GTP hydrolysis, which turns off both G_{α}- and $G_{\beta\gamma}$-mediated signals, is the major determinant of the duration of the response to the ligand.

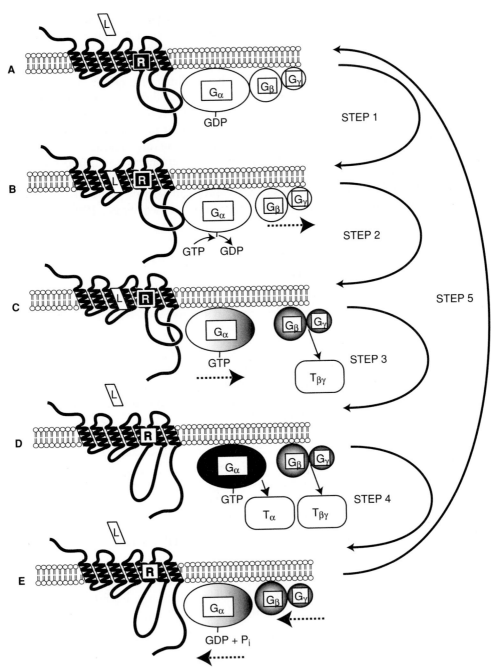

Figure 3-5: Simplified scheme showing five steps in the interactions between a G protein–coupled receptor, its ligand, and the heterotrimeric G proteins. Active states of these proteins are *shaded*. **A:** In the basal state, where the receptor (R) is not bound to its ligand (L), G_α is bound to GDP, the $G_{\beta\gamma}$ dimer, and the receptor in a R-L-G_α-GDP-$G_{\beta\gamma}$ complex. The $G_{\alpha\beta\gamma}$ trimer in this complex increases the ligand-binding affinity of the receptor. **B:** Binding of the ligand to the receptor causes G_α to exchange the bound GDP for GTP, which begins the dissociation of G_α from $G_{\beta\gamma}$. **C:** Dissociation activates $G_{\beta\gamma}$, which interacts with its targets ($T_{\beta\gamma}$). **D:** Dissociation of the G_α-GTP complex from the receptor further activates G_α (*increased shading*), which interacts with its targets (T_α). Dissociation of G_α also reduces the ligand-binding affinity of the receptor, which releases the ligand. **E:** Dissociation of G_α activates its intrinsic GTPase activity, which dephosphorylates the bound GTP to form the inactive G_α-GDP complex. The latter then rebinds both the receptor and $G_{\beta\gamma}$, which increases the ligand-binding affinity of the former and inactivates the latter, thereby returning these signaling proteins to the basal state depicted in **A**. From Katz AM (2006). *Physiology of the Heart*. 4th ed. Philadelphia, Lippincott Williams and Wilkins.

STEP 5: Rebinding of G_α, $G_{\beta\gamma}$, and the receptor to form the receptor-bound $G_{\alpha\beta\gamma}$ complex: The system returns to the basal state when the $G_{\alpha\beta\gamma}$ complex formed by G_α-GDP and $G_{\beta\gamma}$ rebinds the free receptor and increases its affinity for the ligand (Fig. 3-5A).

$$R + G_\alpha\text{-GDP-}G_{\beta\gamma} \rightarrow R\text{-}G_\alpha\text{-GDP-}G_{\beta\gamma} \qquad \text{Eq. 3-6}$$

Overview of the G Protein Cycle

The reactions between the heterotrimeric G proteins and their receptors allow a single ligand to generate two intracellular signals, one carried by G_α-GTP, the other by $G_{\beta\gamma}$, both of which can activate their own downstream targets. At the same time, these reactions help avoid runaway signaling by turning off the cycle; this is due to the instability of the active G_α-GTP complex, which spontaneously hydrolyzes the bound nucleotide to form the inactive G_α-GDP that also rebinds and inactivates $G_{\beta\gamma}$. G protein–mediated signals are also attenuated when dissociation of activated G_α-GTP from the ligand-bound receptor reduces the affinity of the receptor for its ligand. Dependence of the cycle on a continuing supply of GTP can slow G protein–coupled signaling when the GTP/GDP ratio decreases in energy-starved cells.

Regulation of the G Protein Cycle

The key role of signal transduction by G protein-coupled receptors is reflected in the many mechanisms that regulate these systems, a few of which are described in the following paragraphs.

Dephosphorylation of G_α-GTP, the rate-limiting step in the G protein cycle, is regulated by *GTPase-activating* proteins (*GAPs*) that accelerate GTPase activity, and *guanine nucleotide exchange factors* (*GEFs*) that release the GDP bound to G_α. GEFs are inhibited by *guanine nucleotide dissociation inhibitors* (*GDIFs*) that accelerate the cycle by preventing GEFs from inhibiting GDP release.

The risk of runaway signaling is reduced by enzymes that phosphorylate the ligand-bound receptors; these include *G protein–coupled receptor kinases* (*GRKs*) and second messenger–dependent protein kinases like protein kinases A and C. Glycosylation and palmitoylation of the receptors, myristoylation and palmitoylation of the G_α subunits, and interactions of G_α with *GTPase-activating proteins* (*GAPs*) and *regulators of G protein signaling* (*RGSs*) also regulate the G protein cycle. Among the most important of these regulatory mechanisms is *desensitization*, which decreases the number of available β-receptors when adrenergic stimulation is sustained, as occurs in patients with heart failure.

Desensitization

The loss of efficacy that follows prolonged β-adrenergic stimulation is due largely to *desensitization*. This process, which can begin within a few seconds after the receptor binds to its ligand, decreases the number of available receptors by a three-step process: uncoupling, internalization, and digestion (Fig. 3-6).

Uncoupling occurs when activated G protein–coupled receptors are phosphorylated by protein kinases. In *heterologous desensitization*, the receptors are phosphorylated in a single step and need not be bound to a ligand, whereas *homologous desensitization* is a two-step process in which phosphorylation of the ligand-bound

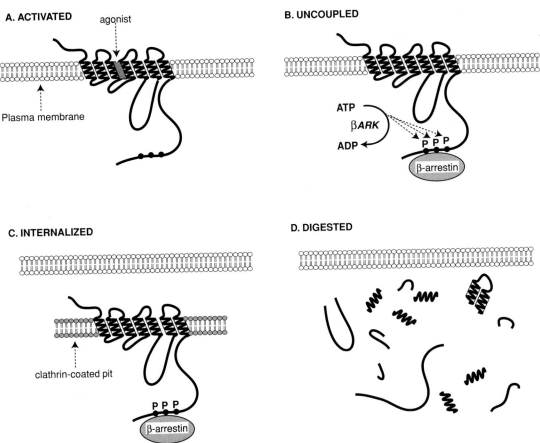

Figure 3-6: β-Adrenergic receptor desensitization. **A:** Activated, ligand-bound receptor. **B:** Prolonged binding of the β-receptor to its agonist stimulates a G protein receptor kinase (GRK) called β-adrenergic receptor kinase (βARK), which phosphorylates the C-terminal intracellular peptide chain of the receptor. The latter then binds a cofactor called β-arrestin that inactivates the receptor. **C:** Transfer of the phosphorylated receptor from the plasma membrane to clathrin-coated pits within the cell internalizes the receptor, which, although structurally intact, can no longer interact with either its agonists or G proteins. Dephosphorylation (not shown) allows the internalized receptors to return to the plasma membrane, which resensitizes the receptor. **D:** Receptors that remain internalized for long periods are digested by intracellular proteolytic enzymes; this step, unlike uncoupling and internalization, is irreversible. From Katz AM (2006). *Physiology of the Heart.* 4th ed. Philadelphia, Lippincott Williams and Wilkins.

receptor by a specific *G protein receptor kinase (GRK)* is followed by binding of the phosphorylated receptor to a cofactor called *β-arrestin* that uncouples the receptor from its G protein (Fig. 3-6B). The GRK that uncouples the β–adrenergic receptor called *βARK (β-adrenergic receptor kinase)*, prevents the receptor from activating its G protein by phosphorylating the intracellular C-terminal peptide chain of the receptor. Uncoupling is readily reversed when the receptor is dephosphorylated by a *G protein–coupled receptor phosphatase,* a process called *resensitization.*

Internalization, the second step in desensitization, removes the phosphorylated β-arrestin–bound receptor from the plasma membrane, after which the receptor (which has already been uncoupled from its G protein) is transferred to a clathrin-coated pit within the cell (Fig. 3-6C). Internalized receptors can no longer interact with their ligands, but initially remain structurally intact so that, like phosphorylation, internalization is reversible if the receptor can be returned to the plasma membrane. A remarkable nuance in signal transduction is the ability of some internalized receptors, which are no longer able to bind to the extracellular messengers that activate functional responses, to participate in proliferative signaling; in the case of internalized β_2-receptors, this occurs when the β_2-receptor–β-arrestin complex forms a "scaffold" that activates mitogen-activated protein kinases (*MAP kinases*) (Luttrell et al., 1999) (see Chapter 4).

Receptors that remain internalized become susceptible to proteolytic *digestion*, the final step in desensitization (Fig. 3-6D). This process, unlike uncoupling and internalization, is irreversible, so that restoration of receptor function requires the synthesis of new receptors.

Denervation Sensitivity

Prolonged administration of β-adrenergic blockers increases the number of available β-receptors, so that sudden withdrawal of the β-blocker finds the heart sensitized to β-adrenergic agonists. This phenomenon, called *denervation sensitivity*, can have fatal consequences in patients who receive prolonged β-blocker therapy because sudden discontinuation of the blocker allows the high levels of norepinephrine generally seen in heart failure to interact with the increased number of β-receptors, which can generate enough cAMP to cause sudden cardiac death (Eichhorn, 1999).

INTRACELLULAR SECOND MESSENGERS

Relatively few neurohumoral signals are mediated by direct coupling of an activated receptor or G protein to an effector (Fig. 3-7A); instead, most intracellular signal transduction pathways generate small molecules, called *second messengers*, that include nucleotides, lipids, phosphosugars, and calcium ions (Table 3-9). Cyclic AMP, the first of these second messengers to be discovered, is generated when norepinephrine-bound β-receptors activate $G_{\alpha s}$, which stimulates adenylyl cyclase to synthesize cAMP from ATP (Fig. 3-7B). Two intracellular messengers mediate the signal generated when norepinephrine binds to α_1-receptors; these are *inositol trisphosphate* (*InsP$_3$*) and *diacylglycerol* (*DAG*), which are released when activated $G_{\alpha q}$ stimulates *phospholipase C* (*PLC*), a lipolytic enzyme, to hydrolyze a membrane phospholipid called *phosphatidylinositol 4,5-bisphosphate* (*PIP$_2$*) (Fig. 3-7C). Other intracellular messengers include cGMP, which can be generated when nitric oxide binds to *guanylyl cyclase* (see subsequent text), and calcium, which enters the cytosol down an electrochemical gradient from the extracellular space or internal stores (see Chapter 5).

Signaling by most intracellular second messengers is regulated by changes in the rates at which they are produced and broken down (Table 3-9); cAMP, for example, is synthesized by adenylyl cyclase and degraded by *phosphodiesterases*, both of which are highly regulated. In the case of *calcium*, an intracellular messenger that obviously cannot be synthesized, signaling begins when this cation enters the cytosol from regions of high concentration in the extracellular space and sarcoplasmic reticulum, and ends when calcium is actively transported out of the cytosol (Chapter 5).

Cyclic AMP

Cyclic AMP, which mediates most of the regulatory cardiovascular responses to sympathetic stimulation, is generated from ATP by adenylyl cyclase (Fig. 3-8),

A. DIRECT (MEMBRANE-DELIMITED) COUPLING

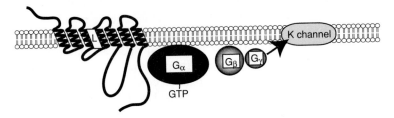

B. INDIRECT (ADENYLYL CYCLASE-MEDIATED) COUPLING

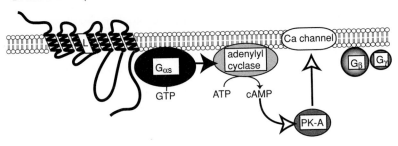

C. INDIRECT (PHOSPHOLIPASE C-MEDIATED) COUPLING

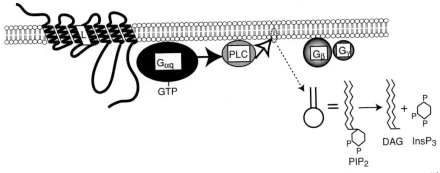

Figure 3-7: Three mechanisms by which ligand binding to a G protein–coupled receptor can modify cell function. **A:** Direct coupling, where an activated G protein interacts directly with a target that alters cell function. This is seen when acetylcholine binding to muscarinic receptors activates $G_{\beta\gamma}$, which then activates a plasma membrane potassium channel. **B** and **C:** Second messenger–mediated coupling, where a G protein–coupled receptor modifies the production of one or more intracellular messengers. **B:** Activation of adenylyl cyclase by $G_{\alpha s}$ increases cAMP production, which increases calcium entry by activating a cAMP-activated protein kinase that phosphorylates plasma membrane L-type calcium channels. **C:** Activation of phospholipase C by $G_{\alpha q}$ stimulates the hydrolysis of phosphatidylinositol, a membrane phospholipid, to generate two second messengers: Diacylglycerol (DAG) and inositol trisphosphate (InsP$_3$). From Katz AM (2006). *Physiology of the Heart.* 4th ed. Philadelphia, Lippincott Williams and Wilkins.

which in the heart is stimulated when $G_{\alpha s}$ is activated by norepinephrine binding to β_1-adrenergic receptors. Most responses to cAMP are mediated by cAMP-dependent protein kinases (PK-A). In addition to increasing contractility, accelerating relaxation, and increasing heart rate, cAMP helps provide substrates needed for the increased energy expenditure by accelerating glycogen breakdown and fatty acid

TABLE 3-9

Major Intracellular Messengers

Second messenger	Initiation of signal	Termination of signal
Cyclic AMP	Synthesized from ATP by adenylyl cyclase	Degraded by to AMP by phosphodiesterases
Cyclic GMP	Synthesized from GTP by guanylyl cyclase	Degraded by to GMP by phosphodiesterases
InsP$_3$	Released from PIP$_2$ by phospholipase C	Dephosphorylated by phosphatases
Diacylglycerol	Released from PIP$_2$ by phospholipase C	Phosphorylated to form a phosphatide or hydrolyzed to form monoglyceride
Calcium	Diffuses into the cytosol from regions of high concentration	Pumped out of cytosol

PIP$_2$, phosphatidylinositol 4,5-bisphosphate; InsP$_3$, inositol 1,4,5-trisphosphate.

metabolism. Cyclic AMP levels are decreased when the intracellular messenger is hydrolyzed by phosphodiesterases.

The major counterregulatory effects of parasympathetic stimulation, whose cardiovascular effects generally oppose those of the sympathetic nervous system, occur when cAMP production is inhibited by G$_{\alpha i}$ (Fig. 3-8).

Cyclic GMP

The counterregulatory responses to natriuretic peptides and nitric oxide (NO) are mediated by cGMP whose effects, which generally oppose those of cAMP, are mediated by cGMP-dependent protein kinases. The mechanisms that stimulate production of this intracellular messenger differ from those that activate adenylyl cyclase.

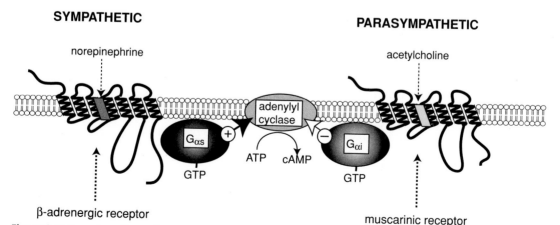

Figure 3-8: Opposing effects of sympathetic (**left**) and parasympathetic (**right**) on cAMP production. Norepinephrine binding to β_1 receptors on the heart activates G$_{\alpha s}$, which stimulates adenylyl cyclase to increase cAMP production, whereas acetylcholine binding to muscarinic receptors activates protein G$_{\alpha i}$, which inhibits adenylyl cyclase. Modified from Katz AM (2006). *Physiology of the Heart.* 4th ed. Philadelphia, Lippincott Williams and Wilkins.

Natriuretic peptides increase cGMP production when they bind to *receptor guanylyl cyclases*, which are plasma membrane enzymes that contain a single membrane-spanning α-helix. Muscarinic receptors on endothelial cells release nitric oxide that, after diffusing to adjacent vascular smooth muscle cells, increases cGMP levels when it binds to the active site of *soluble guanylyl cyclases* in the cytosol (see subsequent text). Cellular levels of cGMP are determined by a balance between guanylyl cyclases and cGMP phosphodiesterases.

Inositol 1,4,5-Trisphosphate and Diacylglycerol

Inositol 1,4,5 trisphosphate ($InsP_3$) and diacylglycerol (DAG), the second messengers generated by phospholipase C (Fig. 3-7C), activate different intracellular signal transduction pathways. $InsP_3$ releases calcium from internal stores by opening $InsP_3$-gated intracellular calcium release channels; the resulting increase in cytosolic calcium constricts vascular smooth muscle, but is of little importance in regulating myocardial contractility because systole is initiated by a much larger calcium flux through a different class of calcium channels that open during excitation–contraction coupling (see Chapter 5). DAG has a weak effect to increase myocardial contractility, and both $InsP_3$-gated calcium release and DAG play an important role in proliferative signaling (see Chapter 4).

Calcium

Calcium, which generally mediates excitatory signals, enters the cytosol by passive downhill fluxes from the extracellular fluid and intracellular stores in the sarcoplasmic reticulum (see Chapter 5). Cellular responses to calcium are influenced by the source of this messenger and how fast it enters the cytosol. In cardiac myocytes, rapid calcium entry through plasma membrane L-type calcium channels activates contraction by opening intracellular calcium release channels in the sarcoplasmic reticulum, whereas slower increases in cytosolic calcium, caused for example by calcium entry through T-type calcium channels or $InsP_3$-gated calcium release channels, participate in proliferative signaling. These distinctions are less important in vascular smooth muscle, whose slow contractions can be initiated when calcium enters the cytosol from both the extracellular space and intracellular stores. In the heart, functional responses to calcium depend on the specific cell type; calcium entry via L-type calcium channels is important for AV conduction and regulation of myocardial contractility, while both L- and T-type calcium channels contribute to pacemaker activity by the SA node. Calcium flux from the sarcoplasmic reticulum into the cytosol does not modify membrane potential because these internal membranes contain anionic channels that neutralize any net charge movements.

SIGNALING ENZYMES

The extracellular messengers listed in Table 3-7 and the intracellular second messengers listed in Table 3-9 often participate in signal transduction by activating enzymes that modify other proteins. For example, ligand-binding to tyrosine kinase receptors activates catalytic sites in these membrane proteins that phosphorylate tyrosine residues in other intracellular proteins, while cAMP-dependent protein kinases phosphorylate serine and threonine residues. Other signaling enzymes transfer chemical groups, such as methyl groups (methylation), fatty acids (acetylation,

TABLE 3-10	
Major Intracellular Protein Kinases	
Protein kinase	**Activated by (second messenger)**
Cyclic AMP-dependent (*protein kinase A*)	cAMP
Cyclic GMP-dependent (*protein kinase G*)	cGMP
Phospholipid-dependent (*protein kinase C*)	Diacylglycerol
Calcium, calmodulin-dependent (*CAM kinase*)	Calcium

myristoylation, and palmitoylation), and sugar residues (glycosylation), to a variety of proteins. Signal transduction ends when these groups are removed by other enzymes.

Protein Kinases

Most of the protein kinases that participate in functional signaling are members of a large family of serine/threonine kinases that phosphorylate serine and threonine residues; these include protein kinase A, protein kinase G, protein kinase C, and calcium, calmodulin-activated (CAM) kinase (Table 3-10). Protein kinase B, also called akt, and tyrosine kinase play an important role in proliferative signaling (see Chapter 4). Signals generated by protein kinases are turned off by *phosphoprotein phosphatases,* which hydrolyze the bonds that link the phosphate moieties to effector proteins.

MAJOR EXTRACELLULAR MEDIATORS OF THE NEUROHUMORAL RESPONSE

The receptors and ligands listed in Table 3-7 play an important role in patients with heart failure. In addition to regulatory functional responses (cardiac stimulation, vasoconstriction, and fluid retention) that help sustain hemodynamic performance, most of these mediators also activate proliferative responses that play a key role in the maladaptive hypertrophy that contributes to the poor prognosis in heart failure (see Chapter 4).

Norepinephrine and Epinephrine

The most powerful components of the neurohumoral response occur when norepinephrine released by the sympathetic nervous system binds to adrenergic receptors (Table 3-11). In the heart, activated β_1-receptors increase contractility, accelerate relaxation, and increase heart rate, while α_1-receptors constrict arteriolar resistance vessels and veins and promote fluid retention by the kidneys.

α-Adrenergic Receptors

Norepinephrine binding to α_1- and α_2-receptors generates different cardiovascular responses; activation of α_1-receptors on blood vessels (Table 3-12) and, to a lesser extent on the heart, generates a regulatory response, whereas α_2-receptors in both the central nervous system and the heart inhibit norepinephrine release, and so are counterregulatory.

TABLE 3-11

Major Receptor Subtypes That Mediate Cardiovascular Actions of Norepinephrine

α_1-Adrenergic Receptors
Functional responses
  Increased myocardial contractility (minor)
  Smooth muscle contraction—vasoconstriction
  Sodium retention by the kidneys
Proliferative responses
  Stimulation of protein synthesis, cell growth, and proliferation

α_2-Adrenergic Receptors
Functional responses
  Central inhibition of sympathetic activity
    Vasodilatation
    Cardiac inhibition

β_1-Adrenergic Receptors
Functional responses
  Cardiac stimulation—positive inotropy, lusitropy, and chronotropy
Proliferative responses
  Stimulation of protein synthesis, cell growth, and proliferation

β_2-Adrenergic Receptors
Functional responses
  Increased myocardial contractility
  Smooth muscle relaxation—vasodilatation
Proliferative responses
  Antiapoptotic
  Regulation of protein synthesis, cell growth, and proliferation (internalized receptor)

TABLE 3-12

Major Regulators of Vascular Tone

Vasoconstrictors	**Vasodilators**
Catecholamine	*Catecholamine*
Norepinephrine (peripheral α_1-adrenergic)	Norepinephrine (central α_2-adrenergic)
Peptide	Epinephrine (β_2-adrenergic)
Angiotensin II	Dopamine
Arginine vasopressin	*Peptide*
Endothelin	Natriuretic peptides
Neuropeptide Y	Bradykinin
Lipid	Adrenomedullin
Thromboxane A_2	*Lipid*
	Prostacyclin, prostaglandin E_2
	Gas
	Nitric oxide (NO)

Binding of norepinephrine to peripheral α_1-receptors activates $G_{\alpha q/11}$, which stimulates signaling pathways that generate InsP$_3$ and DAG. The predominant response in vascular smooth muscle is a powerful vasoconstrictor effect, caused by InsP$_3$-mediated calcium release, while activation of α_1-receptors in human hearts causes a weak positive inotropic effect. DAG also stimulates proliferative signaling by activating protein kinase-C (Chapter 4).

β-Adrenergic Receptors

Norepinephrine binding to β_1-receptors, the major subtype in the human heart, activates $G_{\alpha s}$ which stimulates adenylyl cyclase; the resulting increase in cAMP production initiates powerful inotropic, lusitropic, and chronotropic responses. In addition to these functional responses, β_1-receptor activation mediates hypertrophic responses and causes apoptosis, which contributes to the deterioration of the failing heart. Cardiac β_2-receptors, which are coupled to both $G_{\alpha s}$ and $G_{\alpha i}$, have several effects including $G_{\alpha s}$-mediated regulatory responses that are weaker than those initiated by β_1-receptor activation. Activation of G_{ai} by cardiac β_2-receptors is counterregulatory and has an antiapoptotic effect that is protective in failing hearts, where the proportion of cardiac β_2-receptors relative to β_1-receptors is increased. β_2-Receptors mediate a vasodilator effect in vascular smooth muscle (Table 3-12), but the dominant response of blood vessels to sympathetic stimulation is vasoconstriction caused by α_1-receptor activation. Internalized β_2-receptors also participate in proliferative signaling (see previous discussion).

Dopamine

Dopamine, an intermediate in the biosynthesis of norepinephrine from tyrosine, acts as an extracellular messenger in both the central nervous system and peripheral tissues. At low concentrations, dopamine interacts with peripheral DA$_1$ receptors to exert a physiological counterregulatory effect that relaxes vascular smooth muscle, whereas higher concentrations stimulate norepinephrine release from sympathetic nerve endings and activate β_1-receptors in the heart, both of which have regulatory effects. At still higher concentrations, dopamine cross-reacts with peripheral α_1-receptors to cause vasoconstriction.

Muscarinic (Parasympathetic) and Purinergic Agonists

There is substantial evidence, but not universal agreement, that parasympathetic tone, the number of muscarinic receptors, and $G_{\alpha i}$ are increased in failing hearts (Binkley et al., 1991; Nolan et al., 1992, Vatner et al., 1996; Le Guludec et al., 1997, Wang et al., 2004). These uncertainties reflect the complexity of this signaling system; for example, acetylcholine binds to at least five muscarinic receptor subtypes, called M$_1$ to M$_5$, of which the M$_2$ and M$_3$ receptors mediate the major cardiovascular responses to vagal stimulation. M$_2$-receptor activation shortens the atrial action potential (which reduces atrial contractility) by direct coupling of activated $G_{\beta\gamma}$ to repolarizing potassium channels; acetylcholine-binding to M$_2$ receptors also activates $G_{\alpha i}$, which slows sinus node depolarization, inhibits atrioventricular conduction, and decreases ventricular contractility. In the vasculature, acetylcholine binding to M$_3$ receptors on smooth muscle cells causes vasoconstriction by activating phospholipase C and releasing InsP$_3$, but this regulatory response is normally outweighed by a more powerful counterregulatory effect caused when acetylcholine binding to M_3 receptors on endothelial cells releases NO, a powerful vasodilator (see subsequent text).

Adenosine and other purines can bind to at least seven ligand-gated channels (called P_2X receptors) and eight G protein–coupled receptors (called P_2Y receptors). The major cardiovascular responses, which are mediated by G protein–coupled receptors called A1, A2a, A2b, and A3, are counterregulatory. Activated A1 receptors, which are coupled to $G_{\alpha i}$, inhibit cAMP production and, by a direct interaction, open inward rectifying potassium channels that carry $i_{K.ATP}$; the latter repolarizes smooth muscle cells, and so favors vasodilatation. Opening of $i_{K.ATP}$ channels in the SA node slows heart rate, whereas in the ventricles, where these channels lower resting potential, this response to A1 receptor activation has an energy-sparing effect because excitability is reduced. A2a receptors, which are coupled to $G_{\alpha s}$, increase cAMP production in vascular smooth muscle, which has a vasodilator effect; in the heart, this response has a weak inotropic effect. Some A2b receptors are coupled to both $G_{\alpha s}$ and $G_{\alpha q}$; activation of the latter in smooth muscle causes vasoconstriction by stimulating phospholipase C to release $InsP_3$. A3 receptors, like A1 receptors, are coupled to $G_{\alpha i}$ and so cause vasodilatation and have counterregulatory effects on the heart; in addition, these receptors regulate apoptosis and protect the heart against reperfusion injury. Purinergic responses can also alleviate some maladaptive features of cardiac hypertrophy (see Chapter 4).

The Renin–Angiotensin System

Many of the causal links between Bright's disease, hypertension, and cardiac hypertrophy (see Chapter 1) can be explained by activation of the renin–angiotensin system, which is among the most powerful mechanisms affecting cardiovascular function. The predominant responses are regulatory; functional responses include vasoconstriction, decreased fluid excretion by the kidneys, and a weak inotropic effect on the heart. The renin–angiotensin system also activates counterregulatory functional responses, but the latter are normally overwhelmed by the regulatory effects. This system also evokes important proliferative responses (see Chapter 4).

The extracellular messenger responsible for most of these responses is angiotensin II, a peptide formed by proteolytic reactions in both the circulation and several tissues (Fig. 3-9). The vasoconstrictor substance was initially thought to be *renin*, which is released when the kidneys became ischemic and in response to β-adrenergic stimulation. However, renin turned out to be a protease that forms the active pressor by catalyzing the hydrolysis of an inactive protein called *angiotensinogen*. The story became more complex when *angiotensin I*, a decapeptide generated by renin-catalyzed hydrolysis of angiotensinogen, was found to be the relatively inactive precursor of a more powerful vasoconstrictor peptide released by *angiotensin-converting enzyme* (ACE). The active octapeptide was discovered independently by Page and Helmer (1940) in Cleveland, Ohio, who named it "angiotonin," and by Braun-Menendez et al. (1940) in Argentina, who chose the name "hypertensin"—the term *angiotensin II* was coined 18 years later as a compromise (Braun-Menendez and Page, 1958).

Circulating angiotensin II is synthesized when renin released into the bloodstream by the juxtaglomerular apparatus of the *kidneys* hydrolyzes circulating angiotensinogen made in the *liver* to form angiotensin I that is digested further in the *lung* to form angiotensin II that circulates in the *blood* (Fig. 3-9A). Angiotensin II

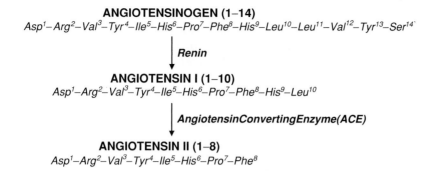

A. THE RENIN-ANGIOTENSIN SYSTEM: "CLASSIC" VERSION

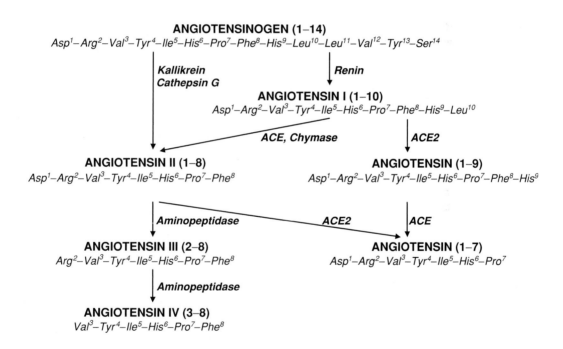

B. THE RENIN-ANGIOTENSIN SYSTEM: UPDATED VERSION

Figure 3-9: Generation of active signaling peptides by the renin–angiotensin system. **A:** The circulating system as originally described includes two proteolytic cleavages, catalyzed by renin and angiotensin-converting enzyme (ACE), which release angiotensin II from angiotensinogen, the inactive precursor. **B:** Additional proteolytic reactions occur in many tissues; these are catalyzed by chymase, cathepsin G, kallikrein, and ACE2, and can form additional biologically active peptides. Modified from Katz AM (2006). *Physiology of the Heart.* 4th ed. Philadelphia, Lippincott Williams and Wilkins.

is also released locally by tissue proteases: directly from angiotensinogen by *kallikrein* and *cathepsin G,* or from angiotensin I by *tissue ACE* and *chymase* (Fig. 3-9B). Additional peptide mediators in the tissue system can be formed by proteolytic cleavage of angiotensin I by *ACE2,* an ACE isoform, which generates the vasoconstrictor nonapeptide *angiotensin (1–9).* Hydrolysis of the latter by ACE forms the heptapeptide *angiotensin (1–7),* which has counterregulatory actions that include vasodilatation and inhibition of proliferative signaling. Further proteolysis of angiotensin II generates the biologically active heptapeptide *angiotensin III* and the hexapeptide *angiotensin IV.* Angiotensin III has proinflammatory actions and binds to AT_1 receptors that cause vasoconstriction.

The circulating and tissue systems appear to serve different functions: The former is probably most important in regulating vasomotor tone, whereas angiotensin II produced in the tissues participates in proinflammatory and proliferative signaling (see Chapter 4). Angiotensin II formed by the circulating system acts on distant targets (endocrine signaling), whereas locally produced angiotensin II binds to adjacent cells (paracrine signaling) and to receptors on the same cell that produce this extracellular messenger (autocrine signaling) (see Table 3-5).

The effects of angiotensin II are mediated by two G protein–coupled receptor subtypes, designated AT_1 and AT_2, that mediate opposing responses (Fig. 3-10). AT_1 receptors, which are regulatory, cause vasoconstriction, have a weak effect to increase myocardial contractility, and stimulate cardiac myocyte hypertrophy; in contrast, AT_2 receptors generally cause counterregulatory responses such as vasodilatation and growth inhibition. Both AT_1 and AT_2 receptors are found in the cardiovascular system; the former predominate in vascular smooth muscle and both are found in the endothelium; an additional receptor subtype, AT_4, binds to angiotensin IV in adult human hearts where it appears to have vasodilator and proinflammatory

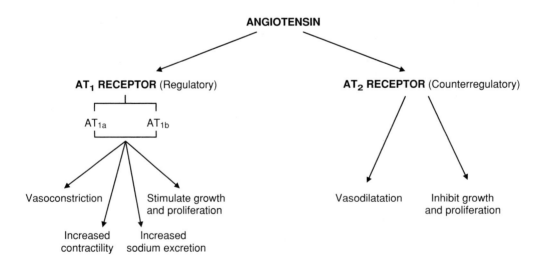

ANGIOTENSIN II RECEPTOR SUBTYPES

Figure 3-10: The responses to these two subtypes differ and in many cases oppose one another. The AT_1 receptors, which include the AT_{1a} and AT_{1b} subtypes, exert regulatory effects, whereas AT_2 receptor stimulation generally evokes counterregulatory responses. Modified from Katz AM (2006). *Physiology of the Heart.* 4th ed. Philadelphia, Lippincott Williams and Wilkins.

effects. The ACE enzyme itself can participate in proliferative and proinflammatory signaling when the intracellular loop of this intrinsic membrane protein activates mitogen-activated protein kinase (MAP kinase) pathways (see Chapter 4).

The renin–angiotensin system, along with other signaling systems, regulates additional mediators of the neurohumoral response (see subsequent text). For example, angiotensin II initiates regulatory amplifications by stimulating the secretion of aldosterone, vasopressin, catecholamines, and endothelin, which worsen many of the vicious cycles seen in patients with heart failure (see Chapters 6 and 7).

Bradykinin and Related Peptides

Kinins are peptides released from inactive protein precursors called *kininogens* by proteolytic enzymes called *kallikreins* (Fig. 3-11). Most kinins cause vasodilatation, are antiproliferative, and often have proinflammatory effects. Levels of *bradykinin,* the octapeptide *Arg-Pro-Gly-Phe-Ser-Pro-Phe-Arg,* and *kallidin* (lysyl-bradykinin) are regulated by the rate at which the peptides are released from their precursors and broken down into inactive fragments. Bradykinin hydrolysis is catalyzed by the same converting enzymes that release angiotensin II (see previous discussion), which means that ACE has a synergistic effect that generates a vasoconstrictor (angiotensin II) and inactivates a vasodilator (bradykinin). Kinins also inhibit maladaptive proliferative signaling (see Chapter 4). Other effects of bradykinin include a cough, noted by some patients who receive ACE inhibitors, and angioneurotic edema, a rare but potentially fatal side effect of this class of drugs (see Chapters 6 and 7).

The biological actions of kinins are mediated by inducible (B_1) and constitutive (B_2) kinin receptors (Fig. 3-12), both of which are G protein–coupled receptors. Most physiological responses are initiated by B_2 receptors; bradykinin and kallidin cause vasodilatation by increasing the production of nitric oxide (NO), cAMP, and prostacyclins. Activation of B_1 receptors, on the other hand, stimulates the synthesis of iNOS, which releases high concentrations of NO that participate in inflammation.

Endothelin

Endothelins (ET), first isolated from endothelial cells, are now known to be released by many cell types; active peptides include ET-1, ET-2 , and ET-3, all of which contain 21 amino acids. Endothelin production is regulated by the rate of synthesis of

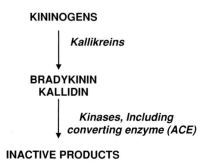

Figure 3-11: Kinin production. Kinins are released from kininogens by plasma and tissue kallikreins, and inactivated by enzymes that include ACE. Modified from Katz AM (2006). *Physiology of the Heart*. 4th ed. Philadelphia, Lippincott Williams and Wilkins.

KININ PRODUCTION AND BREAKDOWN

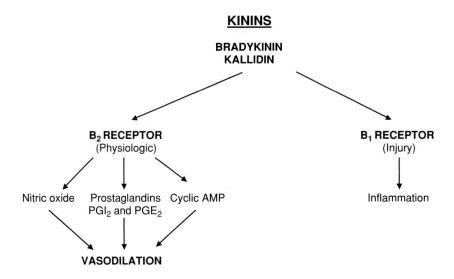

Figure 3-12: Kinin receptor subtypes. The B_2 receptors mediate vasodilator responses that participate in physiologic regulation of the circulation, while B_1 receptors mediate proinflammatory responses. Modified from Katz AM (2006). *Physiology of the Heart*. 4th ed. Philadelphia, Lippincott Williams and Wilkins.

precursors, called *preproendothelins,* and posttranslational processing of preproendothelins by proteolytic enzymes (Fig. 3-13). The initial products of preproendothelin proteolysis, called *proendothelins* or *big endothelins,* are hydrolyzed by *endothelin converting enzyme* to form *endothelin.* Chymases also hydrolyze proendothelins to form endothelins, and can degrade the active peptides. Levels of both big ET1 and ET1 are elevated in patients with heart failure, where the extent of the elevation correlates with the severity of the syndrome.

Figure 3-13: Endothelin production. Expression of endothelin genes produces preproendothelin which is processed by proteolysis to generate proendothelin. Hydrolysis of the latter by endothelin-converting enzymes releases endothelin. Modified from Katz AM (2006). *Physiology of the Heart*. 4th ed. Philadelphia, Lippincott Williams and Wilkins.

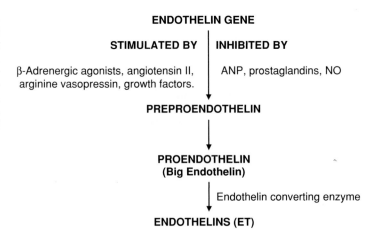

Preproendothelin synthesis is stimulated by several mediators of the neurohumoral response, including angiotensin II, vasopressin, norepinephrine, the cytokine interleukin-1, and peptide growth factors; synthesis is inhibited by ANP, nitric oxide, and prostaglandins. The major cardiovascular isoform, ET-1, is released from blood vessels in response to epinephrine, angiotensin II, cytokines, growth factors, and high shear stress along the endothelium. Endothelin signaling can be inhibited by blocking of both the processing of preproendothelin and the binding of endothelin to its receptors.

Endothelins were initially found to circulate in the plasma, but it is now clear that their major actions are mediated by paracrine signaling. ET-1 binds to two types of G protein–coupled receptor, ET_A and ET_B (Fig. 3-14). Regulatory ET_A receptors, which predominate in vascular smooth muscle and the heart, are coupled to $G_{\alpha q}$ that activates phospholipase C to form $InsP_3$ and DAG. These pathways allow ET_A receptors to mediate regulatory functional responses, notably vasoconstriction and increased myocardial contractility, as well as proliferative and proinflammatory responses. The counterregulatory ET_B receptors, which are found mainly in blood vessels, are coupled to $G_{\alpha i}$ that releases NO and prostacyclin. ET_B receptors are also linked to $G_{\alpha q}$, and so cause vasoconstriction.

Neuropeptide Y, Adrenomedullin, Calcitonin Gene-Related Peptide, Leptin, Ghrelin, and Other Peptides

Neuropeptide Y evokes a variety of functional and proliferative responses when it interacts with at least five different receptor subtypes, called Y_1 to Y_5, in the central nervous system and peripheral tissues. Neuropeptide Y has both regulatory and counterregulatory peripheral effects, notably a powerful centrally mediated regulatory response. In the heart, which has Y_1, Y_2, Y_3, and Y_5 receptors, neuropeptide Y

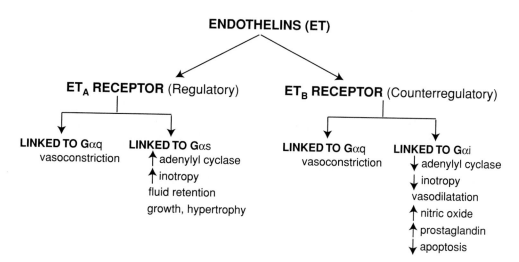

Figure 3-14: Endothelin receptors. ET_A and ET_B receptor subtypes have different affinities for various endothelin isoforms, activate different coupling proteins, and often generate opposing responses. ET_A, which activates $G_{\alpha s}$, usually exerts regulatory effects while most responses to ET_B, which activates $G_{\alpha i}$, are counterregulatory; however, both cause vasoconstriction by activating $G_{\alpha q}$. Modified from Katz AM (2006). *Physiology of the Heart.* 4th ed. Philadelphia, Lippincott Williams and Wilkins.

slows pacemaker activity by reducing the pacemaker current I_f, increases contractility by opening i_{CaL} channels, and modifies both excitability and contractility by reducing the transient outward current i_{to}; some of these responses are due to activation of $G_{\alpha i}$, others to activation of $G_{\alpha q}$. In blood vessels, neuropeptide Y interacts with α_1-adrenergic and angiotensin receptors to potentiate vasoconstriction and stimulate cardiac hypertrophy.

Adrenomedullin, produced in vascular cells, and *calcitonin gene-related* peptide (*CGRP*), a neuropeptide released from sensory nerve endings, are members of the *calcitonin* family of peptides that have counterregulatory effects. Both are powerful vasodilators, and adrenomedullin, whose levels are increased in heart failure, evokes natriuretic and diuretic responses. These peptides bind to a class of G protein–coupled receptors whose activity is regulated in part by *receptor activity modifying proteins* (RAMPs); the latter are single membrane-spanning proteins that regulate trafficking of the receptors to the cell surface. The vasodilator effects of these peptides are mediated by endothelium-dependent and endothelium-independent mechanisms that increase levels of cAMP, cGMP, and NO in responses that can be evoked by ischemia and hypoxia, mechanical stress, glucocorticoids, and cytokines. Adrenomedullin is also proinflammatory and can inhibit proliferative responses.

Ghrelin, an appetite-controlling peptide released from the stomach, binds to a G protein–coupled *growth hormone secretagogue receptor* that decreases sympathetic activity, causes endothelial cell-independent vasodilatation, and has anti-inflammatory effects. These counterregulatory responses explain evidence that ghrelin benefits patients with heart failure (Nagaya and Kanagawa, 2006). *Leptin,* a catabolic peptide related to the cytokines, is released from adipose and other tissues and binds to members of the family of gp130 cytokine receptors whose effects are mediated by the JAK/STAT pathway (see Chapter 4). The cardiovascular effects of leptin include vasoconstriction caused by increased sympathetic activity and endothelial cell-mediated vasodilatation; leptin also evokes a negative inotropic effect that is mediated in part by NO and, like other cytokines, has proinflammatory and proliferative effects. Other peptides, including *corticotrophin-releasing factor* and *α-melanocyte-releasing factor,* have effects similar to those of leptin.

Imidazoline Agonists

A central imidazoline-mediated signaling system with many similarities to the α_2-adrenergic system is activated by several organic molecules including a derivative of arginine called *agmatine* that, in the cardiovascular system, binds to I_1 and I_2 receptors. Counterregulatory effects of I_2 receptor activation resemble those of central α_2-adrenergic activation in that both reduce sympathetic outflow. The ability of α_2-receptor agonists to activate central imidazoline receptors highlights the parallels between these counterregulatory systems, but many details regarding the actions of these receptors are lacking.

Nitric Oxide (NO)

More than 25 years ago, Furchgott and Zawadzki (1980) discovered that the vasodilator responses to several extracellular messengers are not caused by a direct effect on vascular smooth muscle but instead depend on a vasodilator substance derived from endothelial cells. This physiological vasodilator, initially called *endothelial-derived relaxing factor* (*EDRF*), is now known to be *nitric oxide,* a free radical gas whose structural formula is $N=O$, or more simply *NO*. Nitric oxide is released from L-arginine by a family of enzymes called *nitric oxide synthase (NOS)*. Three NOS isoforms are found in the cardiovascular system: Two, *NOS1* (neuronal NOS) and *NOS3* (endothelial NOS), are constitutive enzymes that participate in physiological signaling; the third, *iNOS* (inducible NOS), generates large amounts of NO that act as toxic free radicals during inflammation. In contrast, NOS1 and NOS3, both of which are activated by calcium and calmodulin, play a protective role in failing hearts.

The responses to NO depend on its concentration; low concentrations generally act as autocrine and paracrine regulators, while high concentrations of this free radical gas are toxic and proinflammatory. Two mechanisms account for the effects of low NO concentrations in signal transduction: binding of the free radical to protein-bound metal molecules and nitrosylation of sulfhydryl groups (S-nitrosylation). The first mechanism allows NO to activate guanylyl cyclases, which are heme-containing enzymes that release cGMP; the latter, by activating protein kinase G, causes vasodilatation. Less is known about the effects of S-nitrosylation, which appear to be both regulatory and counterregulatory. In the cardiovascular system, NO causes vasodilatation when it binds to soluble guanylyl cyclases, a negative chronotropic effect that is probably also mediated by cGMP, and a bimodal effect on contractility that includes a positive inotropic response at lower NO concentrations and a negative inotropic response at higher concentrations. High concentrations of nitric oxide have proinflammatory effects that damage cells and, by modifying proliferative signaling, promote left ventricular remodeling (see Chapter 4).

Aldosterone

Aldosterone, a steroid hormone produced by the zone glomerulosa of the adrenal cortex, acts on the distal tubules to increase both sodium reabsorption and excretion of potassium and hydrogen ions by the renal tubules; the latter are important causes of the hypokalemia and metabolic alkalosis often seen in severe heart failure. Aldosterone secretion is regulated differently in normal individuals and patients with heart failure (Fig. 3-15). Low blood volume, an important physiological stimulus, causes the pituitary to release adrenocorticotropic hormone (ACTH) which, when it binds to adrenal cortical receptors, stimulates aldosterone synthesis; ACTH also regulates normal diurnal changes in aldosterone secretion. Hyperkalemia, which promotes aldosterone release, increases potassium excretion by the renal tubules. In heart failure, different mechanisms stimulate aldosterone release. When heart failure is severe, the most important stimulus is the high angiotensin II level, other mediators of the neurohumoral response, notably sympathetic stimulation, vasopressin, and endothelin, also play an important role in stimulating aldosterone secretion in milder, untreated, heart failure. Aldosterone binds to intracellular mineralocorticoid receptors that can also bind to glucocorticoids.

In addition to its role in regulating blood volume and the composition of the blood, aldosterone has important proliferative effects that, by stimulating fibrosis and mediating maladaptive proliferative responses in patients with heart failure, contribute to the poor prognosis in this syndrome (see Chapters 4, 6, 7).

Vasopressin

Vasopressin, the major regulator of water excretion by the kidneys, is an octapeptide that is synthesized in the supraoptic and paraventricular nuclei of the hypothalamus

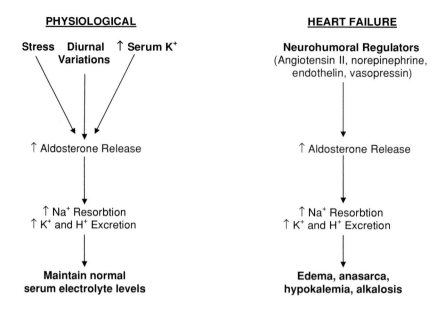

REGULATION OF ALDOSTERONE SECRETION

Figure 3-15: Aldosterone synthesis and release are regulated differently in normal individuals and patients with heart failure. In the former, this steroid serves mainly to maintain normal serum sodium and potassium levels, whereas in heart failure, aldosterone secretion is increased by mediators of the neurohumoral response and promotes fluid retention by the kidneys. Modified from Katz AM (2006). *Physiology of the Heart*. 4th ed. Philadelphia, Lippincott Williams and Wilkins.

and transported to the posterior pituitary where it is stored and released; the human isoform is often called arginine vasopressin because it contains an arginine in position 8. By increasing the water permeability of the renal collecting ducts, vasopressin increases water reabsorption and so inhibits diuresis, which explains why this peptide is also called antidiuretic hormone (ADH). The existence of different classes of vasopressin receptor allows this peptide to act as both a powerful vasoconstrictor and a vasodilator. Most important in cardiovascular regulation are V_{1a} receptors, which mediate the vasoconstrictor response, and V_2 receptors that mediate both water retention and vasodilatation (Fig. 3-16). V_{1a} receptors activate $G_{\alpha q}$ which increases cytosolic calcium, while V_2 receptors increase cAMP levels by activating

Figure 3-16: Vasopressin receptor subtypes. V_{1a} receptors mediate a regulatory vasoconstrictor response, while counterregulatory vasodilatation is mediated by V_2 receptors. Modified from Katz AM (2006). *Physiology of the Heart*. 4th ed. Philadelphia, Lippincott Williams and Wilkins.

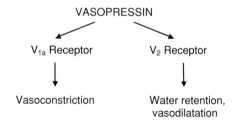

VASOPRESSIN RECEPTOR SUBTYPES

$G_{\alpha s}$ (see subsequent text). The dominant effect of vasopressin on blood vessels is V_{1a} receptor–mediated vasoconstriction; the vasodilator response initiated by V_2 receptor activation probably plays a role in local regulation of renal function.

The most important physiological stimulus of vasopressin secretion is increased plasma osmolarity, which, by stimulating osmoreceptors in the hypothalamus, releases this peptide from the posterior pituitary (Fig. 3-17). This response helps travelers survive a desert crossing because, when plasma osmolarity increases in a water-deprived individual, vasopressin increases water reabsorption by the kidneys and stimulates hypothalamic osmoreceptors that increase thirst, which drives the dehydrated traveler to seek water. The antidiuretic response and thirst are turned off when plasma osmolarity returns to physiological levels. Atrial stretch, which occurs in volume-overloaded patients, inhibits the release of vasopressin by reducing thirst

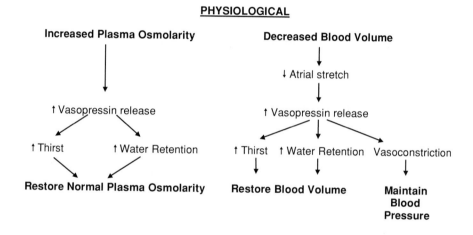

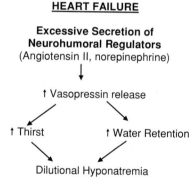

REGULATION OF VASOPRESSIN RELEASE

Figure 3-17: Regulation of vasopressin release. Under physiological conditions, vasopressin secreted in response to increased plasma osmolarity and decreased blood volume promotes water retention by the kidneys, increases thirst, and causes vasoconstriction. These adaptive responses reduce plasma osmolarity, help restore blood volume, and increase blood pressure. In heart failure, where vasopressin release comes under control of the neurohumoral response, inappropriate secretion of this peptide becomes maladaptive when increased thirst and water cause dilutional hyponatremia. Modified from Katz AM (2006). *Physiology of the Heart*. 4th ed. Philadelphia, Lippincott Williams and Wilkins.

and promoting water excretion; conversely, decreased atrial volume releases vasopressin, which by promoting water retention and thirst, helps restore blood volume. Because vasopressin is primarily a vasoconstrictor, this peptide also maintains blood pressure.

Unlike the adaptive responses to increased vasopressin levels, which help restore blood volume and maintain blood pressure in hemoconcentrated and volume-depleted individuals, vasopressin release becomes maladaptive in heart failure (see Chapters 6 and 7). This occurs because the previously described physiological control mechanisms are blunted in these patients, whose vasopressin levels are elevated by reduced arterial filling and a central effect of increased angiotensin II levels. Excessive vasopressin release can be seen in severe heart failure, especially after administration of diuretics (Francis et al., 1985), and can cause a life-threatening dilutional hyponatremia by increasing water reabsorption by the kidneys and thirst.

Natriuretic Peptides

The discovery that the heart is an endocrine organ as well as a pump came about when the density of granules long known to be present in atrial myocardial cells was found to change in response to altered water and electrolyte balance (DeBold, 1979). This observation led to the discovery that natriuretic peptides contained in these granules allow atrial dilatation to evoke a counterregulatory response that, by inducing a diuresis and dilating systemic arterioles, contributes to the defense against volume overload.

Natriuretic peptides are formed when a propeptide is hydrolyzed by a neutral endopeptidase that is similar to the angiotensin-converting enzyme. There are several different natriuretic peptides: *ANP*, which was originally discovered in the atria; *BNP*, first isolated from brain and present in small amounts in adult mammalian ventricles; and *CNP* which is synthesized in the endothelium. All bind to receptor guanyl cyclases that stimulate cGMP synthesis. In addition to its natriuretic and vasodilator actions, ANP has a weak negative inotropic effect.

The gene encoding ANP, which is normally expressed in fetal but not adult ventricles, is re-expressed in failing adult human ventricles; this is an example of the reversion of the overloaded heart to the fetal phenotype (see Chapter 4). BNP production by human ventricles is also increased when the ventricles become hypertrophied, so that measurements of blood BNP levels are useful for identifying patients with heart failure and characterizing the severity of the hemodynamic abnormality (see Chapters 6 and 7).

Prostaglandins and Related Compounds

Two classes of signaling molecules are formed from arachidonic acid, a 20-carbon polyunsaturated fatty acid; *cyclooxygenases (COX)* catalyze the formation of *prostaglandins,* and *lipoxygenases* the formation of *leukotrienes*. Both are short-lived lipid messengers that act locally, gaining access to their target cells by paracrine and autocrine pathways, where they participate in functional, proinflammatory, and proliferative responses. Physiologically active prostaglandins bind to G protein–coupled receptors; most important in cardiovascular regulation are the counter-regulatory mediators *prostacyclin (PGI$_2$)* and *prostaglandin E$_2$ (PGE$_2$)*, which relax vascular smooth muscle and inhibit platelet aggregation and adhesion, and *thromboxane (TxA₂)* a regulatory prostaglandin that causes vasoconstriction, platelet aggregation, and a proliferative response.

Two major COX isoforms synthesize prostaglandins: COX-1, a "housekeeping" protein, helps maintain homeostasis by synthesizing thromboxane, while COX-2 catalyzes production of PGI_2 and PGE_2. These responses are important in the pathophysiology of atherosclerosis, plaque rupture, and clotting, which can lead to myocardial infarction, the major cause of heart failure in developed countries (see Chapter 6).

INTERACTIONS AMONG MEDIATORS OF THE NEUROHUMORAL RESPONSE

The preceding discussion has focused on the individual responses and components of the neurohumoral response to underfilling the arteries. In heart failure, however, the individual components do not operate in isolation but instead interact with one another. The result is a highly organized response in which different components are activated to different extents and at different times as this syndrome progresses. Sympathetic activation is the first to appear in symptomatic heart failure, while the later—and more marked activation of the renin–angiotensin system—is due in part to diuretic therapy (Fig. 3.18). An overview of some of the interactions in the neurohumoral response, which is provided in Figure 3.19, is neither complete nor entirely accurate because the data on which this figure is based were obtained in various animal models as well as patients with heart failure. The importance of the figure, however, is not in the details, but instead in the picture it gives of how these interactions can fine-tune the response.

The neurohumoral response, as noted at the beginning of this chapter, compensates for what Bernard (1878) described as "perpetual changes of external conditions." The latter include short-term stresses, such as altered blood flow distribution caused by changes in body position, that initiate minor adjustments are analogous to the small changes in steering and acceleration that occur when one drives an automobile. In an emergency, such as flight from a predator or after hemorrhage, these mechanisms are amplified, like a driver who swerves to avoid an unexpected obstacle. The need to amplify these responses helps explain why sympathetic stimulation promotes the release of angiotensin II, aldosterone, endothelin, and vasopressin.

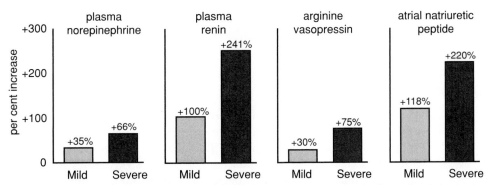

Figure 3.18: Neurohumoral activation in heart failure. Increases in plasma levels of norepinephrine, renin, vasopressin, and atrial natriuretic peptide in patients with early asymptomatic or mildly symptomatic left ventricular dysfunction (mild) and symptomatic heart failure (severe). Data from Francis et al. (1990).

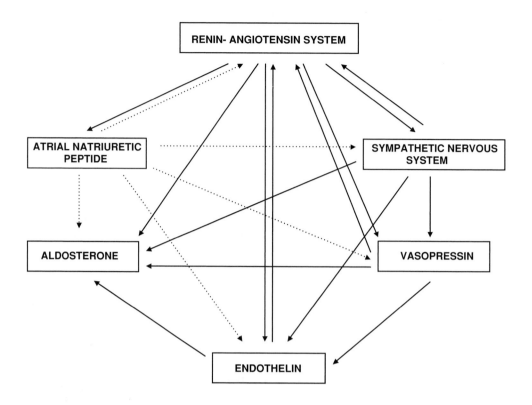

SOME INTERACTIONS AMONG NEUROHUMORAL MEDIATORS

Figure 3.19: Some interactions between key mediators of the neurohumoral response. Stimulation is depicted by *solid arrows*, inhibition by *dotted arrows*. Many interactions between mediators of the neuro-humoral response are omitted, and some interactions depicted here may not apply to all species or to all individuals in one species. The major purpose of this illustration is to provide an overview showing the complexity of these interactions. Modified from Katz AM (2000). *Heart Failure/Pathophysiology, Molecular Biology, and Clinical Management*. Philadelphia, Lippincott Williams and Wilkins.

Conversely, counterregulatory effects help keep these responses under control by preventing "runaway signaling." Understanding of these interactions is essential for physiologically guided therapy in patients with heart failure because most drugs used to treat heart failure modify the signaling systems involved in the neurohumoral response. We return to this subject in Chapter 7, when we discuss the iterative processes needed to optimize care of these patients.

THE "GRAND DESIGN"

The neurohumoral response in heart failure has been described as a "grand design [that maintains] intravascular volume and sufficient perfusion pressure to vital organs" (Francis and McDonald, 1995). This description, which echoes the evolutionary interpretation provided by Harris (1983), defines useful guidelines for understanding the interplay between activation of sympathetic outflow, the renin–angiotensin system, and secretion of vasopressin, the three major regulatory components that cause cardiac stimulation, fluid retention, and vasoconstriction in patients with heart failure. However, there are subtle but important differences between these components. Increased sympathetic outflow acts very rapidly on the heart and vasculature to maintain blood pressure and cardiac output, while slower activation of the renin–angiotensin system and vasopressin secretion has prominent, but delayed, effects that promote fluid retention by the kidneys.

The major regulatory effects of the many components of the neurohumoral response can be both beneficial and deleterious; furthermore, the short-term and long-term consequences generally oppose one another, depending on the specific pathophysiology that initiates these stimuli and the intensity of each response. The fact that the neurohumoral response in heart failure can be both maladaptive and adaptive—and at the same time—provides a challenge because therapy that alters one component of the response can be expected to perturb other components, both directly and indirectly. For these reasons, drugs and devices can have a variety of short-term and long-term consequences that often differ from one patient to another (see Chapters 6 and 7). Therapeutic plans must therefore be designed thoughtfully and monitored carefully in the individual patient to fine-tune the functional components of the neurohumoral response so as to maximize benefit and minimize harm. The complexity of this challenge is increased by the many proliferative components of this response, which are even more complex than those that mediate the functional responses described in this chapter.

BIBLIOGRAPHY

General

Alberts B, Johnson A, Lewis J, et al. *Molecular Biology of the Cell.* 4th ed. New York, Garland.

Braunwald E (2008). Biomarkers in heart failure. New Engl J Med 358:2148–2159.

Brutsaert DL (2003). Cardiac endothelial-myocardial signaling: its role in cardiac growth, contractile performance, and rhythmicity. Physiol Rev 83:59–115.

Devlin T (1997). *Textbook of Biochemistry.* New York, Wiley-Liss.

Francis GS (1990). Neuroendocrine activity in congestive heart failure. Am J Cardiol 66:33D–39D.

Francis GS, Goldsmith SR, Levine TB, et al. (1984). The neurohumoral axis in congestive heart failure. Ann Int Med 101:370–377.

Francis GS, Benedict C, Johnstone DE, et al. (1990). Comparison of neuroendocrine activation in patient with left ventricular dysfunction with and without congestive heart failure. A substudy of the studies of left ventricular dysfunction (SOLVD). Circulation 82: 1724–1729.

Francis GS, McDonald KM (1995). Neurohumoral Mechanisms in Heart Failure. In McCall D, Rahimtoola SH, eds. *Heart Failure.* 91–116. New York, Chapman & Hall.

Landry DW, Oliver JA (2001). The pathogenesis of vasodilatory shock. N Engl J Med 345:588–595.

Olson EN (2004) A decade of discoveries in cardiac biology. Nature Med 10:467–474.

Raine AEG (1992). Renal abnormalities in congestive heart failure. In: Fozzard H, Haber E, Katz AM, et al., eds. *The Heart and Cardiovascular System.* 2nd ed. 1379–1391. New York, Raven Press.

Schrier RW (1988). Pathogenesis of sodium and water retention in high-output and low-output cardiac failure, nephrotic syndrome, cirrhosis, and pregnancy. N Engl J Med 319:1127–1134.

Schrier RW (2006). Water and sodium retention in edematous disorders: role of vasopressin and aldosterone. Am J Med. 119(Suppl 1):S47–S53.

Wencker D (2007). Acute cardio-renal syndrome: Progression from congestive heart failure to congestive kidney failure. Curr Heart Fail Rep 4:134–138.

Extracellular Signaling Molecules; Receptors

Abassi Z, Karram T, Ellaham S, et al. (2004). Implications of the natriuretic peptide system in the pathogenesis of heart failure: diagnostic and therapeutic importance. Pharmacol Ther 102(3):223–241.

Ardaillou R, Chansel D (1997). Synthesis and effects of active fragments of angiotensin II. Kidney Int 52:1458–1468.

Attina T, Camidge R, Newby DE, et al. (2005). Endothelin antagonism in pulmonary hypertension, heart failure, and beyond. Heart 91:825–831.

Banfi C, Ferrario S, De Vincenti O, et al. (2005). P2 receptors in human heart: upregulation of P2X6 in patients undergoing heart transplantation, interaction with TNF alpha and potential role in myocardial cell death. J Mol Cell Cardiol 39:929–939.

Berk BC (1998). Angiotensin II receptors and angiotensin II-stimulated signal transduction. Heart Failure Rev 3:87–99.

Brain SD, Grant AD (2004). Vascular actions of calcitonin gene-related peptide and adrenomedullin. Physiol Rev 84:903–934.

Brodde OE, Bruck H, Leineweber K (2006). Cardiac adrenoceptors: physiological and pathophysiological relevance. J Pharmacol Sci 100:323–337.

Coleman RA, Smith WL, Naruyima S (1994). International Union of Pharmacology Classification of prostanoid receptors: properties, distribution, and structure of the receptors and their subtypes. Pharmacol Rev 46:205–229.

Danilczyk U, Penninger JM (2006). Angiotensin-converting enzyme II in the heart and the kidney. Circ Res 98;463–471.

Diaz-Cabiale Z, Parrado C, Rivera A, et al. (2006). Galanin-neuropeptide Y (NPY) interactions in central cardiovascular control: involvement of the NPY Y receptor subtype. Eur J Neurosci 24:499–508.

Dogné J-M, Hanson J, Pratico D (2005). Thromboxane, prostacyclin and isoprostanes: therapeutic targets in atherosclerosis. Trends Pharm Sci 26:639–644.

Eto T, Kato J, Kitamura K (2003). Regulation of production and secretion of adrenomedullin in the cardiovascular system. Regul Pept 112:61–69.

Fleming I (2006). Signaling by the angiotensin-converting enzyme. Circ Res 98:887–896.

Gavras H (1990). Pressor systems in hypertension and congestive heart failure. Role of vasopressin. Hypertension 16:587–593.

Goldsmith SR, Gheorghiade M (2005). Vasopressin antagonism in heart failure. J Am Coll Cardiol 46:1785–1791.

Kedzierski RM, Yanagisawa M (2001). Endothelin system: the double-edged sword in health and disease. Ann Rev Pharmacol Toxicol 41:851–876.

Konstam MA (2007). Natriuretic peptides and cardiovascular events. JAMA 197:212–214.

Korbonits M, Goldstone AP, Gueorguiev M, et al. (2001). Ghrelin—a hormone with multiple functions. Frontiers Neuroendocrinol 25:27–68.

Kuwasako K, Cao YN, Nagoshi Y, et al. (2004). Adrenomedullin receptors: pharmacological features and possible pathophysiological roles. Peptides 11:2003–2012.

Leeb-Lundberg LM (2004). Bradykinin specificity and signaling at GPR100 and B2 kinin receptors. Br J Pharmacol 143:931–932.

Levin ER (1996). Endothelins. N Engl J Med 333:356–362.

Levin ER, Gardner DG, Samson WK (1998). Natriuretic peptides. N Engl J Med 339:321–328.

Luo JD, Zhang GS, Chen MS (2005). Leptin and cardiovascular diseases. Drug News Perspect 18:427–431.

Marasciulo FL, Montagnani M, Potenza MA (2006). Endothelin-1: the yin and yang on vascular function. Curr Med Chem 13:1655–1665.

Marcondes S, Antunes E (2005). The plasma and tissue kininogen-kallikrein-kinin system: role in the cardiovascular system. Curr Med Chem Cardiovasc Hematol Agents 3:33–44.

Martin P, Mehr AP, Kreutz R (2006). Physiology of local renin-angiotensin systems. Physiol Rev 86:747–803.

Massion PB, Feron O, Dessy C, et al. (2003). Nitric oxide and cardiac function ten years after, and continuing. Circ Res 93:388–398.

Matsumura K, Tsuchihashi T, Fujii K, et al. (2003). Neural regulation of blood pressure by leptins and the related peptides. Regul Pept 114:79–86.

Mizutani S, Ishii M, Hattori A, et al. (2008). New insights into the importance of amino peptidase A in hypertension. Heart Fail Rev 13:273–284.

Mombouli JV, Vanhoutte PM (1992). Heterogeneity of endothelium-dependent vasodilator effects of angiotensin-converting enzyme inhibitors: role of bradykinin generation during ACE inhibition. J Cardiovasc Pharmacol 20(Suppl 9):S974–S982.

Moreau ME, Garbacki N, Molinaro G, et al. (2005). The kallikrein-kinin system: current and future pharmacological targets. J Pharmacol Sci 99:6–38.

Nagaya N, Uematsu M, Kojima M, et al. (2001). Chronic administration of ghrelin improves left ventricular dysfunction and attenuates development of cardiac cachexia in rats with heart failure. Circulation 104:1430–1435.

Protas L, Qu J, Robinson RB (2003). Neuropeptide Y: neurotransmitter or trophic factor in the heart. News Physiol Sci 18:181–185.

Raasch W, Schäfer, Chun J, et al. (2001). Biological significance of agmatine, an endogenous ligand at imidazoline binding sites. Br J Pharmacol 133:755–780.

Remme WJ (2001). Dopaminergic agents in heart failure: rebirth of an old concept. Cardiovasc Drugs Therap 15:107–109.

Ruiz-Ortega M, Lorenzo O, Ruperez M, et al. (2001). Role of the renin-angiotensin system in vascular diseases: expanding the field. Hypertension 38:1382–1387.

Schulze PC, Kratzsch J (2005). Leptin as a new diagnostic tool in chronic heart failure. Clin Chim Acta 362:1–11.

Tang C-M, Insell PA (2004). GPCR expression in the heart. "New" receptors in myocytes and fibroblasts. Trends Cardiovasc Med 14:94–99.

Thibonnier M (2003). Vasopressin receptor agonists in heart failure. Curr Opin Pharmacol 3:683–687.

Tsuruda T, Burnett JC Jr (2002). Adrenomedullin. An autocrine/paracrine factor for cardiorenal protection. Circ Res 90:625–627.

Urata H, Arakawa K (1998). Angiotensin II-forming systems in cardiovascular diseases. Heart Failure Rev 3:119–124.

Villarreal F, Zimmermann S, Makhsudova L, et al. (2003). Modulation of cardiac remodeling by adenosine: in vitro and in vivo effects. Mol Cell Biochem 251:17–26.

Warner TD, Mitchell JA (2004). Cyclooxygenases: new forms, new inhibitors, and lessons from the clinic. FASEB J 18:790–804.

Watanabe T, Barker TA, Berk BC (2005). Angiotensin II and the endothelium: diverse signals and effects. Hypertension 45:163–169.

Wright D H, Abran D, Bhattacharya M, et al. (2001). Prostanoid receptors: ontogeny and implications in vascular physiology. Am J Physiol Regul Integr Comp Physiol 281:R1343–R1360.

Xiao R-P, Zhu W, Zheng M, et al. (2004). Subtype-specific β-adrenoceptor signaling pathways in the heart and their potential clinical implications. Trends Phamacol Sci 25:358–365.

Xiao R-P, Zhu W, Zheng M, et al. (2006) Subtype-specific α_1- and β-adrenoceptor signaling in the heart. Trends Pharmacol Sci 330–337.

Yaar R, Jones MR, Chen J-F, et al. (2005). Animal models for the study of adenosine receptor function. J Cell Phyisol 202:9–29.

Zimmet JM, Hare JM (2006). Nitroso-redox interactions in the cardiovascular system. Circulation 114:1531–1544.

Intracellular Signaling Pathways

Fitzpatrick DA, O'Halloran DM, Burnell AM (2006). Multiple lineage specific expansions within the guanylyl cyclase gene family. BMC Evol Biol 6:26.

Hermans E (2003). Biochemical and pharmacological control of the multiplicity of coupling at G-protein–coupled receptors. Pharmacol Ther 99:25–44.

Lefkowitz RJ, Pitcher J, Krueger K, et al. (1997). Mechanisms of β-adrenergic receptor desensitization and resensitization. Adv Pharmacol 42:416–420.

REFERENCES

Ahlquist PR (1948). A study of the adrenotropic receptors. Am J Physiol 153:586–600.

Bayliss W, Starling E (1902). The mechanism of pancreatic secretion. J. Physiol (London) 28:325–352.

Bernard C (1878). *Leçons sur les phénomènes de la vie communs aux animaux et aux vegetaux*. Paris, Ballièe.

Binkley PF, Nunziata E, Nelson SD, et al. (1991). Parasympathetic withdrawal is an integral component of autonomic imbalance in congestive heart failure: demonstration in human subjects and verification in a paced canine model of ventricular failure. J Am Coll Cardiol 18:464–472.

Braun-Menendez E, Page IH (1958). Suggested revision of nomenclature—angiotensin. Science 127:242.

Braun-Menendez E, Fasciolo E, Leloir JC, et al. (1940). The substance causing renal hypertension. J Physiol (Lond) 98:283–298.

Cannon WB (1932). *The Wisdom of the Body*. New York, WW Norton.

Clapham DE, Neer EJ (1997). G protein βγ subunits. Ann Rev Pharmacol 37:167–203.

DeBold AJ (1979) Heart atria granularity. Effects of changes in water-electrolyte balance. Proc Soc Exp Biol Med 161:508–511.

Eichhorn EJ (1999). Beta-blocker withdrawal: the song of Orpheus. Am Heart J 138:387–389.

Elliott TR (1905). The action of adrenalin. J Physiol (London) 32:401–467.

Francis GS, Siegel R, Goldsmith SR, et al. (1985). Acute vasoconstrictor response to furosemide in patients with chronic congestive heart failure. Ann Int Med 103:1–6.

Francis GS, Benedict C, Johnstone DE, et al. for the SOLVD Investigators (1990). Comparison of neuroendocrine activation in patients with left ventricular dysfunction with and without congestive heart failure. Circulation 82:1724–1729.

Furchgott RF, Zawadzki JV (1980). The obligatory role of endothelial cells in the relaxation of arterial smooth muscle by acetylcholine. Nature 288:373–376.

Harris P (1983). Evolution and the cardiac patient. Cardiovasc Res 17:313–319, 373–378, 437–445.

Laugwitz K-L, Allgeier A, Offermanns S, et al. (1996). The human thyrotropin receptor: a heptahelical receptor capable of stimulating members of all four G-protein families. Proc Acad Sci (USA) 93:116–120.

Le Guludec D, Cohen-Solal A, Delforge J, et al. (1997). Increased myocardial muscarinic receptor density in idiopathic dilated cardiomyopathy. An in vivo PET study. Circulation 96:3416–3422.

Loewi O (1921). Über humorale übertragbarkeit der Herznervenwirkung. I. Mitteilung. Pflügers Arch ges Physiol 189:239–242.

Luttrell LM (2006). Transmembrane signaling by G protein-coupled receptors. Methods Mol Biol 332:3–49.

Luttrell LM, Ferguson SSG, Daaka Y, et al. (1999). β-arrestin-dependent formation of β2 adrenergic receptor-src protein kinase complexes. Science 283:655–661.

Nagaya N, Kanagawa K (2006). Therapeutic potential of ghrelin in the treatment of heart failure. Drugs 66:439–448.

Nolan J, Flapan AD, Capewell S, et al. (1992). Decreased cardiac parasympathetic activity in chronic heart failure and its relation to left ventricular function. Br Heart J 67:482–485.

Oliver G, Schäfer EA (1895). The physiological effects of extracts of the suprarenal capsules. J Physiol (London) 18:230–276.

Page IH, Helmer OM (1940). A crystalline pressor substance (angiotonin) resulting from the reaction between renin and renin activator. J Exp Med 71:29–42.

Vatner DE, Sato N, Galper JB, et al. (1996). Physiological and biochemical evidence for coordinate increases in muscarinic receptors and Gi during pacing-induced heart failure. Circulation 96:102–107.

Wang Z, Shi H, Wang H (2004). Functional M3 muscarinic acetylcholine receptors in mammalian hearts. Br J Pharmacol 142:395–408.

Warren JV, Stead EA Jr (1944). Fluid dynamics in chronic congestive failure. Arch Int Med 73:138–144.

CHAPTER 4

The Hypertrophic Response in Heart Failure: Proliferative Signaling

Arnold M. Katz • Marvin A. Konstam

In virtually every patient with heart failure, the body attempts to compensate for the reduced cardiac function using responses that, while adaptive in the short term, eventually harm both the heart and the patient. This is true for the functional responses described in Chapter 3 and the proliferative responses, discussed in subsequent text, that regulate the size, shape, and composition of hypertrophied and failing hearts. As modern treatment of heart failure generally modifies all of these responses, understanding of the underlying mechanisms has become essential in efforts to optimize the long-term management of this syndrome.

FUNCTIONAL VERSUS PROLIFERATIVE SIGNALING

Functional and proliferative responses were once believed to be controlled by independently regulated, nonoverlapping signaling pathways (Fig. 4-1). However, as described in an elegant editorial by H.R. Bourne (1995), instead of "a few discrete clans" of signaling molecules organized in distinct functional and proliferative pathways, control of these two types of response has emerged as a series of "wheels within wheels! . . . bustling communication networks within and between clans of signaling proteins within the average cell." For example, the G protein–coupled receptors initially identified as regulating cell function also modify growth responses once thought to be under the exclusive control of enzyme-linked tyrosine kinase receptors, and the tyrosine kinase receptors initially viewed as mediating only growth responses influence such functional variables as myocardial contractility and vascular tone. The clinical importance of this cross talk is enormous; it helps explain why direct-acting vasodilators, which improve symptoms over the short term when decreasing peripheral vascular resistance unloads the heart, worsen long-term outcome in heart failure by promoting maladaptive cardiac hypertrophy. Conversely, β-adrenergic blockers, whose ability to reduce contractility has obvious short-term deleterious effects on pump function, improve long-term survival by inhibiting progressive left ventricular dilatation (remodeling). In accord with the principle that what is obvious is not always important, and what is important is not always obvious, it is now clear that formerly overlooked effects of the neurohumoral response and therapy on cell growth are often of greater clinical significance than the more obvious effects on hemodynamics described in Chapter 3.

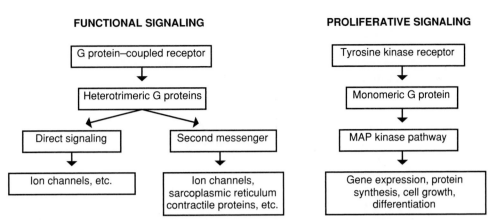

FUNCTIONAL SIGNALING

G protein–coupled receptor
↓
Heterotrimeric G proteins
↙ ↘
Direct signaling | Second messenger
↓ ↓
Ion channels, etc. | Ion channels, sarcoplasmic reticulum contractile proteins, etc.

PROLIFERATIVE SIGNALING

Tyrosine kinase receptor
↓
Monomeric G protein
↓
MAP kinase pathway
↓
Gene expression, protein synthesis, cell growth, differentiation

Figure 4-1: Early view of cell signaling. Two independent systems were once believed to mediate functional and proliferative responses. G protein–coupled receptors, which are linked to heterotrimeric G proteins, were initially discovered as regulators of functional responses, while tyrosine kinase receptors, which are coupled to monomeric GTP-binding proteins, were found to regulate proliferative responses. It is now clear, however, that cross-overs between these systems allow either to initiate both functional and proliferative responses. Modified from Katz AM (2000). *Heart Failure/Pathophysiology, Molecular Biology, and Clinical Management.* Philadelphia, Lippincott Williams and Wilkins.

GENE EXPRESSION

Changes in gene expression brought about by proliferative signaling play an important adaptive role in heart failure, where increased ventricular wall thickness in concentric hypertrophy can normalize wall stress. However, other features of the hypertrophic response can worsen prognosis, for example by causing progressive ventricular dilatation, myocardial cell death, and electrical remodeling that increases arrhythmogenic currents across the plasma membrane in failing hearts. Abnormal proliferative signaling also contributes to the endothelial damage and coronary atherosclerosis that lead to myocardial infarction, the major cause of heart failure in developed countries.

Key to most proliferative responses are changes in the expression of the genes that determine cell composition and structure (Table 4-1). In normal hearts, most of these genes are down-regulated or dormant unless expression of genomic DNA is selectively turned on by transcription factors. Once activated, these genes become a template for the transcription of *messenger RNA (mRNA)* that is transported from the nucleus to the cytosol where it serves as a template for protein synthesis. The mechanisms that control gene expression, protein synthesis, and cell structure and composition are among the most highly regulated of all biological functions.

Promoter, Enhancer, and Repressor DNA Sequences

In addition to the nucleotide sequences that encode proteins, genomic DNA contains sequences that turn genes on and off and control the rate at which genes are transcribed. These regulatory sequences include *promoter* regions located at the 5' end of the gene, upstream from the *start site* where DNA transcription begins, and *enhancer* and *repressor* regions that increase and decrease the rate of gene expression, respectively (Fig. 4-2). One of the most important promoter regions is the *TATA box*, so named because its DNA sequence includes thymidine (T) and adenine (A) in the sequence TATA, which is a weak point in the structure of double-stranded DNA

TABLE 4-1

Regulation of Gene Expression and Protein Composition in the Heart

Protein Synthesis
  DNA transcription
    Selection of the DNA sequence to be read
    Transcription of the selected DNA sequence into a complementary RNA sequence
  RNA processing (alternative splicing)
    Selection and arrangement of exons to be spliced to form messenger RNA (mRNA)
  RNA export
    Control of mRNA transport from the nucleus to the cytoplasm
  Translation
    Control of mRNA translation into protein
  RNA degradation
    Control of mRNA breakdown, which turns off protein synthesis
  Epigenetic mechanisms

Protein Activation and Inactivation (posttranslational control)
    Modification of proteins that increase or decrease their biological activity,
      e.g.,phosphorylation, acetylation
    Protein interactions with other cell components, e.g., myosin-actin interactions,
      troponin C binding to calcium

Protein Breakdown
    Selection and control of proteolysis

where the helix is most easily unwound into the separate single strands used for copying. Basic proteins, called *histones*, that bind to genomic DNA in chromatin also play an important role in regulating gene expression (see subsequent text).

Gene expression is initiated when a transcription factor forms a multiprotein aggregate with other regulatory proteins and an enzyme called *RNA polymerase*. When these complexes bind to the promoter region of a specific gene, the downstream base pair sequence becomes a template for the synthesis of a primary RNA transcript that contains the information encoded in the gene (Fig. 4-2). This information is then transcribed in the messenger RNA that is transported to the cytosol, where it determines the amino acid sequence of a newly synthesized protein.

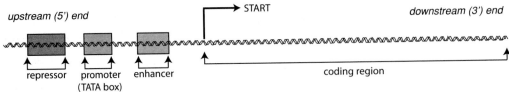

Figure 4-2: Gene transcription. Coding regions of genomic DNA that lie downstream (toward the 3′ end of the DNA sequence) from a start sequence provide templates for the synthesis of the messenger RNA that encodes protein structure. Transcription factors activate gene transcription when they bind to a regulatory sequence located at the 5′-end of the gene, called a *promoter*, such as the *TATA box* that is made up of thymidine (T) and adenine (A) residues. Transcription can be activated by *enhancers* and inhibited by *repressors* that are found upstream from the start site, as shown in the figure, and elsewhere along the gene. From Katz AM (2006). *Physiology of the Heart*. 4th ed. Philadelphia, Lippincott Williams and Wilkins.

RNA Processing and Alternative Splicing

Not all of the RNA encoded by genomic DNA serves as a template for protein synthesis. Some segments of the primary transcript, called *introns*, are eliminated from mRNA before the remaining nucleotide sequences, called *exons*, are assembled into the template that guides protein synthesis (Fig. 4-3). The ability of cells to eliminate introns and rearrange selected exons, called *alternative splicing*, is an important mechanism for providing diversity in proliferative signaling. Figure 4-3 shows how a gene containing three exons can encode four different mRNAs; this illustration is by no means complete as the three exons can be used in additional combinations. Some genes contain dozens of exons, so that alternative splicing can allow many protein isoforms to be generated by a single DNA sequence.

Oncogenes and Protooncogenes

Genes whose activation causes uncontrolled cell growth and proliferation are called *oncogenes*, while *protooncogenes* are normal cellular genes that, when mutated, encode proteins that can induce malignant transformation. The term protooncogene

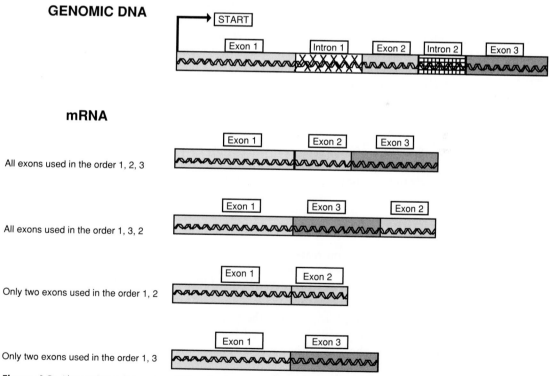

Figure 4-3: Alternative splicing. In addition to the *exons* whose sequence encodes proteins, primary RNA transcripts often include sequences, called *introns*, that are removed before synthesis of messenger RNA (mRNA). Selection and rearrangement of exons after elimination of introns allows a single gene to encode several different mRNAs. The four mRNAs derived from the primary transcript of the three exons shown in this figure are a few of the possible products of alternative splicing that can combine one, two, or all three exons, which can be used in various combinations and sequences. Modified from Katz AM (2006). *Physiology of the Heart*. 4th ed. Philadelphia, Lippincott Williams and Wilkins.

is often used to describe genes, such as *c-myc, c-fos*, and *c-jun*, that are activated rapidly in response to stress (see subsequent text). Oncogenes related to these normal cell regulators are found in some viruses; in the examples just provided, these are called *v-myc, v-fos*, and *v-jun*. Protooncogenes that can induce malignant transformation include many of the genes that encode the signaling molecules discussed in this chapter.

Transcription Factors

Key to proliferative signaling are transcription factors that regulate gene expression by initiating the transcription of specific DNA sequences. Most transcription factors are proteins that bind to promoter regions of the genomic DNA, accelerate gene expression by binding to an enhancer sequence, or modify gene transcription by binding to a repressor sequence (see Fig. 4-2). The ability of transcription factors to select a gene and regulate its expression is made possible by structural motifs that provide the tight "fit" needed to activate a specific target DNA sequence. Most transcription factors operate as homodimers or heterodimers in *helix-turn-helix, helix-loop-helix, leucine zipper*, and *zinc finger* structures (Fig. 4-4), where each subunit binds to one of the two strands of genomic DNA. The subunits in these dimers are held together by noncovalent linkages that include hydrophobic interactions between leucine residues and divalent zinc atoms. Some genes are regulated by steroid hormones that cross the plasma membrane and bind to intracellular *hormone receptor elements* (*HREs*) that enter the nucleus where they regulate gene expression. Cooperative interactions between genes and transcription factors make it possible for a single transcription factor to generate a coordinated growth response by interacting sequentially with several functionally related genes, and for regulatory regions of some genes to modify the actions of a transcription factor.

Transcription factors can be activated in many ways. Most important is *post-translational modification* of an inactive protein, such as by phosphorylation or dephosphorylation. Transcription factor activity can also be regulated when modification of a proliferative signaling cascade activates or inhibits the rate of its synthesis or releases the active protein from an inactive complex.

THE CELL CYCLE

Perhaps the most important reason for the maladaptive consequences of proliferative stimulation of the heart is that the adult human heart is composed of terminally differentiated cardiac myocytes that have little ability to divide. Although these cells have a limited capacity for mitosis when subjected to severe stress, these attempts to proliferate are abortive; for example, the new cells do not form functional connections with neighboring cells but instead become encased in fibrous tissue (Ring, 1950). Because this abortive mitotic response does not regenerate significant amounts of functioning heart muscle (Rumyantsev, 1977), the adult human heart cannot adapt to a sustained overload by increasing cell number (hyperplasia); instead, cardiac myocytes can only become larger (hypertrophy). This response is well suited for the heart, which cannot suspend its pumping to generate new myocytes; as noted by Goss (1966), so that "by giving up the potential for hyperplasia in favor of the necessity for constant function, [the heart has] adapted a strategy that enables [it] to become hypertrophic to a limited extent while doing [its jobs] efficiently". There is, however,

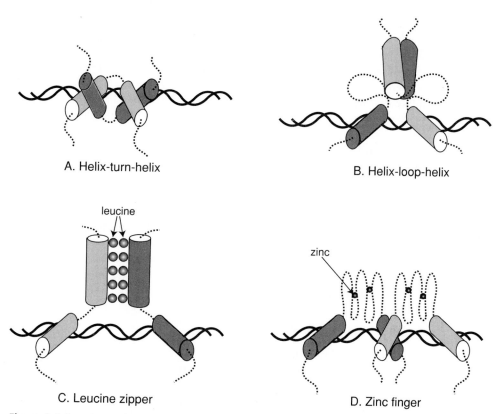

A. Helix-turn-helix

B. Helix-loop-helix

leucine

C. Leucine zipper

zinc

D. Zinc finger

Figure 4-4: Four types of transcription factor. These regulators, which function as dimers, include *helix-turn-helix* and *helix-loop-helix* structures, *leucine zipper* structures in which the two subunits are linked by hydrophobic forces between leucine residues, and *zinc finger* structures where zinc atoms stabilize the structure of the transcription factor dimers. Cylinders represent α-helices. From Katz AM (2006). *Physiology of the Heart*. 4th ed. Philadelphia, Lippincott Williams and Wilkins.

a price: that hypertrophy of these terminally differentiated cells in response to overload and injury, although able to normalize wall stress, is accompanied by molecular changes that shorten myocyte survival.

Terminally differentiated cells, by definition, cannot undergo mitosis because they have withdrawn from the *cell cycle*. The latter is a highly regulated process in which cell enlargement, DNA replication, and nuclear division (*karyokinesis*) are followed by cell division (*cytokinesis*) that produces two daughter cells, each of which contains a set of genes copied from the mother cell. The cell cycle plays a critical role in the survival of *prokaryotes* (the name comes from the absence of a formed nucleus) that lack the internal membrane structures needed to control their *milieu intèrieur*; rapid cell division allows these primitive life forms to survive environmental change by literally growing their way out of trouble. Proliferation of these cells is facilitated by the circular structure of most prokaryotic DNA, which maintains a continually active cell cycle that allows these cells to replicate without pause. Because each prokaryote represents an independent entity with its own complement of genes, when a population of these organisms encounters a major environmental change, selection of cells whose phenotype is best able to withstand the new stress helps some of the population to survive. Even when a vast majority of the cells die, rapid cell cycling allows a few survivors to multiply and fill the new environment. This is evident in bacteria, modern prokaryotes that can divide as rapidly as every 20 minutes, which allows a single individual to generate >4 billion descendants—almost the human population of this planet—within 10 hours.

Cell cycling and DNA replication in eukaryotes (*eukaryote* = discrete nucleus), unlike that in prokaryotes, occurs in spurts; the pauses between mitotic events allow the newly formed daughter cells to carry out their biological functions and rebuild and reorganize their internal structure. The rate of cell cycling in eukaryotic cells varies greatly; pauses average 10 to 20 hours, but can be much longer. In terminally differentiated cells, like adult human cardiac myocytes, the pause lasts forever.

Nuclear division and cell division in cells that undergo mitosis are usually tightly coordinated, so that the cell cycle generates daughter cells that contain a single nucleus. In some cells, however, karyokinesis can occur without cytokinesis, so that the cell cycle generates a *multinucleate* cell. DNA replication without either cytokinesis or karyokinesis generates *polyploid* cells whose nuclei contain more than two sets of chromosomes. In the normal adult human heart, ~ 25% of cardiac myocytes are diploid, and more than half are tetraploid; the degree of ploidy increases with aging and when the heart hypertrophies (Rumyantsev, 1977).

Phases of the Cell Cycle

The cell cycle can be divided into four phases; in two, the cycle is active, while the other two are relatively quiescent. The active phases are the *S phase*, characterized by DNA replication, and the *M phase*, during which the cell divides (Fig. 4-5). These active phases are separated by periods during which processes related to cell division are temporarily suspended to allow cells to enlarge and carry out their physiological functions; these are the G_1 *phase*, between M and S, and the G_2 *phase* between S and M. The G_1 *restriction point*, which occurs late in G_1, represents a major pause in cell cycling (Pardee, 1989). Once this restriction point is passed the cell is committed to dividing, which means that the cell cycle, while still governed by *internal* regulatory mechanisms, has become independent of *external* stimuli.

In terminally differentiated cardiac myocytes, the cells are in a G_1 phase that resists stimuli that would otherwise activate cell cycling. This quiescent state, called G_0 in this text, can be viewed as a detour out of the cell cycle. (The term G_0 is not strictly correct in describing this state in cardiac myocytes because it was initially coined to describe cell cycle arrest associated with low metabolic activity in serum-depleted cultured cells. A more correct characterization of adult cardiac myocytes might be permanent arrest in the G_1 phase, but with apologies to experts, this text uses the simpler term G_0.)

Adult cardiac myocytes do not reenter the cell cycle even when they are exposed to stimuli that would activate mitosis in less differentiated cells; instead, these stimuli can only cause the myocytes to enlarge (hypertrophy). When they are severely stressed, cardiac myocytes make abortive attempts to reverse the transition from G_1 to G_0 so as to reenter the cell cycle, but these efforts turn out badly. In failing hearts, these efforts have deleterious consequences that contribute to a maladaptive growth response that can hasten progression of the hemodynamic disorder, accelerate cell death, and worsen prognosis.

Cyclins, CDK, and Related Proteins

Factors that regulate transitions both within and between the phases of the cell cycle include *cyclin-dependent protein kinases* (CDK) and *cyclins* (Fig. 4-6); the former are serine/threonine kinases, while cyclins regulate CDK activity. Cyclins and CDK

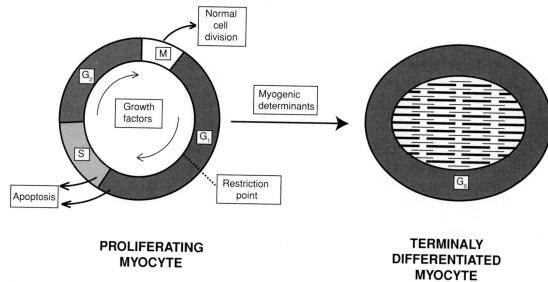

PROLIFERATING MYOCYTE

TERMINALY DIFFERENTIATED MYOCYTE

Figure 4-5: Schematic depiction of the cell cycle and transition to a terminally differentiated cardiac myocyte. **Left:** The cell cycle, seen in the proliferating cells of the embryonic heart, proceeds in a counterclockwise direction. The first gap phase, G_1, occurs after mitosis (M). Cells in the G_1 phase can enlarge and carry out their physiological functions, but from the standpoint of the cell cycle they remain quiescent. Cells in the G_1 phase become committed to the cell cycle when they pass a G_1 restriction point, after which the cell cycle proceeds through a phase of DNA synthesis (S), a second gap phase (G_2), and cell division (M). Susceptibility to programmed cell death (apoptosis) is greatest late in the G_1 phase and during the S phase. **Right:** Myogenic determinants cause cardiac myocytes to withdraw from the cell cycle and enter a prolonged quiescent phase, called G_0, in which they become terminally differentiated, adult myocytes. Modified from Katz AM (2006). *Physiology of the Heart.* 4th ed. Philadelphia, Lippincott Williams and Wilkins.

isoforms form matched pairs in which a specific CDK regulates a given cyclin; cyclin/CDK pairs can stimulate cell growth in G_1, promote DNA replication in S, induce cell division in M, and stimulate transitions from G_2 to M and from G_1 to S. Some cyclin/CDK pairs regulate the activity of transcription factors, such as the myogenic determinants that regulate cell differentiation.

CDKs are enzymatically inactive unless bound to an appropriate cyclin, but cyclins generally cause only partial activation of their corresponding CDKs. Complete activation requires the participation of additional protein kinases, called *CDK-activating kinases (CAK)*, that phosphorylate the cyclin/CDK complexes (Fig. 4-6). Conversely *cyclin-dependent kinase inhibitors (CDKIs)* slow the cell cycle by inhibiting active cyclin/CDK pairs. Additional regulatory proteins, not shown in Figure 4-6, include phosphatases that inhibit cell cycling by dephosphorylating CDKs, and protein kinases that catalyze inhibitory phosphorylations that inactivate cyclin/CDK pairs.

Tumor Suppressor Proteins and E2F

Proliferative signaling is regulated by proteins, whose prototype is the *retinoblastoma protein (pRb)*, that regulate differentiation, DNA repair, and apoptosis; in the heart, the most important member of this family is *p107*. These proteins are often called *tumor suppressor proteins* because they serve as substrates for phosphorylations that inhibit tumor formation; retinal cells that lack both copies of the retinoblastoma gene undergo malignant transformation and can form metastasizing tumors. Tumor suppressor proteins are sometimes called "pocket proteins" because their structure

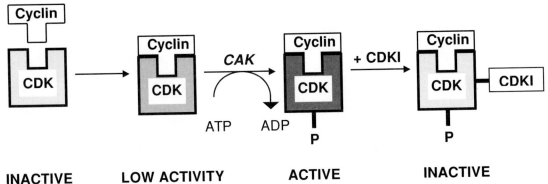

Figure 4-6: Regulation of the cell cycle. Protein kinases called CDK (cyclin-dependent protein kinases) which are inactive in their basal state, are partially activated when they interact with specific cyclins to form cyclin/CDK pairs. Full activation of CDK requires phosphorylation of the cyclin-bound CDKs by another class of protein kinases called CAK (CDK-activating kinases). Inactivators of the phosphorylated cyclin/CDK pairs include CDKIs (cyclin-dependent kinase inhibitors). Additional regulation (not shown) is effected by phosphatases that dephosphorylate the CDKs, and additional proteins. Modified from Katz AM (2006). *Physiology of the Heart.* 4th ed. Philadelphia, Lippincott Williams and Wilkins.

includes a pocket that reversibly binds transcription factors (Fig. 4-7). In the inhibitory (hypophosphorylated) state, where few serine and threonine residues are phosphorylated, these proteins bind and inactivate transcription factors such as E2F (see subsequent text). Serine and threonine phosphorylations convert the tumor suppressor proteins to the activated growth-permissive (hyperphosphorylated) state by "kicking" E2F out of the pocket. The pocket proteins provide a convergence point at which CDK/cyclin pairs, G protein–coupled receptors, tyrosine kinase receptors, steroid receptors, and cytoskeletal proteins regulate proliferative signaling.

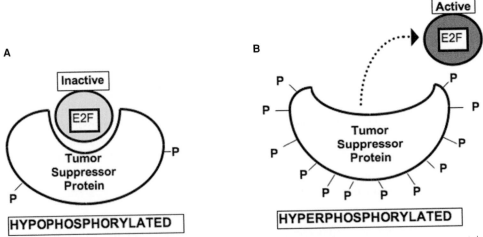

Figure 4-7: Tumor suppressor proteins. **A:** In the hypophosphorylated state, tumor suppressor proteins bind and inactivate transcription factors such as E2F. **B:** Phosphorylation of serine and threonine residues in the tumor suppressor protein reduces their affinity for these transcription factors, which can be released in an active form that regulates gene expression and protein synthesis. Modified from Katz AM (2006). *Physiology of the Heart.* 4th ed. Philadelphia, Lippincott Williams and Wilkins.

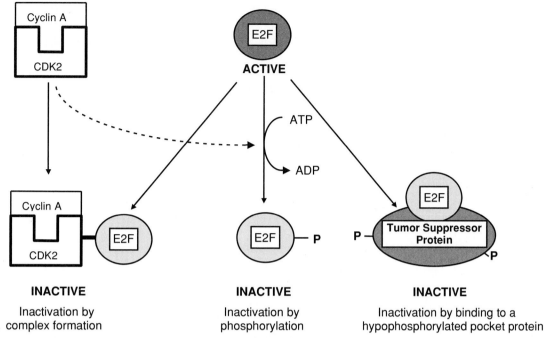

Figure 4-8: Inactivation of E2F. This transcription factor can be inactivated when it forms a complex with the cyclin/CDK pair cyclin A/CDK2 (**left**), by CDK-catalyzed phosphorylation (**center**), and by binding by a hypophosphorylated pocket protein (**right**). Modified from Katz AM (2006). *Physiology of the Heart.* 4th ed. Philadelphia, Lippincott Williams and Wilkins.

The cell cycle is activated when *E2F* is released from hyperphosphorylated tumor suppressor proteins; conversely, binding of E2F to hypophosphorylated tumor suppressor proteins arrests the cell cycle early in the G_1 phase, which favors differentiation and allows cells to enter G_0. Mechanisms that inactivate E2F include phosphorylation and direct binding to the cyclin A/CDK2 pair, and formation of a complex with hypophosphorylated tumor suppressor proteins (Fig. 4-8). E2F activity can also be regulated by changes in the rate at which this transcription factor is synthesized; this mechanism allows increased levels of the mRNA that encodes E2F to stimulate hypertrophy. E2F, which often functions as a heterodimer with a transcription factor called DP-1, can also induce apoptosis.

REGULATION OF PROLIFERATIVE SIGNALING

Proliferative signaling is regulated by many of the extracellular messengers that mediate the functional responses described in Chapter 3, by peptide growth factors and cytokines, and by cytoskeletal signaling molecules that are activated by cell deformation. The role of growth factors became apparent in the middle of the 20th century, when cultured adult cells were found to lose their ability to grow and divide in artificial media even after the addition of all known nutrients, vitamins, and trace elements. The key to these puzzling observations was provided by the observation that inclusion of fetal calf serum in the artificial media allowed these otherwise quiescent cells to proliferate. Efforts to identify the unknown factors that could maintain cell cycling identified the missing ingredients as peptides that came to be called *growth factors.*

A large number of peptides are now known to stimulate proliferative responses. Although initially named for the tissues from which they were first isolated, or whose growth they were initially found to stimulate, most peptide growth factors turned out not to be tissue specific, but instead are able to mediate proliferative signaling in many cell types throughout the body. These include platelet-derived growth factor (PDGF), epidermal growth factor (EGF), fibroblast growth factor (FGF), insulin-like growth factor (IGF), vascular endothelial growth factor (VEGF), and transforming growth factors (TGF), as well as a number of cytokines (Table 4-2). Most receptors for these growth factors contain a latent tyrosine kinase that is activated when the ligand-bound receptors form aggregates. A few, like TGF-β receptors, have latent serine/threonine kinase activity. Cytokine receptors lack an intrinsic protein kinase but instead activate latent tyrosine kinase activity in other membrane-associated proteins with which they form aggregates.

Posttranslational Modification versus Docking Sites

Binding of growth factors to their receptors can activate intracellular signal transduction cascades when a protein kinase or other enzyme modifies an intracellular signaling molecule (Fig. 4-9A), or when the ligand-bound receptor forms an aggregate containing a docking site (scaffold) that binds to additional intracellular signaling molecules (Fig. 4-9B). Activation of proliferative signaling by internalized β_2 receptors (see Chapter 3) is one example of the latter mechanism; other examples are described in subsequent text.

Monomeric G Proteins

Most proliferative signal transduction cascades are coupled by monomeric GTP-binding proteins, such as *Ras, Rho,* and *Rac,* which serve as both molecular switches and timers. Like G_α, their heterotrimeric relative (see Chapter 3), monomeric G

TABLE 4-2

Some Peptide Growth Factors

Tyrosine Kinase Ligands
Platelet-derived growth factor (PDGF)
Epidermal growth factor (EGF)
Fibroblast growth factor (FGF)
Insulin-like growth factor (IGF)
Vascular endothelial growth factor (VEGF)

Serine/Threonine Kinase Ligands
Transforming growth factors (e.g., TGF-β)

Cytokines
Tumor necrosis factor-α
Interleukins 2–7, 9–13
Growth hormone
FAS ligand
Erythropoietin
Granulocyte colony-stimulating factor

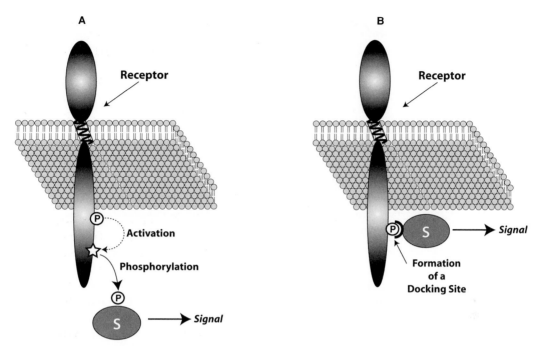

Figure 4-9: Intracellular signal transduction by receptor protein kinases. **A:** Phosphorylation of the receptor activates a protein kinase (star) or other enzyme that modifies an intracellular signaling molecule (S). **B:** Phosphorylation of the receptor creates a docking site, which, by forming an aggregate with an intracellular signaling molecule (S), activates a signal transduction pathway.

proteins are active when bound to GTP and inactivated when the bound GTP is dephosphorylated by an intrinsic GTPase. Unlike G_α, most monomeric G proteins do not interact directly with plasma membrane receptors but instead are activated by intracellular signaling molecules that include enzymes, notably protein kinases, and signaling aggregates formed by docking proteins (see previous discussion). Because monomeric G proteins hydrolyze GTP at a slower rate than G_α, their signals are generally more long lasting. Signaling duration is modified by proteins like *guanine nucleotide exchange factors (GEFs)*, which accelerate the onset of the signal by stimulating exchange of GTP for GDP, and *GTPase-activating proteins (GAPs)*, which shorten signal duration by increasing GTPase. Monomeric G proteins are also regulated by posttranslational modifications such as phosphorylation, methylation, palmitoylation, glutathionylation, and farnesylation.

Fibroblast Growth Factor

Fibroblast growth factors generally respond to mechanical stresses by stimulating cell growth and proliferation, favoring expression of fetal genes, and inhibiting differentiation and apoptosis (Table 4-3). In the heart, FGFs participate in the healing response to injury and the hypertrophic response to overload, while in blood vessels these peptides modify responses to endothelial damage. FGFs, which are often divided into acidic and basic peptides, activate *FGF receptor tyrosine kinases*, which contain a latent tyrosine kinase (Fig. 4-10A). Ligand-binding to these receptors causes the latter to form aggregates with extracellular *FGF receptor heparan sulfate proteoglycans*, which are connective tissue glycoproteins that link cells to one another. Aggregation activates the latent tyrosine kinase, which autophosphorylates

TABLE 4-3
Some Effects of FGF and TGF-β on the Heart

FGF
   Stimulation of myocyte growth
   Inhibition of differentiation and myogenesis
   Expression of the fetal gene program
   Inhibition of apoptosis

TGF-β
   Stimulation of fibrosis
   Stimulation of myocyte differentiation and myogenesis
   Expression of the fetal gene program
   Stimulation of apoptosis

the receptor (Fig. 4-10B); the latter can then activate various intracellular signaling systems including MAP kinases, phospholipase C, and other regulators of proliferative responses (see subsequent text).

In patients with heart failure, FGFs released by angiotensin II, endothelin, and other mediators of the hemodynamic defense reaction activate gene programs that participate in the hypertrophic response to overload. Interactions of FGF receptor heparan sulfate proteoglycans with the extracellular matrix also allow cell deformation to initiate proliferative signals that modify cell size, shape, and composition.

Transforming Growth Factor-β

Transforming growth factor-β plays a major role in tissue responses to injury by stimulating both fibrosis and cell proliferation; TGF-β also stimulates myogenesis and differentiation in embryonic hearts, and in overloaded adult hearts favors expression of fetal genes and activates apoptosis (Table 4-3). In failing hearts this cytokine promotes fibrosis by increasing synthesis of extracellular matrix proteins, inhibiting expression of matrix metalloproteinases, and inducing synthesis of protease inhibitors. Many responses to angiotensin II are mediated by TGF-β_1, the major cardiac isoform of this peptide (see Chapter 3); these include fibrosis and stimulation of proliferative signaling pathways that redirect protein synthesis to favor expression of fetal genes (see subsequent text).

Two classes of TGF-β receptors, called type I and type II, mediate TGF-β signaling. Both contain serine/threonine kinases, but only the type II receptors actually bind TGF-β (Fig. 4-11). Signaling begins when a TGF-β homodimer binds two of the type II receptors to form a ligand-receptor complex that activates the latent serine/threonine kinase in the type II receptors. The latter then phosphorylate two type I receptors that form a complex, which activates their latent protein kinase. The activated type I receptors propagate the TGF-β signal down intracellular signaling cascades by catalyzing serine/threonine phosphorylations in regulatory proteins that include transcription factors called *Smads* (a conflation of the names of two members of this family: "Sma" in the roundworm *Caenorhabditis elegans* and "Mad" in *Drosophila*). Phosphorylated Smads, along with ubiquitin ligases (called *Smurfs* for "Smad ubiquitination regulator factor"), interact with additional signaling proteins like *TGF-β-activated kinase (TAK1)*, which is a mitogen-activated protein kinase kinase (see subsequent text).

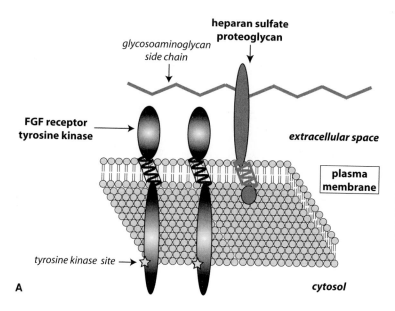

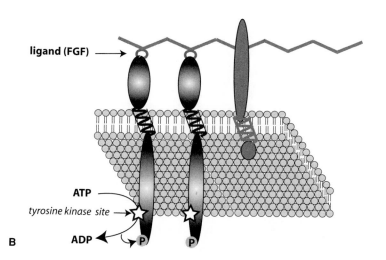

Figure 4-10: FGF signaling. **A:** When the plasma membrane receptor (FGF receptor tyrosine kinase) is not bound to FGF, its latent tyrosine kinase activity is inactive. **B:** Ligand binding to the FGF receptor causes the latter to bind to a heparan sulfate proteoglycan which contains glycosaminoglycan side chains that are linked to the extracellular matrix. Formation of this aggregate activates the latent tyrosine kinase in the receptor, which by autophosphorylating one or more tyrosine residues in the receptor, modifies downstream intracellular signal transduction cascades.

PI3K/PIP₃/Akt Pathways

Insulin, insulin growth factor (IGF), and growth hormone (GH) evoke proliferative responses when they bind to receptor tyrosine kinases that activate *phosphoinositide 3′-OH kinases* (*PI3-kinases* or *PI3K*), which phosphorylate the 3′ hydroxyl group of *phosphatidylinositol trisphosphate* (PIP_3), a membrane phospholipid (Fig. 4-12); PI3-kinases can also be activated by the $G_{\beta\gamma}$ subunits of heterotrimeric G proteins and cytoskeletal deformation. Phosphorylated PIP_3 provides a docking site for a ser-ine/threonine kinase called *Akt* (named for a related transforming component in the T8 strain of AKR/J mice) or, because Akt is homologous to PK-A and PK-C, *protein kinase-B* (*PK-B*). After docking with activated PIP_3, Akt can be phosphorylated by *phosphoinositide-dependent kinase 1* (*PDK1*) which allows Akt to activate *mTOR* (*mammalian target of rapamycin*) and inhibit a proapoptotic serine/threonine kinase called *glycogen synthetase kinase 3β* (*GSK-3β*).

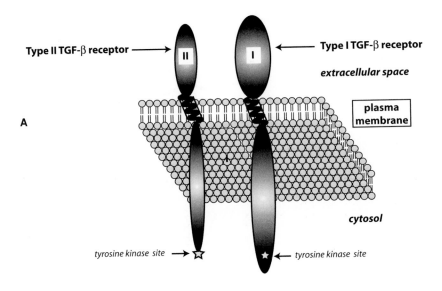

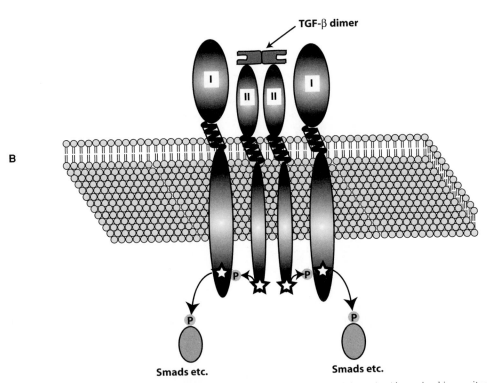

Figure 4-11: TGF-β signaling. **A:** Two types of TGF-β receptor (I and II) contain serine/threonine kinase sites that are inactive when the receptors are not bound to their ligand. **B:** Binding of a TGF-β homodimer to two type II receptors forms a complex that activates the latent serine/threonine kinase, which then phosphorylates the intracellular domains of the type I receptors. This activates the latent protein kinase activity in the type I receptors, which, by phosphorylating one or more serine or threonine residues on the receptor, activates Smads and other intracellular signaling molecules.

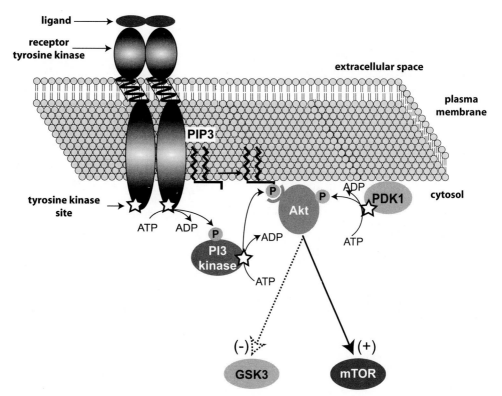

Figure 4.12: PI3K/PIP₃/Akt pathways. Ligand binding to receptor tyrosine kinases activates a latent tyrosine kinase that phosphorylates *phosphoinositide 3'-OH kinase*s (*PI3K*). The latter then phosphorylate the membrane phospholipid *phosphatidylinositol trisphosphate* (*PIP₃*), which, when phosphorylated, provides a docking site that activates *Akt*. Akt is then activated when it is phosphorylated by *phosphoinositide-dependent kinase 1* (*PDK1*). Targets for activated Akt include *glycogen synthetase kinase 3β* (*GSK-3β*), which is inhibited, and *mTOR* (*mammalian target of rapamycin*), which is activated.

Proliferative signaling by PI3K/PIP₃/Akt, unlike most of the other signaling cascades that cause the heart to hypertrophy, tends to favor beneficial rather than deleterious responses. In the heart, adaptive responses mediated by the Akt1 isoform include the *physiological* hypertrophy seen in the athlete's heart, increased capillary density, and an antiapoptotic effect that favors cell survival; however, long-term activation of this signaling pathway can also induce deleterious *pathological* hypertrophy.

G Protein–Coupled Pathways

All of the key regulatory mediators of the neurohumoral response described in Chapter 3 can activate proliferative signaling; these include β-adrenergic receptor agonists, angiotensin II, vasopressin, and endothelin. β-Adrenergic receptor agonists, for example, activate several proliferative signaling pathways (Fig. 4-13) when $G_{\alpha s}$ stimulates cyclic AMP-dependent protein kinases that phosphorylate transcriptional regulators such as *CREB* (*cyclic AMP receptor element–binding protein*) and *CREM* (*cyclic AMP receptor element modulator*), and when $G_{\alpha q}$ stimulates phospholipase C to release InsP₃ and DAG. InsP₃ releases calcium from the endoplasmic reticulum that activates both calcium, calmodulin (CAM) kinases, and *calcineurin* (see subsequent text). Protein kinase C (PK-C), a lipid-dependent protein kinase, catalyzes serine/threonine phosphorylations that activate mitogen-activated protein kinases

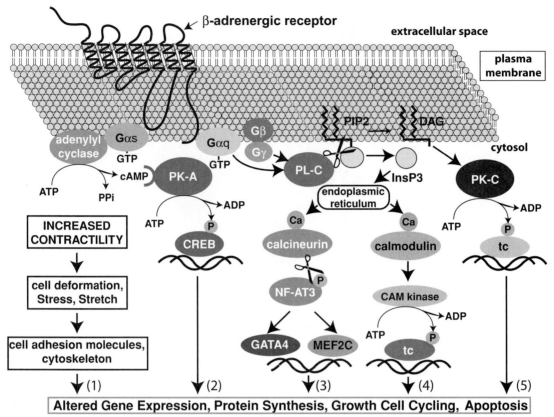

Figure 4-13: Proliferative signaling by β-adrenergic receptors. At least five mechanisms allow β-adrenergic stimulation to modify proliferative signaling; from left to right these are: (1) cytoskeletal signaling that is activated when increased contractility causes cell deformation; (2) activation of PK-A that phosphorylates transcription factors like CREB; (3) calcium released by InsP$_3$ can activate a phosphatase called calcineurin that dephosphorylates and so activates transcription factors such as GATA4 and MEF2C; (4) CAM kinase pathways that activate a number of transcription factors; and (5) activation of PK-C that can phosphorylate transcription factors.

(MAP kinases) and other proliferative signaling pathways. The positive inotropic response to β-adrenergic agonists itself modifies proliferative signaling by causing cell deformations that activate cytoskeletal signaling pathways. Other G protein–coupled receptor agonists, including norepinephrine, angiotensin II, endothelin, and vasopressin, also activate $G_{\alpha q}$ to regulate proliferative responses.

β_2 receptors can generate proliferative signals when they are internalized by prolonged sympathetic stimulation; this occurs when the internalized receptors form scaffolds that activate proliferative signaling systems (see Chapter 3). This shift from functional to proliferative signaling allows a sustained stress to "tell" the heart that reliance on short-term functional responses no longer suffices, so that its myocytes must hypertrophy. Stated simply, this fascinating mechanism recognizes that the time for the stressed heart to run or fight has ended, and that to survive, the heart must grow its way out of trouble!

Parallels and Crossovers between G Protein–Linked and Enzyme-Linked Signaling Pathways

The many parallels and crossovers between proliferative and functional signaling illustrate the integration of these two types of response. One parallel is that both enzyme-linked and G protein–coupled receptors use G proteins to activate downstream

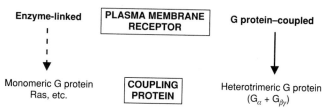

Figure 4-14: Parallels between signals generated by enzyme-linked plasma membrane receptors (**left**), and G protein–coupled receptors (**right**). Both classes of receptor utilize GTP-binding proteins to link receptor activation to downstream signaling. Activation of the monomeric G proteins by enzyme-linked receptors is indirect, and involves several coupling steps (*dashed arrows*), whereas heterotrimeric G proteins interact directly with G protein–coupled receptors (*solid arrow*).

responses (Fig. 4-14; see also Fig. 4-1). However, unlike coupling by *heterotrimeric* G proteins, which interact directly with G protein–coupled receptors, *monomeric* G proteins are activated indirectly by enzyme-linked receptors in reactions that utilize additional signaling proteins. Other parallels include activation of the same or similar downstream signal transduction mechanisms by the two types of receptor; for example, both activate MAP kinases (see subsequent text). In some cases, single ligand, like angiotensin II and some α-adrenergic agonists, activates both G protein–linked and enzyme-linked receptors by a process called *transactivation*. In addition, some G protein-activated receptor agonists stimulate proteases, called *sheddases*, that activate enzyme-linked receptor tyrosine kinases.

Mitogen-Activated Protein (MAP) Kinase Pathways

Among the first systems discovered to regulate cell growth and proliferation were *mitogen-activated protein (MAP) kinase* cascades whose dependence on phosphorylation and dephosphorylation reactions resembles previously described cycles that metabolize carbohydrates (Egan and Weinberg, 1993; Graves et al., 1997). However, as is true of most cell signaling systems, what had originally appeared to be a simple cycle turned out to be several highly regulated pathways in which a sequence of three serine/threonine kinases phosphorylates a MAP kinase that diffuses from the cytosol into the nucleus where it can phosphorylate various nuclear transcription factors (Fig. 4-15).

MAP kinases allow various signals to stimulate protein synthesis, initiate hypertrophy, and in proliferating cells induce mitosis. In the heart, MAP kinases mediate proliferative signals that are responsible for maladaptive hypertrophy and re-expression of fetal genes. In view of the link between cell growth and cell proliferation (see subsequent text), it is not surprising that MAP kinases can also initiate programmed cell death (apoptosis).

The Generic MAP Kinase Pathway

Signaling by MAP kinase pathways resembles an American square dance in which the signal, like a dancer, moves gracefully along a series of partners. The early steps in this dance often take place on a phosphorylated receptor or a scaffold formed by protein aggregates along the inner surface of the plasma membrane (see previous discussion); later in the dance, the action moves through the cytosol, crosses the nuclear membrane, and concludes when the activated MAP kinases phosphorylate transcription factors in the nucleus. Common to all MAP kinase pathways is activation of a *MAP kinase kinase kinase* (MKKK) (Fig. 4-15). These serine/threonine

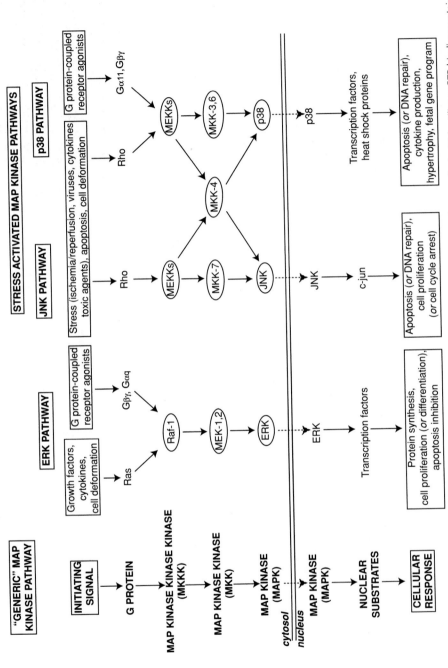

Figure 4-15: MAP kinase pathways. The generic pathway (**left**) lists key steps that are common to these signaling pathways, all of which utilize a GTP-binding protein to activate a sequence of three serine/threonine kinases: MAP kinase kinase kinase (MKKK), which phosphorylates a MAP kinase kinase (MKK), which phosphorylates a MAP kinase. Most of the latter, when phosphorylated, enter the nucleus where they phosphorylate nuclear transcription factors, but a few MAP kinases phosphorylate cytosolic proteins. Three types of MAP kinase pathway are shown the extracellular receptor-activated kinase (ERK) and two stress-activated pathways. The ERK pathway can be coupled by Ras when activated by tyrosine kinase receptors, and by heterotrimeric G proteins, such as $G_{\alpha q}$ and $G_{\alpha \beta}$, when activated by G protein–coupled receptors. The major MKKK in the ERK pathway is Raf-1, MKKs include MEK-1 and MEK-2, and the most important MAP kinase is ERK. The two stress-activated MAP kinase pathways, which phosphorylate JNK and p38, are generally coupled by monomeric G proteins of the *Rho* family and, in the case of the p38 pathway, by $G_{\alpha 11}$ and $G_{\beta, \gamma}$. The MKKs in the stress-activated pathways, called MEKKs, function like Raf-1 to phosphorylate several MKKs that activate JNK and p38. When JNK enters the nucleus it phosphorylates a transcription factor called c-jun, while p38 can phosphorylate nuclear transcription factors and heat shock proteins. Modified from Katz AM (2006). *Physiology of the Heart.* 4th ed. Philadelphia, Lippincott Williams and Wilkins.

kinases then phosphorylate a second kinase, called *MAP kinase kinase* (MKK), which phosphorylates the *MAP kinase*. Most MAP kinases enter the nucleus through large pores in the nuclear membrane where they phosphorylate transcription factors, but some MAP kinase substrates can be cytosolic proteins. Signal diversity is provided by a number of isoforms of the MKKKs, MKKs, and MAP kinases, and by interactions of these pathways with other signal transduction cascades.

Extracellular Receptor Kinase (ERK) Pathways

Extracellular receptor kinase–mediated signals are generally initiated when ligand-binding to tyrosine kinase receptors causes the latter to form aggregates that simulate their latent tyrosine kinase activity (Fig. 4-16). Autophosphorylation of the receptor then creates docking sites that initiate aggregations among additional signaling proteins, much as the partners in our dance join hands to form a square. Aggregation begins when the activated tyrosine kinase receptors phosphorylate adaptor proteins called *shc* (from *Src-homology* because of similarities to the gene *src*) and *grb2* (*growth receptor binding protein*). Scaffolds formed by these multiprotein aggregates

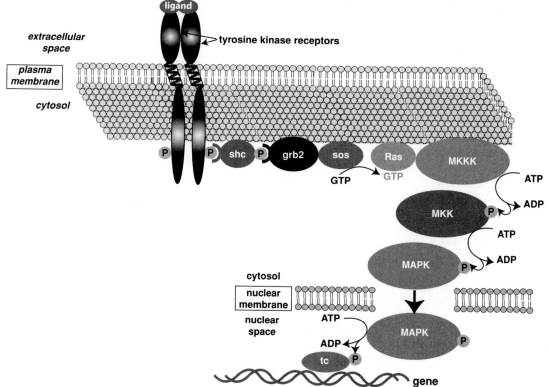

Figure 4-16: Proliferative signaling by an ERK pathway. Binding of the ligand to the receptor forms an aggregate that activates the latent receptor tyrosine kinase. Autophosphorylation of the receptor then creates a "docking site" that binds and phosphorylates the adaptor protein shc to create another docking site in which shc adds grb2 to a multiprotein aggregate assembled along the inner surface of the plasma membrane. This aggregate then activates sos, a guanine nucleotide-exchange factor that exchanges Ras-bound GDP for GTP. The activated Ras-GTP complex stimulates Raf-1, a MAP kinase kinase kinase that phosphorylates and activates the MAP kinase kinase MEK-1, which phosphorylates the MAP kinase ERK-2. Translocation of the latter to the nucleus allows the activated ERK to phosphorylate nuclear transcription factors (tc) that interact with specific DNA sequences.

along the inner surface of the plasma membrane interact with a guanine nucleotide-exchange factor called *sos* (named after the drosophila mutant *son-of-sevenless*), which activates Ras by exchanging its bound GDP for GTP in a reaction that is analogous to activation of G_α by ligand-bound G protein–coupled receptors (see Chapter 3). Activation of Ras by other phosphorylated receptors, protein kinase C, and cytoskeletal components allows additional proliferative signals to activate MAP kinase pathways. The Ras-GTP complex in the ERK pathway activates a MKKK called *Raf-1* that phosphorylates and activates the MKKs, which are the next partners in the dance; the latter include *MEK-1* and *MEK-2* (MEK is an abbreviation for *MAP kinase/ERK kinase*) that phosphorylate a MAP kinase called *extracellular receptor kinase* (*ERK*), which moves to the nucleus where it can phosphorylate various transcription factors. G protein–coupled receptors also activate the ERK pathway when G_α, $G_{\beta\gamma}$, or $G_{\alpha q}$ allows mediators of the hemodynamic defense reaction, like norepinephrine, angiotensin II, and endothelin, to induce maladaptive hypertrophy in failing hearts.

Stress-Activated MAP Kinase Pathways

Two stress-activated MAP kinase pathways are activated by inflammatory cytokines, cell deformation, and injury caused by such insults as viral infection, radiation, and toxins. There are many similarities between stress-activated MAP kinases and the ERK pathway described previously, but the JNK and p38 pathways are regulated differently and activate *c-Jun amino-terminal kinase* (*Jun kinase* or *JNK*) and *p38*, respectively. Stress-activated MKKKs include several *MEKK* (*MEK Kinase*) isoforms, whose function is analogous to that of Raf-1, and MKKs that are analogous to MEK-1. The latter include MKK-7, which mediates JNK signaling, MKK-3 and MKK-6, which operate in the p38 pathway, and MKK-4 which is active in both. Phosphorylation of JNK activates the transcription factor *c-jun*, while p38 is itself a transcription factor. Responses to stress-activated MAP kinase include maladaptive hypertrophy and apoptosis, which play an important role in determining prognosis in patients with heart failure.

Calcium

Increased levels of cytosolic calcium are generally linked to such functional responses as contraction and secretion (see Chapter 3), but it is clear that this cation also mediates proliferative signaling. The response to calcium depends in part on the rate of rise of cytosolic calcium (Berridge, 1997); in contrast to functional signals, like excitation–contraction coupling, which are activated by rapid but brief increases in cytosolic calcium, proliferative responses are typically initiated by the small sustained elevations of cytosolic calcium that occur after opening of plasma membrane T-type calcium channels and $InsP_3$-gated intracellular calcium release channels.

A number of cytosolic proteins mediate the proliferative responses to calcium, these include calcium/calmodulin-dependent protein kinases (CAM kinases) that phosphorylate regulatory proteins like histone deacetylases (HDACs) (see subsequent text) and transcription factors such as cyclic AMP-response element binding protein (CREB). Calcium also activates *calcineurin*, a phosphatase that stimulates cardiac hypertrophy by dephosphorylating the inactive form of a transcription factor called *NF-AT3* (*nuclear factor of activated T cells* or *NFAT*). Phosphorylation allows NFAT to bind to and activate transcription factors called *GATA4* and *MEF2C* that mediate pathological hypertrophy. NFAT can distinguish between the short-term calcium pulses that activate functional responses like contraction and the more prolonged elevations of cytosolic calcium that stimulate proliferative responses because NFAT translocates to the nucleus only after cytosolic calcium has remained elevated for several minutes (Timmerman et al., 1996). Like a high-frequency electronic filter, therefore, NFAT responds only to sustained elevations of cytosolic calcium.

EPIGENETICS

Phenotype is determined largely when transcriptional regulation selects specific genes for expression or suppression, or when alternative splicing modifies gene transcripts. More recently, another type of regulatory mechanism, called *epigenetics*, has also been found to play an important role in translating genotype to phenotype. As defined most broadly, epigenetics refers to non-Mendelian mechanisms of inheritance that influence phenotype without changing the information encoded in the base pair sequences in genomic DNA (Waddington, 1942).

The mechanisms that allow epigenetics to modify gene transcription differ from the more familiar genetic mechanisms in that the primary targets of epigenetic regulation are neither the transcription factors that use the double-stranded DNA helix to determine RNA sequence, nor alternative splicing of exons that transcribes the information encoded in genomic DNA to synthesize different protein isoforms. At least three types of mechanism play a role in epigenetic control (Table 4-4). The first are changes in DNA that include mobile genetic elements that regulate gene expression, interactions between *trans*-gene alleles, and covalent modification of genomic DNA by cytosine methylation. The second group of epigenetic mechanisms use small sequences of RNA, called *RNAi*, to inhibit ("silence") RNA translation. The third, which modify chromosome structure, include posttranslational covalent modifications of basic DNA-binding nuclear proteins called *histones* that alter the accessibility of genomic DNA to transcriptional regulators, ATP-dependent histone modifications, and alterations in chromatin and chromosomal architecture. One way to contrast genetics and epigenetics is to view the former as using the information encoded in genomic DNA to determine how cells, organs, and overall body plan *can* appear, whereas epigenetics provides additional mechanisms that determine how this genetic information is used to determine what actually *does* appear.

Among the most remarkable features of epigenetic regulation is its ability to allow environmental change, including toxic molecules, temperature, nutritional state, and even maternal nurturing, to induce heritable changes in phenotype that can be passed down successive generations (Jirtle and Skinner, 2007). This ability of epigenetic changes to modify the germ line marks a return toward the 19th century Lamarckian view that environment can modify inherited traits, and so represents a paradigm shift in modern biology.

Operating together, genetics and epigenetics have participated in the evolution of the eukaryotic tree of life, in embryonic development, and in causing human disease. In cardiology, epigenetic mechanisms help regulate impulse conduction, contribute to molecular changes in failing hearts, cause several inherited cardiomyopathies, and influence the clinical manifestations of specific gene mutations.

DNA Modification

Mobile Genetic Elements (Transposons): Site-Specific Recombination

In both genetic and epigenetic control, movements of DNA segments through the genome allow a single genotype to generate different phenotypes (Table 4-4). The most familiar genetic mechanisms are DNA rearrangements between pairs of

---

TABLE 4-4

Some Epigenetic Phenomena

DNA Modifications
Modifications by mobile genetic elements (*transposons*)
Communications between *trans*-gene alleles and homologous DNA sequences
(*paramutations*)
Methylation and demethylation

RNA Modifications
RNA interference (RNAi)

Chromosomal Changes
Histone modifications
Covalent modifications
Acetylation, methylation, phosphorylation ubiquitination, ADP-ribosylation,
and other modifications of ϵ-amino lysyl groups
ATP-dependent histone remodeling

Chromatin modifications
Changes in nuclear conformation
Gene compartmentalization and interactions among chromatin loops
Organization of chromosomes at various sites within the nuclei
Localization of chromosomes within and at the periphery of the nucleus
Altered positioning of chromosomes during anaphase
Modifications of chromatin structure

---

homologous genes that occur during mitosis, called *general* or *homologous recombination*. More than 50 years ago, a novel epigenetic mechanism was discovered by McClintock (1950), who observed that a given gene could appear at various loci in the maize genome. This form of genetic instability, which occurs when DNA sequences move between nonhomologous regions of the genomic DNA, was initially referred to as "jumping genes" and is now called *site-specific recombination*. The mobile genetic elements, called *tranposons*, make up almost half of the human genome and include segments of DNA that range in size from hundreds to tens of thousands of nucleotide pairs. Many transposons, called *cryptic elements*, are suppressed within chromatin and so remain silent. Another epigenetic phenomenon, called *parental* or *genomic imprinting*, or *parent-of-origin regulation*, occurs when various mechanisms inactivate large segments of either the X or Y chromosomes.

Paramutation

Interactions between *trans*-regions of paired or homologous DNA sequences can initiate gene silencing by a process called *paramutation* that can utilize several epigenetic mechanisms to inhibit both transcription and translation of the information in genomic DNA (Fig. 4-17). These differ from genetic mechanisms because they are brought about by mechanisms such as DNA methylation and RNA inhibition (see subsequent text). The ability of the silenced alleles to inhibit expression of other alleles can allow environmentally induced responses to be inherited through several generations.

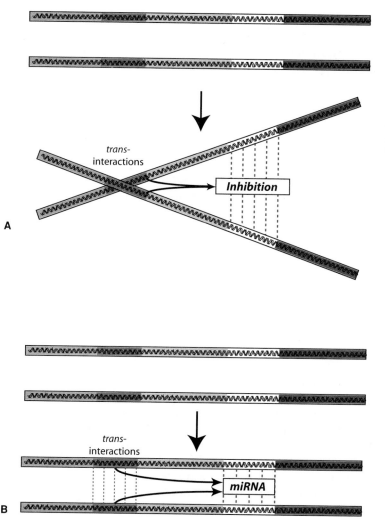

Figure 4-17: Epigenetic regulation by paramutation. **A:** Pairing model in which communications between *trans* regions of homologous genes initiates reactions, like DNA methylation, that inhibit transcription. **B:** RNA-silencing model where interactions between *trans* regions of homologous genes silence gene expression by initiating the formation of miRNA.

DNA Methylation and Demethylation

Covalent modification of DNA by methylation and demethylation occurs in both prokaryotes and eukaryotes and is among the most ancient of the epigenetic mechanisms. DNA methylation, which generally locks genes in a silent state, appears to have evolved to prevent transcription of foreign DNA introduced by invading microbes; this occurs when organisms methylate their own DNA, which protects the genome against hydrolysis by an endonuclease that can hydrolyze only the non-methylated DNA in the foreign genes (Hendrich and Tweedle, 2003). In modern eukaryotes, both hypomethylation and hypermethylation of cytosine in genomic DNA provide epigenetic mechanisms that regulate gene expression.

DNA is methylated by enzymes called *DNA methyl transferases* that can add methyl groups to both cytosine and adenine in prokaryotes, but cytosine is the only base that is methylated in eukaryotes. Demethylation is catalyzed by *DNA demethylase*, while *methyl-CpG binding proteins* identify and initiate responses to the methylated bases. Methylated cytosine is commonly found in repeats of the dinucleotide 5'-CpG-3' (CpG), which occurs in groups often called "tandem repeats."

In developing animals, widespread demethylation of the genome occurs after fertilization in a process that, by favoring gene transcription, is essential for embryogenesis. Differential methylation of selected parental chromosomes, notably X or Y, plays an important role in phenotypic expression and sexual development by selecting some genes for transcription and silencing others ("imprinting," see previous discussion).

Changes in cytosine methylation contribute to several human diseases. Hypomethylation of genomic DNA in malignant cells can activate genes inappropriately, while hypermethylation contributes to the survival of abnormal cells by down-regulating apoptosis. Differences in the extent of cytosine methylation also appears to contribute to the increased phenotypic differences seen during aging of monozygotic twins. Cytosine methylation is being recognized in the pathogenesis of a growing number of human diseases including syndromes as diverse as Huntington's disease and systemic lupus erythematosus, as well as several myopathies including myotonic dystrophy type 1, spinocerebellar ataxia, facioscapulohumeral muscular dystrophy, and Friedreich's ataxia (Robertson, 2005; Rodenhiser and Mann, 2007). Some of the latter, which can affect the heart (see Chapter 5), have been linked to cytosine methylation-induced instability of CpG tandem repeats.

RNA Modifications

RNA Interference

RNA interference (RNAi), which is emerging as one of the most important epigenetic mechanisms that regulate gene transcription, occurs when short (19–25 nucleotide) segments of noncoding double stranded RNA sequences inhibit gene expression. The inhibitory RNAs can be derived from various sources, both exogenous and endogenous. The former, called *small interfering (si)RNAs*, are readily synthesized *in vitro* and show considerable promise in treating infectious and autoimmune diseases by silencing specific genes. Endogenous mechanisms, in which small *micro RNAs (miRNAs)* inhibit posttranslational gene expression (Fig. 4-18), play an important role in cardiac development. In adult hearts, specific miRNAs have recently been found to regulate both conduction velocity (Zhao et al., 2007) and expression of connexin and the inward rectifying potassium channel i_{K1} (Yang et al., 2007), to inhibit overexpression of the β-myosin heavy chain isoform in the response to pressure overloading (van Rooij et al., 2007), and to inhibit the development of cardiac hypertrophy (Carè et al., 2007; Tatsuguchi et al., 2007).

MicroRNA interference is a physiological mechanism that utilizes fragments cleaved from RNA precursors that are synthesized in the nucleus (Fig. 4-18). After the latter are transported to the cytoplasm as ~70 nucleotide pre-miRNAs, they are hydrolyzed by a highly conserved enzyme called *dicer* to form shortened double-stranded RNAs that are processed to form the miRNAs that silence specific RNA sequences. This occurs after further cleavage liberates ~22 nucleotide miRNAs, which then form complexes (called RISCs) with additional regulatory proteins that bind with high specificity to ribosomal RNA sequences where they inhibit protein synthesis.

Epigenetic regulation by RNA inhibition can utilize RNA both to transmit genetic information and serve as a catalyst. This is especially fascinating because RNA is a primitive nucleotide that, in the distant past, appears to have served many functions now carried out by DNA and proteins, both of which appeared later in evolution.

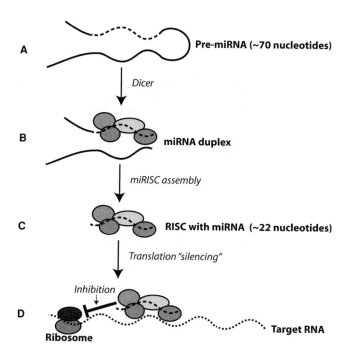

A Pre-miRNA (~70 nucleotides)

Dicer

B miRNA duplex

miRISC assembly

C RISC with miRNA (~22 nucleotides)

Translation "silencing"

Inhibition

D

Ribosome   Target RNA

Figure 4-18: Epigenetic regulation by micro-RNA (miRNA) interference. **A:** Precursors of microRNAs, called pre-miRNA are cleaved from ~70 nucleotide primary miRNAs that are synthesized in the nucleus and transported to the cytoplasm as pre-miRNAs. **B:** The pre-miRNAs are further processed by a highly conserved enzyme called *dicer* to form a duplex that contains a shortened double-stranded RNA. **C:** One of these strands forms the miRNA that binds to regulatory proteins for processing and assembly that includes further cleavage to form RNA-induced silencing complexes (RISCs), which contain short, ~22 nucleotide strands of RNA called miRNA (*dashed lines*). **D:** Binding of RISCs to ribosomal RNA sequences (target RNA) allows the miRNA to silence (inhibit) translation of the latter.

Today, DNA has assumed the primary role in storing genetic information because it is more stable than RNA, and proteins took over as enzymes because of their superior catalytic properties.

Chromosomal Changes

Histone Modifications

Basic DNA-binding proteins called *histones* stabilize DNA within chromosomes by forming structures called *nucleosomes* in which the two strands of genomic DNA are wound tightly around the protein cores to form structures in which the DNA is not readily accessible to transcription factors. Addition of anionic groups to ϵ-amino lysyl residues in histone by acetylation, methylation, phosphorylation ubiquitination, and ADP ribosylation neutralizes the positive charge of these basic proteins, which, by unwinding the tightly packed nucleosomes, can activate gene transcription. In this way, *histone acetyltransferases* (*HATs*) that catalyze histone acetylation stimulate proliferative signaling by exposing active sites on the DNA (Fig. 4-19). Conversely, this stimulatory effect is lost when *histone deacetylases* (*HDACs*) remove the acetyl groups from histones which causes DNA to condense in chromatin where it becomes inaccessible to transcriptional regulation.

HATs and HDACs are members of extended protein families that can be regulated by many of the signaling cascades described in this chapter. Some HDACs are activated when they are phosphorylated by calcium/calmodulin (CAM) kinases and PK-C. Class II HDACs have beneficial actions in animal models of heart failure because they inhibit the responses to transcription factors, like MEF2/*SRF*, that promote pathological hypertrophy. Less is known of the effects of class I and class III HDACs, which are also expressed in adult mammalian hearts.

Figure 4-19: Epigenetic regulation of DNA transcription by histone acetylation. **A:** Deacetylated histone forms tightly packed nucleosomes in which DNA transcription sites (*closed circles*) cannot interact with transcription factors. **B:** Acetylation of histone by histone acetyltransferases (HATs) inhibits chromatin condensation by unwinding histone-bound DNA, which allows the DNA transcription sites (*open circles*) to interact with transcription factors. The activated DNA transcription sites are inactivated when histone is deacetylated by histone deacetylases (HDACs).

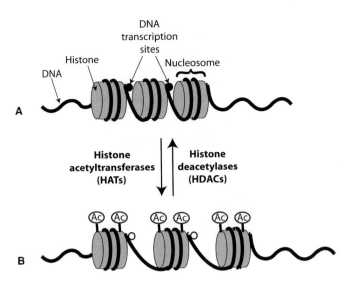

Epigenetically mediated changes in gene expression can also occur during histone remodeling and DNA repair. These highly regulated processes require loosening of the bonds linking DNA to histone, separation of the two strands of DNA, excision of the damaged DNA, resynthesis of the deleted nucleotide sequence using the complementary DNA strand as a template, ligation of the repaired strand, and restoration of chromatin structure. These reactions require the participation of histone-modifying enzymes which can cause epigenetic changes in chromatin structure that modify gene expression.

Conformational and Other Chromatin Modifications

Several epigenetic mechanisms regulate gene expression by modifying nuclear architecture. These chromosomal changes provide opportunities for spatial organization of genes and transcriptional regulators that can create environments for epigenetic transcriptional regulation (Fig. 4-20). The latter include compartmentalization of regions of genomic DNA in specialized chromatin loops, functional organization of chromosomes in various degrees of proximity at adjacent and remote sites, localization of chromosomes within and at the periphery of the nucleus, and changes in chromosome positioning relative to the nucleolus during anaphase. The latter are especially important because the nucleolus is a major site for the processing of RNA, its assembly into ribosomes, and protein synthesis. The ability of epigenetic mechanisms to localize DNA at spatially defined "hot spots" along with RNA polymerases and transcription factors can form "replication factories" (Cook, 2002).

Role of Epigenetics in Human Disease

Appreciation of the importance of epigenetic mechanisms in modifying the clinical manifestations of human disease is still in its infancy. However, it is already clear that some familial cardiomyopathies have an epigenetic etiology (Robertson, 2005) and that epigenetics influences the manifestations in various conditions

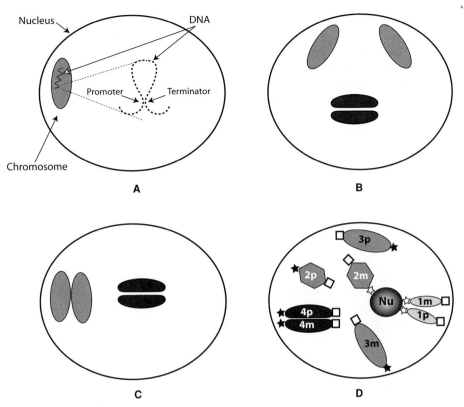

Figure 4-20: Some epigenetic mechanisms by which chromatin structure and nuclear architecture can organize genes and transcriptional regulators. **A:** Compartmentalization of DNA in specialized chromatin loops can bring interacting functional regions into proximity. **B:** Organization of chromosomes in varying proximity relative to one another at different sites in the nucleus. **C:** Localization of chromosomes within and at the periphery of the nucleus. **D:** Positioning of paternal (p) and maternal (m) chromosomes during anaphase showing centromeres (*stars*), telomeres (*squares*), and their relationship to the nucleolus (Nu). Both of the chromosomes 1 and the maternal chromosome 2 are linked to *nucleolar organizing regions* in the nucleolus by centromeres (*open stars*) while centromeres in paternal chromosome 2 and both of the chromosomes 3 (*closed stars*) are not associated with each other or with the nucleolus. Chromosomes 4 are paired even though they are not associated with the nucleolus. Panel **D** modified from Cook PR (2002). Predicting three-dimensional genome structure from transcriptional activity. Nat Genet 32:347–352.

including arrhythmias, heart failure, and the development of cardiac hypertrophy (see previous discussion). The role of epigenetics in determining the phenotypic expression of a given gene abnormality may also help explain variations in the severity ("penetrance") of the clinical syndromes that can result from specific mutations (see Chapter 5). For these reasons, it is likely that this new science will have a major impact on the diagnosis and treatment of heart failure.

SIGNALING BY THE CYTOSKELETON

Cardiac myocytes and other cells are not simply fluid-filled bags in which enzymes and cell organelles like myofilaments and mitochondria float freely in the cytosol; instead, a complex cellular architecture is maintained by a protein framework called the *cytoskeleton*. Like the girders in a modern building, these structural proteins hold cell constituents in place, organize functionally related proteins, and facilitate mechanical interactions with adjacent cells and the extracellular matrix. In addition to these structural functions, the cytoskeleton makes a major contribution to proliferative regulation; these proteins, therefore, not only provide a system of girders that maintain cell architecture, but like a phone system play a key role in cell signaling!

Cytoskeletal signaling allows cell deformation and mechanical stress to adapt form to function by modifying the size, shape, and molecular composition of the heart. This role is especially important in disease, where cytoskeletal signaling contributes to hypertrophic responses. In heart failure, for example, proliferative regulation by cytoskeletal proteins contributes to the progressive ventricular dilatation (remodeling) that shortens survival (see Chapter 1). Activation of specific signaling pathways by various types of cytoskeletal deformation also makes an important contribution to the appearance of different phenotypes of cardiac hypertrophy and helps explain why pressure overload causes concentric hypertrophy (seen in aortic stenosis, where *systolic* stress is increased) and volume overload causes eccentric hypertrophy (as occurs in aortic insufficiency, where *diastolic* stress is increased) (see Chapter 1).

The mechanical and signaling functions of the cytoskeleton are made possible by interactions among literally dozens of proteins. Some of these proteins are largely structural, while other proteins associated with the cytoskeleton, such as protein kinases and phosphatases, function mainly in signal transduction. Because many cytoskeletal proteins serve both mechanical and signaling functions, any attempt at classification is arbitrary. In many ways these proteins are like the front wheels of an automobile, which both hold the vehicle to the road and participate in steering.

The cytoskeleton includes three types of intracellular fiber: *microfilaments*, which consist of actin; *intermediate filaments*, which contain desmin; and *microtubules*, which are made up of tubulin. The microfilaments and intermediate filaments in cardiac myocytes maintain sarcomere structure, connect the sarcomeres to one another and to adjacent cells, and participate in multiprotein complexes that bridge the plasma membrane to connect cells to each other and to the extracellular matrix. Key structures that link cells to the extracellular matrix are the dystrophin glycoprotein complex and the integrins. The major structures that hold cells together are the fascia adherens and desmosomes in the intercalated discs.

Cytoskeletal Proteins Associated with the Myofilaments

The *Z-lines* (or *Z-discs*) separate adjacent sarcomeres and link the myofilaments to the cell surface (Fig. 4-21). These structures include bands, often called *costameres* that, like the staves of a barrel, encircle the myofilaments which they link to adjacent cells and extracellular matrix through desmin and actin microfilaments. *Actin*, the backbone of the thin filament (see Chapter 5), can be viewed both as a contractile protein (*sarcomeric actin*) and as part of the cytoskeleton (*cortical actin*). *Desmin* serves mainly a mechanical role as do α-*actinin*, which weaves the thin filaments into the Z-line, and *nebulette* which runs alongside the thin filaments near the Z-lines. *Titin* and *t-cap* (*telethonin*) link the Z-lines to the thick filaments. *Ankyrin* connects the cytoskeleton to adhesion molecules that cross the plasma membrane and, in concert with *obscurin*, connects the Z-lines to the sarcoplasmic reticulum through linkages that help orient the cytoskeleton, myofilaments, and sarcoplasmic reticulum to one another. The thin filaments are capped by cytoskeletal proteins that regulate thin filament length and interact with proteins that participate

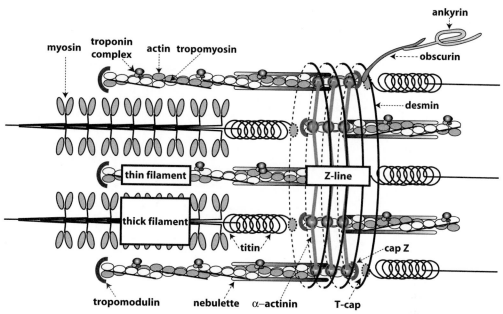

Figure 4-21: Cytoskeletal proteins of the Z-lines and thin filaments that provide mechanical linkages. Desmin and α-actinin link the Z-lines to desmosomes in the intercalated discs, T-cap binds the Z-lines to titin in the thick filaments, and obscurin, along with ankyrin, connects the Z-lines to the sarcoplasmic reticulum and plasma membrane. Thin filament length is regulated by two "capping" proteins: tropomodulin and cap Z; the latter, along with α-actinin and nebulette, connects the thin filaments to the Z-lines. Modified from Katz AM (2006). *Physiology of the Heart.* 4th ed. Philadelphia, Lippincott Williams and Wilkins.

in proliferative signaling; the ends within the Z-lines are covered by *cap Z* (*β-actinin*), while the ends that interdigitate with the thick filaments are capped by *tropomodulin.*

Z-line proteins that function mainly in proliferative signaling include *protein kinases, CARP* (cardiac ankyrin repeat protein); the *myopalladin–mytolin–paladin* complex that forms a signaling scaffold; a tumor suppressor called *myopodin; calcineurin* and the calcineurin-binding protein *calcarcin*; the docking protein *filamin*; a calcium-binding protein that regulates myogenesis called *S100; atrogin,* which is a ubiquitin ligand that regulates proteolysis; and a regulatory subunit of plasma membrane voltage-gated potassium channels called *minK* (Fig. 4-22). Among the most important cytoskeletal signaling proteins are the *LIM proteins* (named for *lin-11* and *mec-3* found in *Caenorhabditis elegans* and Isl-1, an insulin binding protein) that contain zinc fingers that form homodimers and heterodimers. Other LIM proteins, including *cypher1, FHL2, PDZ-3, enigma,* and *muscle-specific LIM,* regulate myofilament assembly, link cytoskeletal elements to one another, and connect myocardial cells at the intercalated discs. Some LIM proteins regulate cyclic AMP-dependent protein kinases that phosphorylate CREM and CREB, while others are transcription factors that interact with DNA.

The thick filaments, like the thin filaments, contain a number of cytoskeletal proteins. *Titin,* a huge protein with a molecular weight of ~3,000,000 that extends from the Z-lines to the center of the thick filament (Fig. 4-23), supports sarcomeric structure and contributes to the high resting stiffness of the myocardium. *Myosin-binding protein C (C protein),* which binds to both myosin and titin, forms transverse fibers that connect adjacent thick filaments near the centers of the sarcomeres;

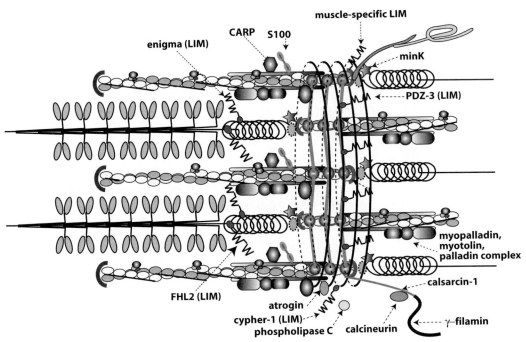

Figure 4-22: Some of the cytoskeletal proteins of the Z-lines and thin filaments that participate in signal transduction. The locations of these proteins, which are labeled in this figure, are approximations because these signaling proteins can move from one location to another. Modified from Katz AM (2006). *Physiology of the Heart.* 4th ed. Philadelphia, Lippincott Williams and Wilkins.

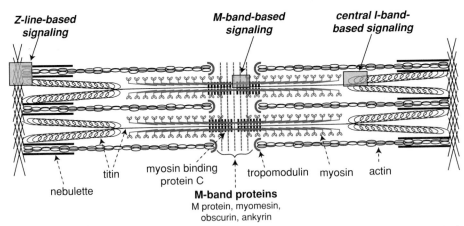

Figure 4-23: Cytoskeletal proteins of the thick filaments. Proteins that provide mechanical linkages include the giant protein *titin*, which extends from the Z-band into the thick filament where it is connected to myosin by *myosin-binding protein C* near the center of the A-band. The portions of the titin molecule that lie within the A-band are quite rigid, while the regions in the I-band are more elastic. Several proteins make up the M-bands that link the thick filaments in the center of the A-band; these include *M protein, myomesin, obscurin, ankyrin,* and the *MM isoform* of the enzyme creatine phosphokinase. *Nebulette* and *tropomodulin,* which bind to the thin filaments, are also shown. Regions that are active in signal transduction (*shaded rectangles*) are labeled "Z-line signaling," "M-band-based signaling," and "Central I-band-based signaling." From Katz AM (2006). *Physiology of the Heart.* 4th ed. Philadelphia, Lippincott Williams and Wilkins.

these fibers, along with *M protein* and *myomesin*, provide lateral mechanical stability to the sarcomere and help organize interactions between titin and the thick filaments. Other proteins, including obscurin and ankyrin, link the M-bands and the sarcoplasmic reticulum. Many of the cytoskeletal proteins associated with the thick filaments participate in cell signaling. Titin, for example, contains three "hot spots" that contain many signaling proteins that appear to participate in the proliferative responses initiated by mechanical stress; one hot spot interacts with the signaling proteins of the Z-line, the second is located in the center of the I-band, while the third interacts with signaling proteins in the center of the M-band (Fig. 4-24).

Cytoskeletal Proteins Associated with the Plasma Membrane

The cytoskeletal proteins that link intracellular structures to the plasma membrane, like those described previously, serve both structural and signaling functions. In addition to desmin and cortical actin, these proteins include ankyrin and spectrin.

Ankyrins link actin microfilaments to sarcoplasmic reticulum and plasma membrane proteins (Fig. 4-25); the latter include receptors, cell adhesion molecules, ion channels, ion pumps, ion exchangers, and clathrin. Ankyrins play an important role in integrating the actions of functionally related proteins, for example by coordinating sodium fluxes across the plasma membrane when they colocalize voltage-gated sodium channels, the sodium pump ATPase, and the sodium/calcium exchanger. Ankyrins also organize interactions between plasma membrane calcium channels (dihydropyridine receptors) and the intracellular calcium release channels in the sarcoplasmic reticulum (ryanodine receptors) (see Chapter 5). Actin- and plasma membrane-binding domains in ankyrins can form aggregates with additional proteins that participate in proliferative signaling. Some ankyrins contain a "death domain" that plays a role in apoptosis.

Spectrins, which link ankyrin to the actin microfilaments (Fig. 4-25), function as heterodimers made up of two subunits (α and β). Some spectrins contain a calcium-binding domain and an amino acid sequence similar to that found in regulatory tyrosine kinases that allows them to participate in cell signaling.

Cytoskeletal Proteins That Link Cells to Each Other

Intercalated Discs

The intercalated discs contain two structures that transmit tension developed by the contractile proteins from one cardiac myocyte to another; these are the *fascia adherens* (also called *adherens junctions* or *focal adhesions*) (Fig. 4-26) that bind to cortical actin microfilaments and *desmosomes* that bind to intermediate filaments. Both contain *cadherins* that link cells to one another; the cadherins in the fascia adherens bind to actin microfilaments (Fig. 4-26A), while other members of the cadherin family called *desmoglein* and *desmocollin* link the intermediate (desmin) filaments to the desmosomes (Fig. 4-26B). Cadherin oligomers, which are held together by calcium-dependent linkages, bind to complexes made up of α, β, and γ *catenins* (the latter is also called *plakoglobin*) that function as anchoring proteins. The cadherin-containing complexes in the fascia adherens are linked to actin microfilaments by *α-actinin* and *vinculin*, while desmocollin in the desmosomes binds to catenin γ (plakoglobin) and desmoglein in a complex that, along with a cytosolic protein called *desmoplakin*, is connected to desmin in the intermediate filaments. These and other cytoskeletal proteins in the fascia adherens and desmosomes participate in cell signaling.

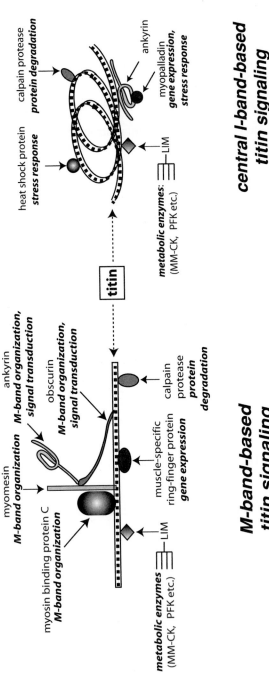

**M-band-based
titin signaling**

*central I-band-based
titin signaling*

metabolic enzymes
(MM-CK, PFK etc.)
— LIM

myosin binding protein C
M-band organization

myomesin
M-band organization

ankyrin
*M-band organization,
signal transduction*

obscurin
*M-band organization,
signal transduction*

muscle-specific
ring-finger protein
gene expression

calpain
protease
*protein
degradation*

titin

calpain protease
protein degradation

heat shock protein
stress response

ankyrin

myopalladin
*gene expression,
stress response*

metabolic enzymes:
(MM-CK, PFK etc.)
— LIM

Figure 4-24: Signaling "hot spots" in titin. M-band–based signaling (**left**): The thick filaments are organized in the M-band by myomesin, myomesin-binding protein C, and obscurin, which link titin and myosin. These proteins, along with additional M-band proteins (labeled) also participate in cell signaling and, in the case of the LIM protein, organize metabolic enzymes that participate in energy-production. Central I-band–based signaling (**right**): Titin-linked proteins in the center of the I-band that participate in cell signaling are labeled. From Katz AM (2006). *Physiology of the Heart.* 4th ed. Philadelphia, Lippincott Williams and Wilkins.

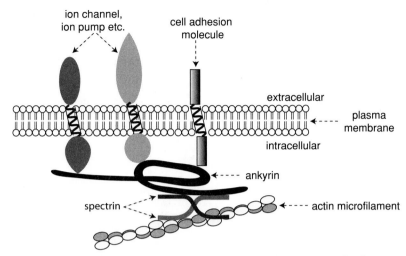

Figure 4-25: Ankyrin and spectrin heterodimers bind actin microfilaments to cell adhesion molecules, organize functionally related membrane proteins, and participate in proliferative signaling. Modified from Katz AM (2006). *Physiology of the Heart*. 4th ed. Philadelphia, Lippincott Williams and Wilkins.

The Dystrophin Glycoprotein Complex

The plasma membrane is anchored to cortical actin by the dystrophin glycoprotein complex, which connects actin microfilaments to extracellular matrix proteins (Fig. 4-27). *Dystrophin* anchors the actin microfilaments to *dystroglycan*, which spans the plasma membrane to bind such extracellular matrix proteins as *fibronectin* and *laminin*; within the cytosol, dystrophin and dystroglycan form a signaling complex with *dystrobrevin* and *syntrophins*. Dystroglycan also binds to a family of six

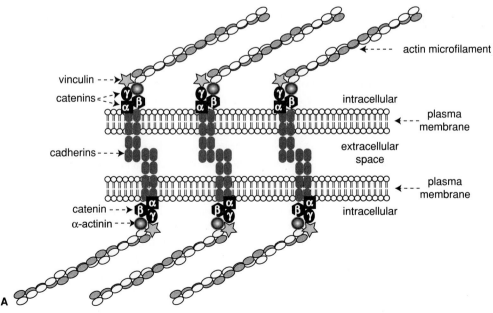

Figure 4-26: Structures that connect adjacent cardiac myocytes in the intercalated discs. **A:** Cadherins in the fascia adherens link actin microfilaments of adjacent cells through α, β, and γ catenins, α-actinin, and vinculin. (*continued*)

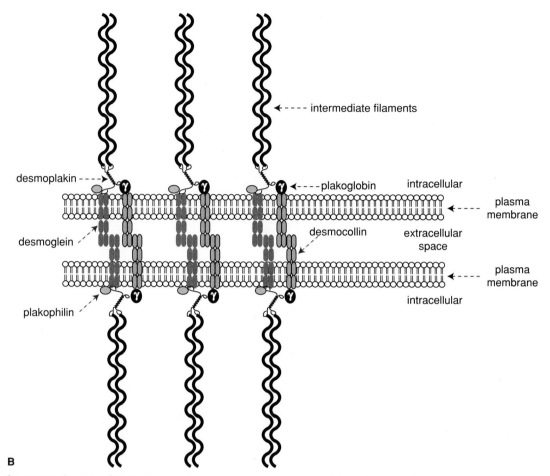

B

Figure 4-26: (*Continued*) **B:** Cadherins in the desmosomes, called desmoglein and desmocollin, are linked to intermediate microfilaments through a complex that includes plakoglobin (γ catenin), plakophilin, and desmoplakin. From Katz AM (2006). *Physiology of the Heart.* 4th ed. Philadelphia, Lippincott Williams and Wilkins.

membrane-spanning glycoproteins called *sarcoglycans*, whose assembly is regulated by *sarcospan* in a complex that, along with the syntrophins and dystrobrevin, links dystrophin to the plasma membrane.

The dystrophin glycoprotein complex participates in several signaling systems. Dystrobrevin is a substrate for regulatory phosphorylations, contains a calcium-binding domain, and, along with *caveolin-3*, regulates nitric oxide production by *nitric oxide synthetase* (*NOS*). Caveolin-3 integrates the activities of functionally related signaling molecules and mediates signal transduction across the plasma membrane when it interacts with dystroglycan in the dystrophin glycoprotein complex. Mutations in dystrophin, dystroglycan, and other proteins in this complex can cause dilated cardiomyopathies by destabilizing cell-matrix linkages, and dystrobrevin mutations have been implicated in *noncompaction* of the left ventricular wall. Disruption of dystrophin linkages appears to exacerbate progressive dilatation in failing hearts.

Integrins

Integrins, which link cells to the extracellular matrix, form heterodimers that include different α- and β-subunits whose properties determine the binding

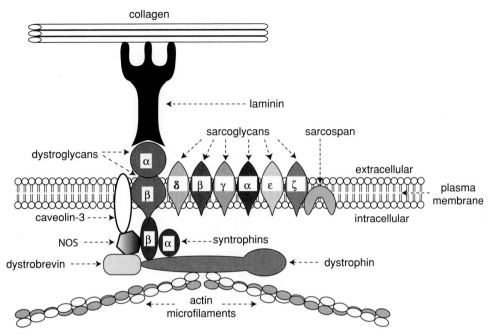

Figure 4-27: Major proteins of the dystrophin glycoprotein complex. Dystrophin links actin filaments to the plasma membrane through a protein complex that includes syntrophins α and β, and dystrobrevin. The latter are bound to the plasma membrane by dystroglycans α and β, six isoforms of sarcoglycan, and sarcospan that are linked to dystrophin, laminin, and other extracellular matrix proteins. These cytoskeletal proteins participate in cell signaling, for example by interacting with caveolin-3 and nitric oxide synthase (NOS). From Katz AM (2006). *Physiology of the Heart.* 4th ed. Philadelphia, Lippincott Williams and Wilkins.

specificity and signaling effects of this cell adhesion molecule. The intracellular domains of the integrins bind to actin microfilaments through adaptor proteins that include *α-actinin, vinculin, tensin,* and *talin; paxillin,* another intracellular protein that can bind to this complex, is a substrate for regulatory phosphorylations. Integrins bind to extracellular matrix proteins including *fibronectin, laminin,* and *vitronectin,* which along with *proteoglycans* such as heparan, link the integrins to *collagen* (Fig. 4-28A).

In addition to their structural role, integrins participate in several proliferative signaling pathways (Fig. 4-28B). Although integrins lack enzymatic activity, these cell adhesion molecules allow mechanical stresses to regulate all three of the *MAP kinase pathways* described previously. Many of these proliferative effects are mediated by nonreceptor protein kinases that are linked to the cytoskeleton; these include the tyrosine kinases *focal adhesion-associated kinases (FAKs), proline-rich tyrosine kinase 2 (PYK2),* and *c-Src-kinase (CSK)* along with serine/threonine kinases such as *integrin-linked kinase (ILK), p21-activated kinase (PAK),* and protein kinase Cε *(PKCε).* Integrin-linked signaling proteins that play a protective role in overloaded hearts include *melusin,* which activates the Akt pathway, and several LIM proteins that participate in the hypertrophic response and regulate apoptosis in failing hearts.

INFLAMMATORY RESPONSES: CYTOKINES

When living organisms first discovered that their neighbors could provide a source of food, they evolved means to attack and eat each other. This, of course, led to the development of defenses to ward off attack, and even better, to turn the tables by

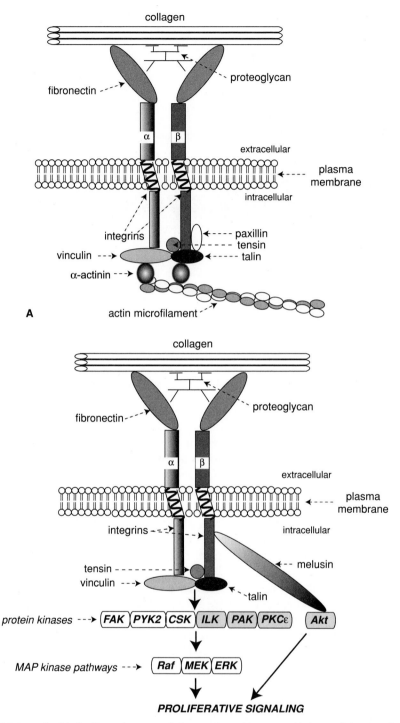

Figure 4-28: Integrins bind cells to the extracellular matrix and interact with intracellular signaling pathways. **A:** Integrins are heterodimers made up of α- and β-subunits that can bind to fibronectin, laminin, proteoglycans, and other matrix proteins that are linked to collagen. Within the cell, integrins bind to actin microfilaments through a protein complex that includes talin, tensin, vinculin, paxillin, and α-actin. **B:** Integrin signaling occurs when these proteins interact with intracellular signaling molecules that include talin, tensin, and vinculin, which activate tyrosine kinases such as FAK, PYK2, and CSK (*unshaded*) and serine/threonine kinases like ILK, PAK, and PKCϵ (*shaded*) that stimulate Raf, MEK, and ERK MAP kinase pathways. Integrin signals are also mediated when melusin activates the serine/threonine kinase Akt.

killing and eating the attacker! The best defense—and offense—was to secrete a noxious chemical (Beck and Habicht, 1991). Today, this cellular violence is controlled by an extended family of peptides, the *cytokines*, which probably arose from a limited number of ancestral proteins, and possibly only a single protein (Shields et al., 1995). By gene duplication and subsequent divergence, this family has grown to include many signaling peptides (Table 4-5) that have a wide variety of biological actions (Table 4-6). This text focuses on the inflammatory cytokines, which can be viewed as coordinating a counterattack as well as a defense.

Adaptations of the primitive defense/counterattack mechanism are seen in the inflammatory responses that attack invading microorganisms and other foreign materials that enter the body (see Chapter 3). Moreover, many of the signaling molecules that mediate inflammation stimulate reactions that are involved in cell growth and healing as well as providing tools for a counterattack. Unfortunately, release of these powerful molecules is not always beneficial because they can attack self rather than other, as in autoimmune diseases. In chronic heart failure, the inflammatory response has both deleterious and beneficial effects because cytokines, in addition to causing damage, stimulate hypertrophy and promote cellular repair and healing, which are not illogical elements of an adaptive mechanism in these patients.

Inflammatory Responses in Heart Failure

Heart failure is accompanied by inflammatory responses that operate both systemically and locally. The systemic response, which attacks tissues throughout the body, plays an important role in causing *cardiac cachexia*, a wasting response that can be especially severe in end-stage heart failure. This systemic inflammatory response probably contributes to the skeletal muscle myopathy responsible for the fatigue and muscle weakness that occur in this syndrome (see Chapter 3). Although systemic and local cytokine release also contribute to myocardial cell death, and so can accelerate the progressive deterioration of these patients, stimulation of

---

TABLE 4-5

Some Members of the Cytokine Family

Tumor necrosis factor α
Interleukins 2–7, 9–13
Interferons
Lymphotoxin
Transforming growth factor-β
Growth hormone
Prolactin
Erythropoietin
Thrombopoietin
Leukemia inhibitory factor
Granulocyte colony-stimulating factor

Selected and compiled from Beck G, Habicht GS (1991). Primitive cytokines: harbingers of vertebrate defense. Immunol Today 12:180–183;.and Shields DC, Harmoin DL, Nunez F, et al. (1995). The evolution of haematopoietic cytokine/receptor complexes. Cytokine 7:679–688.

TABLE 4-6

Selected Actions of the Cytokines

Cellular Effects
Inflammation
Cell proliferation
Cell transformation
Apoptosis (programmed cell death)

Signal Transduction
Activate tyrosine kinases, e.g., janus kinase (JAK)
Activate protein kinases A and C
Activate stress-activated MAP kinases
Activate phospholipases A_2 and C
Increase levels of cyclic AMP and diacylglycerol
Activate signal transducer and activator of transcription
(STAT)
Activate NF-κB
Activate immediate-early genes

Induce Synthesis of
Inflammatory mediators including other cytokines
Inducible nitric oxide synthase (iNOS)
Growth factors: e.g., PDGF, GM-CSF
Receptors: e.g., EGF receptor, IL-2 receptor
Cytoskeletal molecules
Heat shock proteins

proliferative responses by cytokines provides an adaptive response by promoting hypertrophy in damaged or overloaded hearts (see subsequent text).

Cardiac Cachexia

Wasting in patients with dropsy, which was noted by Hippocrates >2,500 years ago (see Chapter 1), is an important complication of end-stage heart failure. Fifty years ago one of the authors, as a medical student, helped care for a young woman who, shortly before she died of rheumatic mitral insufficiency (which was then inoperable), exhibited the severe wasting typical of terminal malignancy; it came as a surprise when a resident pointed out that cachexia is also common in end-stage heart failure. Until recently, this loss of body tissue was assumed to be caused by a combination of inactivity, inadequate caloric intake, and excessive metabolic demands, sometimes complicated by digitalis-induced nausea and anorexia (Pittman and Cohen, 1964). It is now clear, however, that cardiac cachexia differs from that caused by malnutrition, where wasting is due mainly to loss of adipose tissue, rather than the decreased lean tissue mass seen in patients with heart failure (Thomas et al., 1979; Freeman and Roubenoff, 1994). Loss of muscle mass is probably not due mainly to disuse atrophy because the skeletal muscle abnormalities caused by inactivity differ from those seen in heart failure (Simonini et al., 1996; Vescovo et al, 1996). Instead, elevated cytokine levels, which are well known to cause cachexia and weakness in many chronic diseases, play an important role in this complication of severe heart failure.

Cytokines and the Failing Heart

The modern era in our understanding of cardiac cachexia began less than two decades ago, when circulating levels of *tumor necrosis factor α (TNF-α, or cachectin)* were found to be elevated in patients with heart failure (Levine et al., 1990). In addition to this systemic response, hemodynamic overloading releases TNF-α and other cytokines from cells within the heart, where they play a role in the pathophysiology of heart failure.

Although TNF-α is not normally expressed in adult mammalian cardiac myocytes, this cytokine is commonly found in diseased hearts. In myocarditis, these inflammatory mediators are brought to the heart by mononuclear cells that are attracted by infectious agents and tissue injury; cytokines are also synthesized by cardiac myocytes at the edges of a myocardial infarct. Hemodynamic overload causes the myocardium to release chemotactic and other activating factors that recruit monocytes which carry cytokines to the heart and stimulate cytokine synthesis by myocardial cells. For example, aortic banding in rats elevates levels of the mRNA encoding TNF-α within 30 minutes, and after an hour, TNF-α protein levels increase more than tenfold in both myocytes and nonmyocytes (Kapadia et al., 1997). These and other findings indicate that overload stimulates a local inflammatory response in which cytokines released by invading monocytes and produced locally by stressed cardiac myocytes can damage the heart and so contribute to the poor prognosis in heart failure. However, there is also evidence that cytokines can be beneficial, at least in the short term.

Although best known for their proinflammatory effects, cytokines also regulate proliferative responses and apoptosis. Cytokine-activated proliferative signaling pathways can participate in both adaptive and maladaptive cardiac hypertrophy, but it is not clear which predominates in heart failure. Inhibiting the response to cytokines in a mouse model of heart failure has been found to have serious deleterious consequences (Uozumi et al., 2001), and adverse effects of anticytokine therapy in human heart failure (see Chapter 6) suggest that these proinflammatory peptides can evoke important beneficial responses that may be due in part to stimulation of adaptive hypertrophy.

Cytokines, like peptide growth factors, bind to plasma membrane receptors. Unlike the receptor tyrosine kinases described previously, cytokine receptors do not contain protein kinase moieties but instead activate protein kinases farther downstream in their signaling cascades. Cytokine receptors are specific for individual members of this family of signaling peptides, but a single class of cytokines can bind to more than one receptor. Signal transduction by cytokines begins when the ligand-bound receptors form aggregates that can include an additional coupling protein called *gp130* (Fig. 4-29). Most responses to cytokines are mediated by phosphorylation of tyrosine, and less frequently serine and threonine; substrates include the cytokine receptors gp130 and protein kinases that can interact with both cytokine receptors and gp130.

Among the most important mediators of cytokine signaling is the JAK/STAT pathway, where cytokine-bound receptors activate intracellular tyrosine kinases called *JAK* (this acronym, which originally stood for "just another kinase," has been redefined to mean *Janus kinase* because like Janus—the two-faced Roman god of doorways who looks both outward and inward—JAKs respond to binding of cytokines outside the cell by phosphorylating proteins within the cell). The major substrates for JAK-catalyzed phosphorylations are transcription factors called *signal transducer and activator of transcription (STAT)* that, when phosphorylated by JAK, move to the nucleus to regulate gene expression. Cytokine signaling is also mediated by stress-activated MAP kinases (see previous discussion) and signaling cascades that activate a transcription factor called NF-κB. In the latter, cytokine binding to the receptor forms a trimer that aggregates with adaptor proteins to initiate a series of

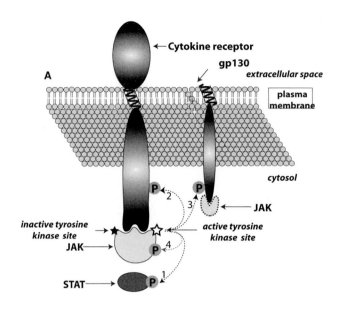

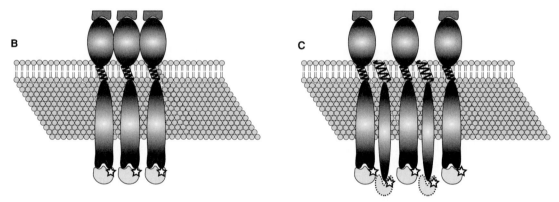

Figure 4-29: Cytokine signaling: The JAK/STAT pathway. **A:** Components include the cytokine receptors, the coupling protein gp130, tyrosine kinases called JAK, and the transcription factor STAT. Cytokine receptors lack protein kinase activity; instead, activated receptors stimulate JAK to phosphorylate (1) the STAT transcription factors, (2) the receptor, (3) gp130, and/or (4) itself (autophosphorylation). JAK is activated when ligand binding causes cytokine receptors to form trimeric aggregates (**B**) that can include gp130 (**C**).

reactions that, after phosphorylating, ubiquitylating, and then digesting an inhibitory cofactor called IκB, releases the active form of NF-κB (Fig. 4-30). The cytoplasmic domain of some cytokine receptors contain an amino acid sequence, referred to as a death domain, that stimulates apoptosis (see subsequent text). Cytokine signaling can be turned off by inhibitors of cytokine-induced phosphorylation pathways and phosphatases that dephosphorylate the activated signaling proteins.

Cytokine receptors are also found in a soluble form whose circulating levels, although low in normal individuals, are elevated in the blood of patients with infectious and autoimmune diseases and in some patients with heart failure. Soluble cytokine receptors can be produced when limited proteolysis of the membrane-bound receptors releases the extracellular ligand-binding domain of the molecule in a process called *shedding*; soluble receptors can also be synthesized *de novo* from mRNAs that encode only the ligand-binding portion of the receptor molecule.

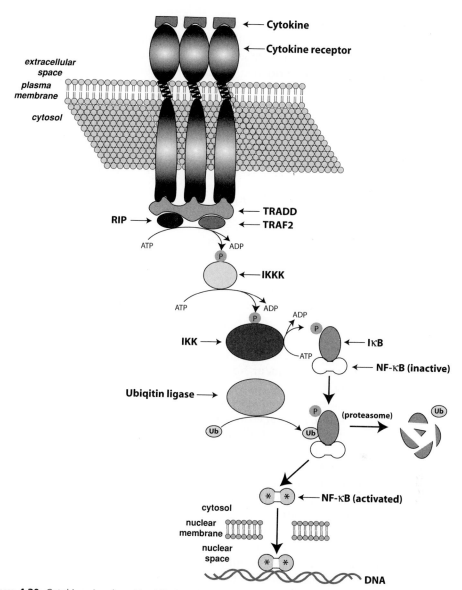

Figure 4.30: Cytokine signaling. The NF-κB pathway. Binding of TNF-α and other cytokines to their receptors (**top**) forms a trimer that aggregates with adaptor proteins such as TNF-associated death-domain protein (TRADD), TNF-receptor associated factor 2 (TRAF2), and receptor-interacting protein kinase (RIP) that can phosphorylate IκB kinase kinase (IKKK). The latter phosphorylates IκB kinase (IKK), which in turn phosphorylates IκB in a complex with the inactive transcription factor NF-κB. A ubiquitin ligase transfers ubiquitin (Ub) to IκB, which dissociates from NF-κB; this activates NF-κB while IκB is degraded by proteasomes. Translocation of activated NF-κB to the nucleus allows this transcription factor to regulate gene expression.

Soluble cytokine receptors form complexes with their ligands that serve regulatory functions similar to those of the membrane-bound receptor and can protect the bound cytokines from proteolysis; conversely, soluble receptors can inhibit cytokine actions.

THE MYOCARDIAL RESPONSE TO STRESS

Gene expression is rapidly modified when cardiac myocytes are subjected to stresses such as injury, ischemia, diastolic stretch (increased preload), or high systolic tension (increased afterload). The first genes to be upregulated, called *immediate-early response genes*, are not normally transcribed in the resting (G_0) phase of the cell cycle. The rapidity with which these genes become activated, often within minutes after a cardiac myocyte is overloaded, indicates that their activation does not require protein synthesis; instead, most immediate-early genes are activated by phosphorylations and other posttranslational modifications. However, if the stress is sustained, additional *late-response genes* become activated in reactions that do require the synthesis of new proteins. Many late-response genes are activated by transcription factors whose synthesis is stimulated by the immediate-early genes. Both immediate-early and late-response genes play a pathogenic role in cardiac hypertrophy and heart failure.

Immediate-Early Response Genes

When the heart becomes damaged or is overloaded, proliferative signaling pathways initiate an immediate-early response in which >100 different genes are activated and deactivated. Genes whose expression is increased include nuclear transcription factor regulators like *c-myc*, *c-fos*, and *c-jun*, along with *ras*, which encodes the monomeric GTP-binding protein Ras, and *hsp-70*, which encodes a heat shock protein. The sequential appearance and disappearance of the mRNA encoded by these stress genes demonstrates that instead of responding in a monotonic fashion, the many genes that participate in the immediate-early response are activated at different times during the first minutes and hours after the onset of the stress and then inactivated at different rates over the subsequent hours and days. In addition to these temporal heterogeneities, there are spatial heterogeneities in the immediate-early response; for example, overload causes mRNAs encoding specific contractile protein isoforms to be upregulated at different times in various regions of the heart (Schiaffino et al., 1989).

The rich control of the immediate-early response can be seen in the behavior of *c-Myc*, a nuclear transcription factor expressed in proliferating cells (Henriksson and Lüscher, 1996). Because c-Myc induces the transcription of genes whose protein products regulate the cell cycle, it is not surprising that levels of the c-Myc protein are low and its mRNA (*c-myc*) is virtually undetectable in G_0, the quiescent state of the cell cycle. Increased c-Myc levels are associated with continuous cell cycling in malignant cells. In adult cardiac myocytes, which do not divide, overload-induced increases in c-Myc stimulate hypertrophy, activate apoptosis, and lead to preferential expression of fetal genes. Because c-Myc inhibits expression of adult genes during skeletal muscle myogenesis (Miner and Wold, 1991), reversion to the fetal phenotype in overloaded hearts is probably due in part to the ability of c-Myc, along with other mediators of the immediate-early response, to inhibit synthesis of protein isoforms that characterize the adult phenotype seen normally in terminally differentiated cardiac myocytes.

Heat Shock Proteins

Genes that encode *heat shock* proteins are among the first to be activated by stress; the rapidity of the upregulation of these genes is remarkable as even a single stretch of the adult rat heart can greatly increase their expression (Knowlton et al., 1991)! Heat shock proteins (the term reflects their rapid appearance shortly after cells are exposed to elevated temperatures) are also called *molecular chaperones* because of their ability to stabilize hydrophobic surfaces that become exposed in partially denatured proteins. Like an elderly relative who protects a susceptible youngster from associating with undesirable companions, heat shock proteins prevent the irreversible aggregations that denature damaged proteins in stressed cells. Heat shock proteins also promote refolding of damaged proteins, facilitate the natural folding of newly synthesized proteins, and regulate proliferative signaling by modifying the activity of several transcription factors. In the heart, upregulation of Hsp-70 heat shock proteins (so named because their molecular weight is about 70 kD) during the immediate-early response to pressure overload plays a protective role by inhibiting maladaptive growth; in addition, some smaller heat shock proteins have an antiapoptotic effect.

Late-Response Genes

The immediate-early response, which is transient, is followed by sustained activation of a different complement of genes called *late-response genes*. Unlike the genes expressed in the immediate-early response, late-response genes encode newly synthesized proteins, including mitochondrial components, cytoskeletal and myofibrillar proteins, enzymes, and transcriptional regulators like cyclins and CDKs. In response to overload, many of these newly activated genes encode fetal proteins and protein isoforms normally found during development of the fetal heart. Late-response proteins that stimulate the cell cycle probably play an important maladaptive role in patients with heart failure when efforts to push terminally differentiated cardiac myocytes out of G_0 increase their susceptibility to apoptosis.

Reversion to the Fetal Phenotype

A remarkable feature of the proliferative response seen in overloaded hearts is the reappearance of the patterns of gene expression normally seen in fetal life. This preferential expression of the fetal phenotype in stressed cardiac myocytes can be viewed simplistically as part of a failed effort of these terminally differentiated cells to proliferate. The functional consequences of this reversion of the heart to the fetal phenotype are complex. For example, increased expression of a low ATPase fetal myosin heavy chain, which replaces the higher ATPase myosin normally found in the adult heart (see Chapter 5), has detrimental effects because it reduces contractility by slowing the turnover of myosin cross-bridges, thereby worsening the hemodynamic abnormalities caused by chronic overloading (see Chapter 2). At the same time, however, this isoform shift reduces the rate of ATP hydrolysis by the heart's contractile machinery, which has a beneficial energy-sparing effect in the overloaded heart (see Chapter 5). Another important feature of reversion to the fetal phenotype is a decrease in the content of sarcoplasmic reticulum that reduces contractility, slows relaxation, and increases the heart's dependence on calcium derived from the extracellular fluid. Because both calcium entry and calcium efflux across the plasma membrane are accompanied by depolarizing currents, this feature of the reversion to the fetal phenotype contributes to the arrhythmias and sudden death commonly seen in end-stage heart failure (see Chapter 5).

STRUCTURAL CHANGES

A large number of architectural phenotypes can be found in human hearts (Table 4-7; see also Chapter 1). Those that appear and then disappear during embryonic development are not abnormal, nor is the physiological hypertrophy (the athlete's heart) that is induced by training. In contrast, the phenotypes that appear when the heart is damaged or chronically overloaded are pathological because they are accompanied by maladaptive changes that include reversion to the fetal phenotype, progressive dilatation, myocyte death, and fibrosis.

TABLE 4-7

Examples of Different Cardiac Myocyte Phenotypes

Normal Embryonic Phenotypes

Normal Adult Phenotypes

  Working myocardial cells
    Atrial myocardium
    Ventricular myocardium
  Specialized cells
    Nodal cells
    His-Purkinje cells

Physiologic Hypertrophy Phenotype
  The athlete's heart: exercise-induced hypertrophy

Pathological hypertrophy phenotypes

  Eccentric hypertrophy
    Volume overload (e.g., aortic and mitral regurgitation)
    Myocyte damage (e.g., viral or toxic myocarditis)
    Myocyte stretch caused by myocardial infarction
    Dilated cardiomyopathies

  Concentric hypertrophy
    Pressure overload (e.g., aortic stenosis, hypertension)
    Hypertrophic cardiomyopathies

Cellular Phenotypes

The possibility that changes in myocyte size and shape contribute to the abnormal architecture in overloaded hearts was suggested more than 40 years ago by Grant et al. (1965), who postulated that eccentric hypertrophy (dilatation) occurs when sarcomeres are added to cardiac myocytes in series, which causes cells to become longer, whereas parallel addition of sarcomeres in concentric hypertrophy causes the myocytes to become thicker (Fig. 4-31). This insight has been confirmed by studies of the size and shape of cardiac myocytes isolated from hypertrophied human hearts; in concentric hypertrophy, myocyte size is increased largely by a greater cross-sectional area, whereas cell length is increased in myocytes isolated from eccentrically hypertrophied hearts (Gerdes et al., 1994). The progressive dilatation (remodeling) seen in *chronic* systolic heart failure results from a combination of myocyte elongation and myocyte death, rather than changes in sarcomere length, because sarcomere length remains normal in both eccentric and concentric hypertrophy. Side-to-side slippage between adjacent cardiac myocytes, another explanation for ventricular dilatation, occurs in *acute* dilatation and contributes to the infarct expansion sometimes seen immediately after a large myocardial infarction.

    The different cardiac myocyte phenotypes in eccentric and concentric hypertrophy appear to be due to the ability of diastolic stretch to cause new sarcomeres to be added at the ends of these cells, which increases cell length, whereas increased systolic stress causes new sarcomeres to be added throughout the myocytes, which

Eccentric hypertrophy (remodeling)

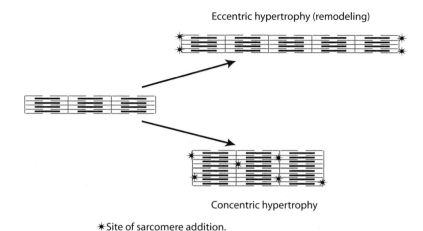

Concentric hypertrophy

✳ Site of sarcomere addition.

Figure 4-31: Cellular basis for eccentric and concentric hypertrophy. Eccentric hypertrophy, which leads to progressive dilatation (remodeling), occurs when sarcomeres are added in series at the ends of cells, which increases myocyte length. Sarcomere addition in concentric hypertrophy occurs throughout the cell, which increases myocyte width. From Katz AM (2006). *Physiology of the Heart*. 4th ed. Philadelphia, Lippincott Williams and Wilkins.

increases their width (Russell et al., 2000). Support for this view comes from evidence that different patterns of cellular hypertrophy are controlled by different signaling pathways. For example, cardiotrophin-1, a cytokine, induces cell elongation in neonatal cardiac myocytes whereas the α-adrenergic agonist phenylephrine causes the cells to become thicker (Wollert et al., 1996). Furthermore, different MAP kinases are activated when cardiac myocytes are stretched during diastole and during systole (Yamamoto et al., 2001), and activation of the MEK1-ERK1/2 pathways leads to concentric hypertrophy (Bueno et al., 2000) whereas activation of the MEK5 pathway induces eccentric hypertrophy (Nicol et al., 2001).

Molecular Changes

The possibility that heart failure is accompanied by molecular abnormalities in the contractile proteins was suggested almost 50 years ago, when the molecular weight of cardiac myosin was reported to increase threefold in an animal model of heart failure (Olson and Piatnek, 1959); however, subsequent studies showed that these data were flawed. The first solid evidence of a molecular change in failing hearts was published by Alpert and Gordon (1962), who found that myofibrils isolated from failing hearts have low ATPase activity. This abnormality, which provided a potential explanation for the depressed contractility in these patients, opened a new field of research that led to the discovery of molecular changes in most of the myofibrillar proteins, as well as in many of the membrane proteins that regulate cardiac function and several metabolic enzymes (see Chapter 5).

Fibrosis and Connective Tissue Deposition

At least two mechanisms can cause fibrosis of the walls of the failing heart: stimulation of matrix production when fibroblasts and other connective tissue cells are activated by FGF and other receptor tyrosine kinase ligands, and collagen deposition secondary to cardiac myocyte necrosis (see subsequent text). Both mechanisms probably contribute to the increased connective tissue content found in most failing hearts.

In addition to an increased amount of collagen, the type of collagen changes in failing hearts. During the initial hypertrophic response, the more elastic embryonic type III collagen is synthesized preferentially, whereas when the overload becomes chronic type III collagen is replaced by type I collagen, which has a higher tensile strength (Chapman et al., 1990; Marijianowski et al., 1995). Physiological hypertrophy, unlike pathological hypertrophy, is not accompanied by abnormal fibrosis (Weber and Brilla, 1991), which is one reason that the former lacks adverse long-term effects.

Proliferation of the extracellular matrix and fibrosis has both maladaptive and adaptive consequences. The increased connective tissue content impairs filling by reducing diastolic compliance, injures myocardial cells, and, by slowing impulse conduction, provides a substrate for arrhythmias. On the other hand, connective tissue proliferation can also slow progressive dilatation.

MYOCARDIAL CELL DEATH

Myocardial cell death is a calamity because the heart has little or no ability to replace its terminally differentiated myocytes. For this reason, myocyte death increases the work that must be done by the surviving myocytes, and so establishes a vicious cycle in which cell death increases overload, which intensifies the hypertrophic response, which accelerates cell death, which increases overload, and so on.

Cardiac myocytes can die in three fundamentally different ways: they can be programmed to die by highly regulated signal transduction systems that cause *apoptosis* (programmed cell death) and *autophagy* (programmed self-digestion), both of which are normal processes, or they can be killed by extrinsic factors (*necrosis* or accidental cell death). Stated briefly, apoptosis and autophagy can be viewed as cell suicide, whereas necrosis represents cell murder. All occur in failing hearts. Apoptosis and autophagy, which are coordinated with each other, share a number of regulatory components that also operate in proliferative signaling. Causes of cardiac myocyte necrosis include energy-starvation and possibly membrane damage caused by fatty acid accumulation. Energy-starvation is especially important in failing hearts because it increases cytosolic calcium, which can establish vicious cycles that increase energy demand and impair energy production (see Chapter 5); in addition, increased cytosolic calcium is pro-apoptotic.

The hallmark of necrosis, which can be viewed as a "catastrophic failure of cellular homeostasis" (Raffray and Cohen, 1997), is cell rupture, which is generally preceded by cell swelling and breakdown of the plasma membrane barrier. Because plasma membrane rupture releases reactive cellular contents that evoke an intense inflammatory response, necrosis generally leads to fibrosis. Increased plasma membrane permeability exposes the heart's contractile proteins to high calcium concentrations that cause explosive interactions between the myofilaments that literally tear cells apart (*contraction-band necrosis*). In apoptosis, on the other hand, the dying cells shrink, and their contents become condensed in fragments that undergo phagocytosis, which allows the cells to vanish without scarring. Although these extremes differ markedly, there are gradations between necrosis and apoptosis, and similar mechanisms can operate in both; for these reasons, it is not always possible to distinguish between these two forms of cell death. Autophagy, like apoptosis, allows cells to self-destruct, but does not involve phagocytosis.

Apoptosis

Before describing *apoptosis*, we cannot refrain from commenting on its pronunciation—and frequent mispronunciation. This term is derived from two Greek words, *apo* (away) and *ptosis* (falling), and there are defensible reasons to pronounce or not to pronounce the second "p" *(apoptosis' or apotosis')*. However, there is no basis for the mispronunciation *a · pop' · tosis,* which combines parts of the two words to create a third, nonsense, syllable. For this reason, there is no "pop" in apoptosis!

Apoptotic cell death is increased in end-stage heart failure, so that this normally rare cause of myocardial cell death contributes to the progressive deterioration of these patients. Apoptosis can be triggered by injury, such as caused by viruses, toxins, energy starvation, reactive oxygen free radicals, as well as by various proliferative signals. The concurrence between proliferation and apoptosis is apparent in rapidly dividing tissues, where programmed cell death eliminates cells for which the need has ended. Apoptosis helps prevent malignant transformation by killing cells with a tendency for unchecked growth, and is essential for embryonic development; for example, as many as half of the neurons that appear in the embryo are eliminated after they form synaptic connections with their target cells (Raff et al., 1993). If unneeded cells could not be eliminated during embryogenesis without provoking fibrosis, we would all be born a mass of scar tissue with gills, tails, and webs between our fingers and toes!

Apoptosis is highly controlled—death, after all, is irreversible. The process begins when a "decision" is made that a cell must die; these decisions can be initiated by activation of programs that lead to programmed cell death, or when withdrawal of apoptosis-inhibitory factors allows a preprogrammed death process to kill the cell. Apoptosis is mediated by regulatory programs that cause cells to shrink and eventually break up into membrane-surrounded fragments that often contain bits of condensed chromatin called *apoptotic bodies* (Fig. 4-32). Maintenance of plasma membrane integrity until late in the apoptotic process prevents release of reactive cellular contents; instead, fragments of the dying cell are engulfed by macrophages. In this way, apoptosis differs from necrosis, which is characterized by cell swelling and rupture. Another distinction between necrosis and apoptosis is the way DNA is degraded; in necrosis the DNA is broken down into randomly sized fragments, whereas DNA breakdown in apoptosis releases regularly sized fragments that resemble a ladder when they are fractionated on gels. The ability of phagocytes to ingest the cell fragments formed during apoptosis without provoking the inflammatory response seen when "raw" indigestible cell contents are spilled into tissues is like preparation of an elegant meal in which meats are boned, tenderized, and cut into bite-sized pieces; shells are removed from lobsters, shrimp, and clams; and fruits and vegetables are cored and peeled. In necrosis, according to this culinary analogy, the same ingredients are presented in raw form, often still alive, which causes the diner a stomachache that is analogous to the inflammation and scarring that characterize necrosis.

Control of Apoptosis

Signals that initiate apoptosis include *extracellular* messengers, such as G protein–coupled receptor agonists, growth factors, and cytokines, and *intracellular* mechanisms that are activated in injured cells. Some extracellular stimuli cause *adaptor proteins* to form a *death-inducing signaling complex* (DISC) with precursors called *procaspases.* The latter release cysteine proteases called *caspases* that hydrolyze tumor suppressors, cytoskeletal and nuclear regulatory proteins, and enzymes that participate in RNA splicing, cell division, and DNA repair and replication. Other caspases participate in regulatory signaling cascades. Some caspases contain a *death domain* that activates apoptosis when it binds to homologous death domains in adaptor proteins.

Extracellular proapoptotic pathways can be triggered when plasma membrane receptors called *Fas* bind to peptides, such as *Fas ligand (FasL)* (Fig. 4-33). The latter, which are cytokines that occur in both membrane-bound (mFasL) and soluble (sFasL)

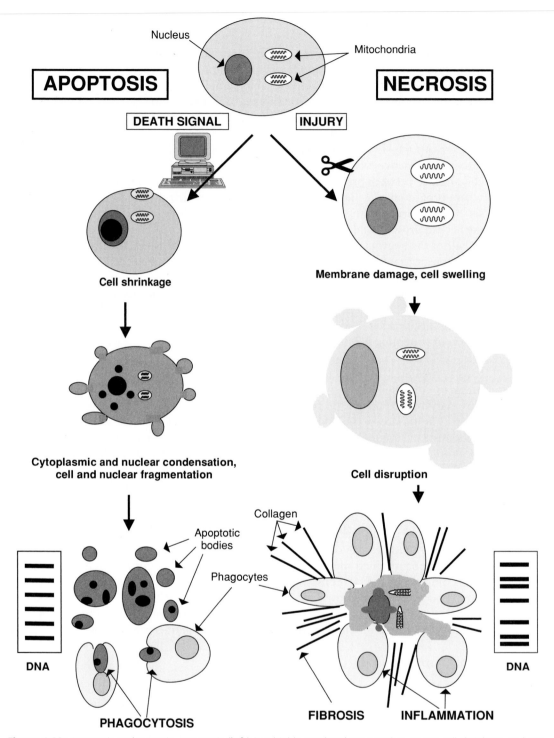

Figure 4-32: Apoptosis and necrosis. Apoptosis (**left**) is a highly regulated process that causes cell shrinkage and condensation of the cytosol and nucleus; this yields cell fragments, called apoptotic bodies that, because they are surrounded by plasma membrane, can be engulfed and digested by phagocytes without evoking an inflammatory reaction. DNA breakdown in apoptosis releases regularly sized fragments that, when fractionated on gels, resemble ladders. Necrosis (**right**) is generally caused when plasma membrane damage impairs its ability to serve as a permeability barrier, which causes cells to swell and eventually burst. The resulting release of cell contents initiates an inflammatory reaction that leads to fibrosis and scarring. DNA breakdown into random-sized fragments prevents the appearance of the ordered laddering seen in apoptosis. From Katz AM (2006). *Physiology of the Heart.* 4th ed. Philadelphia, Lippincott Williams and Wilkins.

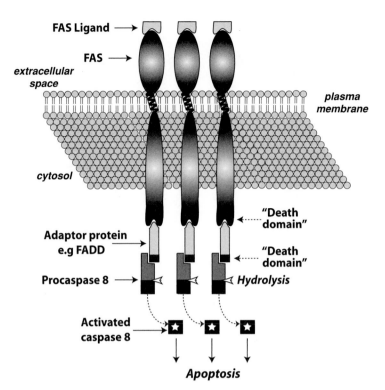

FAS Ligand

FAS

extracellular
space

plasma
membrane

cytosol

"Death
domain"

Adaptor protein
e.g FADD

"Death
domain"

Procaspase 8

Hydrolysis

Activated
caspase 8

Apoptosis

Figure 4-33: Extracellular proapoptotic pathways. Cytokines called Fas ligands (FasL) bind to Fas, which are plasma membrane receptors that contain FASL-binding and death domains. Binding of FasL to Fas causes the latter to form a trimeric aggregate in which the death domains interact with adaptor proteins like FADD, which also contain death domains, and procaspase 8. These aggregates activate caspase 8 and other enzymes that break down various cell constituents.

forms, initiate apoptosis by activating a sequence of 70–90 amino acids in the Fas receptor called a *death domain*; additional death domains are found in other cytokine receptors, caspases, and several regulatory proteins. When bound to their ligands, Fas receptors form trimers in which the death domains bind to adaptor proteins, such as *FADD (Fas-associated death domain protein)* that contain additional death domains. Peptides that activate apoptosis can be synthesized when cells interact with activated cytokine receptors and gp130. Triggers for apoptosis include functional mediators like norepinephrine, angiotensin II, and endothelin, along with cytoskeletal deformation and many of the proliferative signaling pathways described in this chapter. Some extracellular signaling molecules, including activators of the PI3K-Akt pathway and a cytosolic protein called *FLIP* (Fas ligand inhibitory protein), inhibit apoptosis.

Intracellular proapoptotic pathways play an important role in causing programmed cell death when the heart is damaged, becomes energy starved, or is calcium overloaded. All can open pores in the mitochondrial inner membrane that release *cytochrome C*, an electron carrier that participates in oxidative phosphorylation (Fig. 4-34). These pathways are controlled by members of a peptide family called Bcl-2 (an abbreviation for *B-cell lymphoma/leukemia 2 gene*) that can be both proapoptotic and antiapoptotic: Some, like *Bak, Bax, Bad, Bid, Bim, Bmf,* and *Nix* promote cell death, while others (e.g., *Bcl-2* and *Bcl-x$_L$*) compete at the mitochondrial surface to suppress this process (Fig. 4-34). Once in the cytosol, cytochrome c binds to *procaspase 9* and *Apaf-1 (apoptotic protease activating factor-1)*, an adaptor protein whose function is similar to that of FADD, to form an *apoptosome* containing activated *caspase 9* that can initiate, accelerate, and amplify apoptotic pathways.

The transcription factor *p53*, a major regulator of cell survival, has been called the "master watchman" of the genome because it regulates cell cycling in normally proliferating cells but is proapoptotic in damaged cells (Saini and Walker, 1998). These effects allow p53 to help decide the fate of an injured cell. When the damage

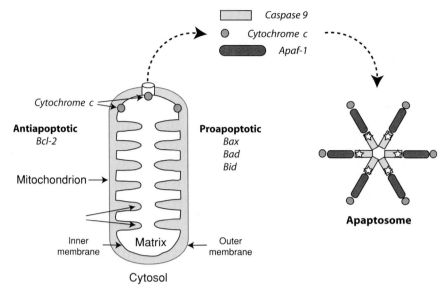

Figure 4-34: Intracellular proapoptotic pathways. Opening of pores in the mitochondrial inner membrane releases cytochrome C, which interacts with Apaf-1 and procaspase 9 to form apoptosomes that contain activated caspase 9. These pathways are controlled by Bcl-2 and related peptides, some of which favor cell death (e.g., Bax, Bad, and Bid), while others (e.g., Bcl-2) are antiapoptotic.

is mild, p53 favors DNA repair by shutting down the cell cycle, whereas when an injury is so severe that the DNA damage cannot be repaired, its proapoptotic effects kills the cell. In proliferating tissues, the proapoptotic effect of p53 helps prevent malignant transformation by eliminating severely damaged, potentially transformed cells. In terminally differentiated cells like cardiac myocytes, where malignant transformation is rare, p53 serves mainly to kill badly damaged cells.

Autophagy

Autophagy, which can be viewed as a highly regulated process of cellular self-digestion, has been suggested to be an adaptive mechanism that helps preserve viability in stressed cells; for example, this process allows breakdown of cell organelles in single-celled organisms to provide amino acids and energy during periods of energy-starvation. Autophagy can also be cytoprotective by stabilizing DNA and by removing damaged proteins and cell organelles. Although this mechanism appears to be of transient benefit in overloaded hearts, autophagy, like apoptosis, eventually becomes maladaptive by destroying the terminally differentiated cardiac myocytes.

Adaptive and Maladaptive Hypertrophy

The hypertrophic response, which had dominated studies of heart failure in the 19th century (see Chapter 1), attracted little notice during the first half of the 20th century. It was not until the 1960s, when overload-induced hypertrophy was found to normalize wall stress in the hearts of patients with valvular disease (Sandler and Dodge, 1963; Hood et al., 1968; Grossman et al., 1975), that this proliferative response was proven to be adaptive. At the same time, however, evidence that overload-induced hypertrophy is associated with shortened survival (Meerson, 1961) indicated that hypertrophy can also be maladaptive. Further support for the importance of maladaptive hypertrophy was provided when ACE inhibitors, unlike most other vasodilators, were found to prolong survival in patients with heart failure. Along with evidence that angiotensin II can stimulate proliferative signaling, this clinical finding suggested that inhibition of hypertrophic responses to angiotensin II might explain some of the benefits of these drugs (Katz, 1990a). These and other observations led to the hypothesis that mechanisms that cause the heart to hypertrophy initiate a "cardiomyopathy of overload" that reduces long-term survival in patients with heart failure (Katz, 1990b). Additional support for the view that maladaptive features of the hypertrophic response contribute to the poor prognosis in heart failure is provided by the ability of most mediators of the neurohumoral response to initiate proliferative responses (see Chapter 3 and previous discussion). Perhaps the strongest evidence that maladaptive effects of proliferative signaling shorten survival in this syndrome is the finding that β-blockers, in spite of a negative inotropic action that initially worsens the hemodynamic abnormality, improve prognosis in part by slowing, and sometimes reversing, the progressive dilatation of the failing heart (see Chapter 7).

Signaling Pathways That Mediate Cardiac Hypertrophy

Several of the important proliferative signaling mechanisms that mediate cardiac hypertrophy are summarized in Figure 4-35. However, this figure is incomplete because some pathways are omitted and many connections between pathways are not shown. Extensive cross talk between signaling cascades makes it impossible to assign a specific role to any pathway, but in spite of these and other complexities it is becoming clear that some signaling systems tend to cause pathological hypertrophy (progressive dilation and concentric hypertrophy), while others favor physiological hypertrophy (the athlete's heart). Pathways that evoke mainly maladaptive hypertrophy are activated by G protein–coupled receptors, mitogen-activated protein kinases, and histone deacetylases; adaptive and maladaptive signaling are more balanced in the case of the cytokine-activated pathways, while the hypertrophic response to activation of the PI3K/PIP$_3$/Akt pathway appears to be largely adaptive.

OVERVIEW AND SUMMARY

It seems appropriate to conclude this chapter with a few generalizations that highlight the role of proliferative signaling in the failing heart. Most important is that terminally differentiated cardiac myocytes normally have few options other than to contract and relax. Like stolid oxen, cardiac myocytes spend their lifetimes pulling a burden. The remarkable durability of these cells, which can survive for decades—and sometimes for a century—is due in part to the fact that, as long as their activity is restricted to the task of contracting and relaxing, they can last a lifetime. However, this durability carries a price, which is that efforts to modify this routine can have fatal consequences. If, for example, a heart is paced continuously at a rapid rate, it begins to fail and cells begin to die; similarly, sustained mechanical overload shortens cardiac myocyte survival. Thus, even though cardiac myocytes normally contract without pause for decades, their activity must remain within limits because forcing the cardiac pump to exceed its limits triggers responses that, while initially compensatory, eventually destroy the heart.

Another feature of proliferative signaling highlighted in this chapter is that even the simplest intervention that modifies cellular function evokes a multiplicity of responses. A stimulus as simple as an increase in diastolic volume not only evokes an immediate change in cardiac function (Starling's law of the heart), but because stretch

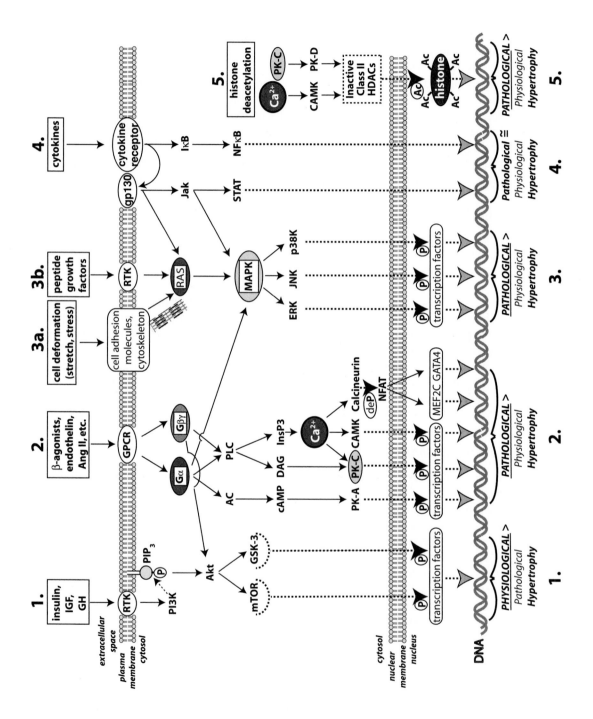

Figure 4-35: Major proliferative signaling pathways that mediate cardiac hypertrophy are divided into five groups; reading from left to right these are: (1) PI3K/PIP$_3$/Akt pathways, (2) G protein–coupled receptor (GPCR) pathways, (3) mitogen-activated protein kinase (MAPK) pathways, (4) cytokine-activated pathways, and (5) histone deacetylases (HDACs). The major response to the GPCR, MAPK pathways, and HDAC is *pathological* hypertrophy, whereas the major response to the PI3K/PIP$_3$/Akt pathways is *physiological* hypertrophy; cytokines appear to mediate both *physiological* and *pathological* hypertrophy. The PI3K/PIP$_3$/Akt pathway is activated when insulin, insulin growth factor (IGF) and growth hormone (GH) bind to receptor tyrosine kinases (RTK); the cascade involves phosphorylation of phosphatidylinositol trisphosphate (PIP$_3$) by phosphoinositide 3'-OH kinases (PI3K), which activates a protein kinase called Akt that activates a regulator of proliferative signaling called mammalian target of rapamycin (mTOR) and inhibits an inhibitory serine/threonine kinase called glycogen synthetase kinase 3 (GSK-3); the major response is physiological hypertrophy. Mediators of the hemodynamic defense reaction, such as β-adrenergic receptor agonists, angiotensin II (Ang II), and endothelin, activate mainly pathological hypertrophy when the activated GPCR interacts with the heterotrimeric G proteins to activate G_α and $G_{\beta\gamma}$, which participate in a number of signaling pathways. Binding of β-adrenergic agonists to $G_{\alpha s}$ activates adenylyl cyclase (AC) to form cyclic AMP (cAMP), which stimulates protein kinase A (PKA) to phosphorylate several transcription factors. Other G_α isoforms, notably $G_{\alpha q}$, along with $G_{\beta\gamma}$, activate phospholipase C (PLC) to form diacylglycerol (DAG) and inositol trisphosphate (InsP$_3$). DAG activates protein kinase C (PKC), which phosphorylates additional transcription factors. Calcium released from intracellular stores by InsP$_3$ activates protein kinase C and calcium/calmodulin kinase (CAMK), both of which phosphorylate transcription factors. Calcium also activates calcineurin, a protein phosphatase that dephosphorylates and activates the nuclear factor of activated T cell (NFAT), which activates the transcription factors MEF2C and GATA4 which lead to pathological hypertrophy. Pathological hypertrophy can also be stimulated when peptide growth factors bind to receptor tyrosine kinases (RTK) and when cell deformation activates cytoskeletal signaling pathways. Many of the latter are mediated by Ras, a monomeric G protein that stimulates mitogen-activated protein kinase (MAPK) pathways that include extracellular receptor-mediated kinases (ERK) and two stress-activated pathways, c-Jun kinase (JNK) and p38 kinase (p38K), all of which phosphorylate transcription factors that favor pathological hypertrophy. Cytokine-bound receptors regulate proliferative signaling when they release an inhibitory effect of IκB on the transcription factor NFκB; cytokine receptors also activate gp130-mediated signaling pathways that stimulate janus kinase (Jak) to activate transcription factors called signal transducer and activator of transcription (STAT) as well as MAP kinases. Cytokines appear to induce both *physiological and pathological* hypertrophy. Calcium and protein kinase C can also stimulate hypertrophy by inactivating class II histone deacetylases (HDACs), which by increasing histone acetylation, reduce an inhibitory effect on DNA transcription that favor pathological hypertrophy. Key: *Thin solid arrows* indicate signaling pathways, *dashed arrows with solid arrowheads* indicate phosphorylations (P), dephosphorylations (deP), and acetylations (Ac) that activate transcription factors. Factors that regulate transcription are indicated by *dotted arrows with shaded arrowheads*. Modified from Katz AM (2006). *Physiology of the Heart.* 4th ed. Philadelphia, Lippincott Williams and Wilkins.

deforms the cytoskeleton, it also activates a multigene response. Increased rest length has been known to increase the ability of a muscle to do work since the discovery of the length–tension relationship in the mid-19th century. Elucidation of the signaling function of the cytoskeleton has made this story vastly more complex as it is now clear that stretch also generates signals that modify cell size, shape, and composition.

Another generalization apparent in this and the preceding chapters is that cell signaling rarely proceeds in a straight line; instead, most stimuli generate an impressive array of cellular responses. An important corollary to this principle, which applies to patients with heart failure, is that efforts to modify cell signaling that are intended to do good, almost always do some harm. That the harm can exceed the benefit is apparent in the counterintuitive results of many of the clinical trials discussed in Chapter 7. Signal transduction should therefore be viewed as a floodlight rather than a spotlight. Although compensatory responses help the patient with heart failure stay on the safest path and avoid the many pitfalls and dangers that lurk alongside the road, the beam of these "compensatory torches" is often so broad that it not only helps the patient avoid danger but also attracts dormant monsters whose awakening can prove fatal. For these reasons, the challenges of modern therapy, much of which operates to modify cell signaling, require an understanding of both the benefits and the dangers that can accompany the responses in a given patient. In heart failure, this is best accomplished by the use of physiologically based medicine, where informed and thoughtful use of drugs and interventions, along with monitoring the individual responses, can reduce suffering and prolong survival without attracting demons that can injure these patients. Unfortunately, this is not an easy task because, as we are learning from the clinical trials that provide the basis for evidence-based medicine, what helps the average patient can harm specific individuals.

BIBLIOGRAPHY

General

Alberts B, Bray D, Lewis J, et al. (2002). *Molecular Biology of the Cell*. 4th ed. New York, Garland.

Bugaisky L, Gupta M, Gupta MG, et al. (1992). Cellular and molecular mechanisms of hypertrophy. In: *The Heart and Cardiovascular System*. 2nd ed. Fozzard H, Haber E, Katz A, eds. 1621–1640. New York, Raven Press.

Frey N, Katus HA, Olson EN, et al. (2004). Hypertrophy of the heart. A new therapeutic target. Circulation 109:1580–1589.

Gerdes AM (2002). Cardiac myocyte remodeling in hypertrophy and progression to failure. J Card Failure. 8(6 Suppl):S264–268.

Hill JA, Olson EN (2008). Cardiac plasticity. New Engl J Med 358:1370–1380.

Hoshijima M, Chien KR (2002). Mixed signals in heart failure: cancer rules. J Clin Invest 1098:849–855.

Izumo S (2004). Molecular basis of heart failure. In: Mann DL, ed. *Heart Failure*. Philadelphia, Saunders.

Lodish H, Berk A, Zipursky SL, et al. (2000). *Molecular Cell Biology*. 4th ed. New York, Freeman.

Mercadier JJ (2006). Determinants of left ventricular hypertrophy. Immun Endoc Metab Agents Med Chem 6:343–365.

Morita H, Seidman J, Seidman CE (2005). Genetic causes of human heart failure. J Clin Invest 115:518–526.

Novartis Foundation Symposium 274 (2006). *Heart Failure: Molecules, Mechanisms and Therapeutic Targets*. Chichester UK, Wiley.

Olson EN (2004). A decade of discoveries in cardiac biology. Nature Med 10:467–474.

Swynghedauw B (1999). Molecular mechanisms of myocardial remodeling. Physiol Rev 79:215–262.

Gene Expression, Cell Cycle

Bartek J, Bartkova J, Lukas J (1997). The retinoblastoma protein pathway in cell cycle control and cancer. Exp Cell Res 237:1–6.

Bernards R (1997). E2F: a nodal point in cell cycle regulation. Biochim Biophys Acta 1333:M33–M40.

Chiarugi V, Magnelli L, Cinelli M (1997). Complex interplay among apoptosis factors: RB, P53, E2F, TGF-β, cell cycle inhibitors and the Bcl-2 gene family. Pharmacol Res 35:257–261.

Dannenberg JH, te Riele HP (2006). The retinoblastoma gene family in cell cycle regulation and suppression of tumorigenesis. Results Probl Cell Differ 42:183–225.

Field LJ (2004). Modulation of the cardiomyocyte cell cycle in genetically altered animals. Ann N Y Acad Sci 1015:160–170.

Ford HL, Pardee AB (1999). Cancer and cell cycling. J Cell Biochem 75(S32):166–172.

Herwig S, Strauss M (1997). The retinoblastoma protein: a master regulator of cell cycle, differentiation, and apoptosis. Eur J Biochem 246:581–601.

Ravitz MJ, Wenner CE (1997). Cyclin-dependent kinase regulation during G1 phase and cell cycle regulation by TGF-β. Adv Cancer Res 71:165–207.

Scheuer J, Buttrick P (1985). The cardiac hypertrophic responses to pathologic and physiologic loads. Circulation 75(1 Pt 2):I63–I68.

Springer J, Filippatos G, Akashi YJ, et al. (2006). Prognosis and therapy approaches of cardiac cachexia. Curr Opin Cardiol 21:229–233.

Yurkova N, Shaw J, Blackie K, Weidman D, Jayas R, Flynn B, Kirshenbaum LA (2008). The cell cycle factor E2F-1 activates Bnip3 and the intrinsic death pathway in ventricular myocytes. Circ Res 102;472–479.

Proliferative Signaling

Akazawa H, Komuro I (2003). Roles of cardiac transcription factors in cardiac hypertrophy. Circ Res. 92:1079–1088.

Backs J, Olson EN (2006). Control of cardiac growth by histone acetylation/deacetylation. Circ Res 98:15–24.

Bueno OF, Molkentin JD (2002). Involvement of extracellular signal-regulated kinases 1/2 in cardiac hypertrophy and cell death. Circ Res 91:776–781.

Ceci M, Ross J Jr, Condorelli G (2004). Molecular determinants of the physiological adaptation to stress in the cardiomyocyte: a focus on AKT. J Mol Cell Cardiol 37:905–912.

Ceconi C, Curello S, Bachetti T, et al. (1998). Tumor necrosis factor in congestive heart failure: a new mechanism of disease for the new millennium? Prog CV Dis 41:25–30.

Chien KR, Knowlton KU, Zhu H, et al. (1991). Regulation of cardiac gene expression during myocardial growth and hypertrophy: molecular studies of an adaptive physiologic response. FASEB J 5:3037–3046.

Clapham DE, Neer EJ (1997). G protein $\beta\gamma$ subunits. Ann Rev Pharmacol 37:167–203.

Clerk A, Sugden PH (2006). Ras: the stress and the strain. J Mol Cell Cardiol 41:595–600.

Detillieux KA, Sheikh F, Kardami E, et al. (2003). Biological activities of fibroblast growth factor-2 in the adult myocardium. Cardiovasc Res 57:8–19.

Diwan A, Dorn GW II (2006). Decompensation of cardiac hypertrophy: cellular mechanisms and novel therapeutic targets. Physiology 22:56–64.

Dorn GW II, Force T (2005). Protein kinase cascades in the regulation of cardiac hypertrophy. J Clin Invest 115:527–537.

Downward J (2004). PI 3-kinase, Akt and cell survival. Sem Cell Develop Biol 15:177–182.

Gratton J-P, Bernatchez P, Sessa WC (2004). Caveolae and caveolins in the cardiovascular system. Circ Res 94:1408–1417.

Hefti MA, Harder BA, Eppenberger HM, et al. (1997). Signaling pathways in cardiac myocyte hypertrophy. J Mol Cell Cardiol 29:2873–2892.

Ichijo H (1999). From receptors to stress-activated MAP kinases Oncogene 18:6087–6093.

Kardami E, Jiang Z-S, Jimenez SK, et al. (2004). Fibroblast growth factor 2 isoforms and cardiac hypertrophy. Cardiovasc Res 63:458–466.

Khan R, Sheppard R (2006). Fibrosis in heart disease: understanding the role of transforming growth factor-beta in cardiomyopathy, valvular disease and arrhythmia. Immunology 118:10–24.

Liang Q, Molkentin JD (2003). Redefining the roles of p38 and JNK signaling in cardiac hypertrophy: dichotomy between cultured myocytes and animal models. J Mol Cell Cardiol 35:1385–1394.

Lips DJ, deWindta LJ, van Kraaij DJW, et al. (2003). Molecular determinants of myocardial hypertrophy and failure: alternative pathways for beneficial and maladaptive hypertrophy Europ Heart J 24:883–896.

McKinsey TA, Olson EN (2005). Toward transcriptional therapies of the failing heart: chemical screens to modulate genes. J Clin Invest 115:538–546.

Molkentin JD, Dorn GW II (2001). Cytoplasmic signaling pathways that regulate cardiac hypertrophy. Annu Rev Physiol 63:391–426.

Natarajan K, Berk BC (2006). Crosstalk coregulation mechanisms of G protein-coupled receptors and receptor tyrosine kinases. Methods Mol Biol 332:51–77.

O'Neill BT, Abel ED (2005). Akt1 in the cardiovascular system: friend or foe? J Clin Invest 115:2059–2064.

Ono K, Han J (2000). The p38 signal transduction pathway: activation and function. Cell Signaling 12:1–13.

Petrich BG, Wang Y (2004). Stress-activated MAP kinases in cardiac remodeling and heart failure: new insights from transgenic studies. Trends Cardiovasc Med 14:50–55.

Prasad SVN, Perrino C, Rockman HA (2003). Role of phosphoinositide 3-kinase in cardiac function and heart failure. Trends Cardiovasc Med 13:206–212.

Rao A, Luo C, Hogan PG (1997). Transcription factors of the NFAT family. Regulation and function. Annu Rev Immunol 15:707–747.

Rosenkranz S (2004). TGF-β1 and angiotensin networking in cardiac remodeling. Cardiovasc Res 63:423–432.

Sekiguchi K, Li X, Coker M, et al. (2004). Cross-regulation between the renin-angiotensin system and inflammatory mediators in cardiac hypertrophy and failure. Cardiovasc Res 63:433–442.

Selvetella G, Hirsch E, Notte A, et al. (2004). Adaptive and maladaptive hypertrophic pathways: points of convergence and divergence. Cardiovasc Res 63:373–380.

Seo D, Hare JM (2007). The transforming growth factor β/Smad 3 pathway: coming of age as a key participant in cardiac remodeling. Circulation 116:2096–2098.

Simpson PC (1999). β-protein kinase C and hypertrophic signaling in human heart failure. Circulation 93:334–337.

Steinberg SF (2004). β_2-Adrenergic receptor signaling complexes in cardiomyocyte caveolae/lipid rafts. J Mol Cell Cardiol 37:407–415.

ten Dijke P, Hill CS (2004). New insights into TGF-β–Smad signalling. Trends Biochem Sci 29:265–273.

van Biesen T, Luttrell LM, Hawes BE, et al. (1996). Mitogenic signaling via G protein-coupled receptors. Endoc Rev 17:698–714.

van Bilsen M, van der Vusse GJ, Reneman RS (1998). Transcriptional regulation of metabolic processes: implications for cardiac metabolism. Pflügers Arch - Eur J Physiol 437:2–14.

Walsh K (2006). Akt signaling and growth of the heart. Circulation 113:2032–2034.

Wang Y (2007). Mitogen-activated protein kinases in heart development and disease. Circulation 116:1413–1423.

Widmann C, Gibson S, Jarpe MP, et al. (1999). Mitogen-activated protein kinase: conservation of a three kinase module from yeast to human. Physiol Rev 79:143–180.

Yano M, Ikeda Y, Matsuzaki M (2005). Altered intracellular Ca^{2+} handling in heart failure. J Clin Invest 115:556–564.

Zhang T, Brown JH (2004). Role of Ca^{2+}/calmodulin-dependent protein kinase II in cardiac hypertrophy and heart failure. Cardiovasc Res 63:476–86.

Epigenetics

Ataian Y, Krebs JE (2006). Five repair pathways in one context: chromatin modification during DNA repair. Biochem Cell Biol 84:490–504.

Chandler VL, Stam M (2004). Chromatin conversions: mechanisms and implications of paramutation. Nat Rev Genetics 5:532–544.

Couture J-F, Trievel RC (2006). Histone-modifying enzymes: encrypting an enigmatic epigenetic code. Curr Opinion Struct Biol 16:753–760.

Ducasse M, Brown MA (2006). Epigenetic aberrations and cancer. Mol Cancer 5:60.

Goldberg AD, Allis CD, Bernstein W (2007). Epigenetics: a landscape takes shape. Cell 128:635–638.

Gopisetty G, Ramachandran K, Singal R (2006). DNA methylation and apoptosis. Mol Immunol 43:1729–1740.

Henikoff S (2005). Rapid changes in plant genomes. Plant Cell 17;2852–2855.

Holmes R, Soloway PD (2006). Regulation of imprinted DNA methylation. Cytogenet Genome Res 113:122–129.

Kaminsky Z, Wang S-C, Petronis A (2006). Complex disease, gender, and epigenetics. Ann Med 38:530–544.

Klose RJ, Bird AP (2006). Genomic DNA methylation: the mark and its mediators. Trends Biochem Sci 31:89–97.

Mishima Y, Stahlhut C, Giraldez AJ (2007). miR-1-2 gets to the heart of the matter. Cell 128:247–249.

Mistelli T (2007). Beyond the sequence: cellular organization of genome function. Cell 128:787–800.

Rama TM (2007). Illuminating the silence: understanding the structure and function of small RNAs. Nature Rev Mol Cell Biol 8:23–36.

Richards EJ (2006). Inherited epigenetic variation—revisiting soft inheritance. Nature Rev Genetics 7:395–401.

Slotkin RK, Martienssen R (2007). Transposable elements and the epigenetic regulation of the genome. Nat Rev Genetics 8:272–285.

Wilson AS, Power BE, Molloy PL (2007). DNA hypomethylation and human diseases. Biochim Biophys Aca 1775:138–162.

Yang PK, Kuroda MI (2007). Noncoding mRNAs and intranuclear positioning in monoallelic gene expression. Cell 128:777–786.

Zaratiegui M, Irvine DV, Martienssen RA (2007). Noncoding RNAS and gene silencing. Cell 128:763–776.

Zufall RA, Robinson T, Katz LA (2005). Evolution of developmentally regulated genome arrangements in eukaryotes. J Exp Zool 304B:448–455.

Cytoskeleton

Assoian RK, Zhu X, Giancotti FG (1997). Cell anchorage and the cytoskeleton as partners in growth factor dependent cell cycle progression. Curr Opin Cell Biol 9:93–98.

Bennett V, Baines AJ (2001). Spectrin and ankyrin-based pathways: metazoan inventions for integrating cells into tissues. Physiol Rev 81:1353–1392.

Bennett V, Chen L (2001). Ankyrins and cellular targeting of diverse membrane proteins to physiological sites. Curr Opin Cell Biol 13:61–67.

Brancaccio M, Hirsch E, Notte A, et al. (2006). Integrin signalling: the tug-of-war in heart hypertrophy. Cardiovasc Res 70:422–433.

Flashman E, Redwood C, Moolman-Smook J, et al. (2004). Cardiac myosin binding protein C. Its role in physiology and disease. Circ Res 94:1279–1289.

Goldsmith EC, Borg TK (2002). The dynamic interaction of the extracellular matrix in cardiac remodeling. J Cardiac Failure 8(Suppl):S314–S318.

Granzier HL, Labeit S (2004). The giant protein titin. A major player in myocardial mechanics, signaling and disease. Circ Res 94:284–295.

Gustafsson AB, Gottlieb RA (2004). Mechanisms of apoptosis in the heart. J Clin Immunol 23:447–459.

Hillis GS, MacLeod AM (1996). Integrins and disease. Clin Sci 91:639–650.

Hoshijima M (2006). Mechanical stress-strain sensors embedded in cardiac cytoskeleton: Z disk, titin, and associated structures. Am J Physiol Heart Circ Physiol 290: 1313–1325.

Hsueh WA, Law RE, Do YS (1997). Integrins, adhesion, and cardiac remodeling. Hypertension 31:176–180.

Hu H, Sachs F (1997). Stretch-activated ion channels in the heart. J Mol Cell Cardiol 29:1511–1523.

Katz AM. Cytoskeletal abnormalities in the failing heart: out on a LIM?. Circulation 2000;101:2672–2673.

Komoro I, Yazaki Y (1994). Intracellular signaling pathways in cardiac myocytes induced by mechanical stress. Trends in Cardiovasc Med 4:117–121.

Kontrogianni-Konstantopoulos A, Catino DH, Strong JC, et al. (2006). Obscurin modulates the assembly and organization of sarcomeres and the sarcoplasmic reticulum. FASEB J 20:2102–2111.

Kudoh S, Akazawa H, Takano H, et al. (2003). Stretch-modulation of second messengers: effects on cardiomyocyte ion transport. Prog Biophys Mol Biol 82:57–66.

Lapidos KA, Kakka R, McNally EM (2004). The dystrophin glycoprotein complex signaling strength and integrity for the sarcolemma. Circ Res 94:1023–1031.

Ozawa E, Mizuno Y, Hagiwara Y, et al. (2005). Molecular and cell biology of the sarcoglycan complex. Muscle Nerve 32:563–576.

Pyle WG, Solaro RJ (2004). At the crossroads of myocardial signaling. The role of Z-discs in intracellular signaling and cardiac function. Circ Res 94:296–305.

Ross RS (2002). The extracellular connections: the role of integrins in cardiac remodeling. J Cardiac Failure 8(Suppl):S326–S331.

Ross RS, Borg TK (2001). Integrins and the myocardium. Circ Res 88:1112–1119.

Sadoshima J, Izumo S (1997). The cellular and molecular response of cardiac myocytes to mechanical stress. Annu Rev Physiol 59:551–571.

Saffitz JE, Kléber AG (2004). Effects of mechanical forces and mediators of hypertrophy and remolding of gap junctions in the heart. Circ Res 94:585–591.

Samarel AM (2005). Costameres, focal adhesions, and cardiomyocyte mechanotransduction. Am J Physiol Heart Circ Physiol 289:2291–2301.

Sussman MA, McCulloch A, Borg TK (2002). Dance band on the Titanic. Biomechanical signaling in cardiac hypertrophy. Circ Res 91:888–898.

Tarone G, Lembo G (2003). Molecular interplay between mechanical and humoral signalling in cardiac hypertrophy. Trend Mol Med 9:376–382.

Cytokines

Hall G, Hasday JD, Rogers TB (2006). Regulating the regulator: NF-κB signaling in the heart. J Mol Cell Cardiol 41:580–591.

Libera LD, Vescovo G (2004). Muscle wastage in chronic heart failure, between apoptosis, catabolism and altered anabolism: a chimaeric view of inflammation? Curr Opin Clin Nutr Metab Care 7:435–441.

Mann DL (2003). Stress-activated cytokines and the heart: from adaptation to maladaptation. Annu Rev Physiol 65:81–101.

McFalls EO, Liem D, Schoonerwoerd K, et al. (2003). Mitochondrial function: the heart of myocardial preservation. J Lab Clin Med 142:141–149.

Stroud RM, Wells JA (2004). Mechanistic diversity of cytokine receptor signaling across cell membranes. Sci STKE (231):re7.

Apoptosis and Autophagy

Baehrecke EH (2005). Autophagy: dual roles in life and death? Nat Rev Mol Cell Biol 6:505–510.

Crow MT, Mani K, Nam Y-J, Kitsis RN (2004). The mitochondrial death pathway and cardiac myocyte necrosis. Circ Res 95:957–970.

Foo RS-Y, Mani K, Kitsis RN (2005). Death begets failure in the heart. J Clin. Invest 115:565–571.

Giordano FJ (2005). Oxygen, oxidative stress, hypoxia, and heart failure. J Clin Invest 115:500–508.

Haunstetter A, Izumo S (1998). Apoptosis: basic mechanisms and implications for cardiovascular disease. Circ Res 82:1111–1129.

Hetts SW (1998). To die or not to die: an overview of apoptosis and its role in disease. JAMA 279:300–307.

Kidd VJ (1998). Proteolytic activities that mediate apoptosis. Ann Rev Physiol 60:533–573.

Kitsis RN, Narula J (2008). Introduction—cell death in heart failure. Heart Failure Rev 13:107–109.

Levine B, Kroemer G (2008). Autophagy in the pathogenesis of disease. Cell 132:27–42.

Manjo G, Joris I (1995). Apoptosis, oncosis, and necrosis. An overview of cell death. Am J Pathol 146:3–15.

Marín-García J, Goldenthal MJ (2008). Mitochondrial centrality in heart failure. Heart Failure Rev 13:137–150.

Mizushima N, Levine B, Cuervo AM, Klionsky DJ (2008). Autophagy fights disease through cellular self-digestion. Nature 451:1069–1075.

Movassagh M, Foo R S-Y (2008). Simplified apoptotic cascades. Heart Failure Rev 13:111–119.

Mowat MRA (1998). p53 in tumor progression: Life, death and everything. Adv Cancer Res 74:25–48.

Saini KS, Walker NI (1998). Biochemical and molecular mechanisms regulating apoptosis. Mol Cell Biochem 178:9–25.

van Empel VPM, De Windt LJ (2004). Myocyte hypertrophy and apoptosis: a balancing act. Cardiovasc Res 63:487–499.

Wyllie AH (1997). Apoptosis: an overview. Br Med Bull 53:451–465.

Stress Proteins

Bukau B, Horwich AL (1998). The Hsp70 and Hsp60 chaperone machines. Cell 92:351–366.

Chi NC, Karliner JS (2004). Molecular determinants of responses to myocardial ischemia/reperfusion injury: focus on hypoxia-inducible and heat shock factors. Cardiovasc Res 61:437–447.

Knowlton AA (1995). The role of heat shock proteins in the heart. J Mol Cell Cardiol 27:121–131.

Pratt WB, Toft DO (2003). Regulation of signaling protein function and trafficking by the hsp90/hsp70-based chaperone machinery. Exp Biol Med 228:111–133.

Sun Y, MacRae TH (2005). The small heat shock proteins and their role in human disease. FEBS J 272: 2613–2627.

REFERENCES

Alpert NR, Gordon MS (1962). Myofibrillar adenosine triphosphatase activity in congestive heart failure. Am J Physiol 202:940–946.

Beck G, Habicht GS (1991). Primitive cytokines: harbingers of vertebrate defense. Immunol Today 12:180–183.

Berridge M (1997). The AM and FM of calcium signaling. Nature 386:759–760.

Bourne HR (1995). Team red sees blue. Nature 376:727–729.

Bueno OF, De Windt LJ, Tymitz KM, et al. (2000). The MEK1-ERK1/2 signaling pathway promotes compensated cardiac hypertrophy in transgenic mice. EMBO J 19:6341–6350.

Carè A, Catalucci D, Felicetti F, et al. (2007). MicroRNA-133 controls cardiac hypertrophy. Nat Med 13:613–618.

Chapman D, Weber KT, Eghbali M (1990). Regulation of fibrillar collagen types I and III and basement membrane type IV collagen gene expression in pressure overloaded rat myocardium. Circ Res 67:787–794.

Cook PR (2002). Predicting three-dimensional genome structure from transcriptional activity. Nat Genet 32:347–352.

Egan SE, Weinberg RA (1993). The pathway to signal achievement. Nature 365:781–783.

Freeman LM, Roubenoff R (1994). The nutrition implications of cardiac cachexia. Nutr Rev 52:340–347.

Gerdes AM, Kellerman SE, Malec KB, et al. (1994). Transverse shape characteristics of cardiac myocytes from rats and humans. Cardioscience 5:31–36.

Goss RJ (1966). Hypertrophy versus hyperplasia. Science 153:1615–1620.

Grant C, Greene DG, Bunnell IL (1965). Left ventricular enlargement and hypertrophy. A clinical and angiocardiographic study. Am J Med 39:895–904.

Graves LM, Bornfeldt KE, Krebs EG (1997). Historical perspectives and new insights involving the MAP kinase cascades. Adv Second Messenger Phosphoprotein Res 31:49–61.

Grossman W, Jones D, McLaurin LP (1975). Wall stress and patterns of hypertrophy in the human left ventricle. J Clin Invest 56:56–64.

Hendrich B, Tweedie S (2003). The methyl-CpG binding domain and the evolving role of DNA methylation in animals. Trends genet 19:269–277.

Henriksson M, Lüscher B (1996). Proteins of the Myc network: essential regulator of cell growth and differentiation. Adv Cancer Res 68:109–182.

Hood WP Jr, Rackley CE, Rolett EL (1968). Wall stress in the normal and hypertrophied human left ventricle. Am J Cardiol 22:550–558.

Jirtle RL, Skinner MK (2007). Environmental epigenomics and disease susceptibility. Nat Rev Genet 8:253–262.

Kapadia S, Oral H, Lee J, et al. (1997). Hemodynamic regulation of tumor necrosis factor-α gene and protein expression in adult feline myocardium. Circ Res 81:187–195.

Katz AM (1990a). Angiotensin II: hemodynamic regulator or growth factor? J Mol Cell Cardiol 22:739–747.

Katz AM (1990b). Cardiomyopathy of overload. A major determinant of prognosis in congestive heart failure. N Engl J Med 322:100–110.

Knowlton AA, Eberli FR, Brecher P, et al. (1991). A single myocardial stretch or decreased systolic fiber shortening stimulates the expression of the heat shock protein 70 in the isolated, erythrocyte-perfused rabbit heart. J Clin Invest 88:2018–2025.

Levine B, Kalman J, Mayer L, et al. (1990). Elevated circulating levels of tumor necrosis factor in severe chronic heart failure. N Engl J Med 323:236–241.

Marijianowski MMH, Teeling P, Mann J, et al. (1995). Dilated cardiomyopathy is associated with an increase in the type I/type III collagen ratio: a quantitative assessment. J Am Coll Cardiol 25:1263–1272.

McClintock B (1950). The origin and behavior of mutable loci in maize. Proc Nat Acad Sci 36:344–355.

Meerson FZ (1961). On the mechanism of compensatory hyperfunction and insufficiency of the heart. Cor et Vasa 3:161–177.

Miner JH, Wold BJ (1991). c-myc inhibition of MyoD and myogenin-initiated myogenic differentiation. Mol Cell Biochem 11:2842–2851.

Nicol RL, Frey N, Pearson G, et al. (2001). Activated MEK5 induces serial assembly of sarcomeres and eccentric cardiac hypertrophy. EMBO J 20:2757–2767.

Olson RE, Piatnek DA (1959). Conservation of energy in cardiac muscle. Ann N Y Acad Sci 72:466–478.

Pardee AB (1989). G1 events and regulation of cell proliferation. Science 246:603–608.

Pittman JG, Cohen P (1964). The pathogenesis of cardiac cachexia. N Engl J Med 271: 403–409, 453–460.

Raff MC, Barres BA, Burne JF, et al. (1993). Programmed cell death and the control of cell survival: lessons from the nervous system. Science 262:695–700.

Raffray M, Cohen GM (1997). Apoptosis and necrosis in toxicology: a continuum or distinct modes of cell death? Pharmacol Ther 75:153–177.

Ring PA (1950). Myocardial regeneration in experimental ischaemic lesions of the heart. J Path Bact 62:21–27.

Roberts SGE, Green MR (1995). Dichotomous regulators. Nature 375:105–106.

Robertson KD (2005). DNA methylation and human disease. Nat Rev Genet 6:597–610.

Rodenhiser D, Mann M (2007). Epigenetics and human disease: translating basic biology into clinical applications. Canad Med Assn J 174:341–348.

Rumyantsev PP (1977). Interrelations of the proliferation and differentiation of processes during cardiac myogenesis and regeneration. Int Rev Cytol 51:187–273.

Russell B, Motlagh GHG, Ashley WW (2000). Form follows function: how muscle shape is regulated by work. J Appl Physiol 88:1127–1132.

Saini KS, Walker NI (1998). Biochemical and molecular mechanisms regulating apoptosis. Mol Cell Bioochem 178:9–25.

Sandler H, Dodge HT (1963). Left ventricular tension and stress in man. Circ Res 13: 91–104.

Schiaffino S, Samuel JL, Sassoon D, et al. (1989). Nonsynchronous accumulation of α-skeletal actin and β-myosin heavy chain mRNAs during early stages of pressure-overload–induced cardiac hypertrophy demonstrated by in situ hybridization. Circ Res 64:937–948.

Shields DC, Harmoin DL, Nunez F, et al. (1995). The evolution of haematopoietic cytokine/receptor complexes. Cytokine 7:679–688.

Simonini A, Long CS, Dudley GA, et al. (1996). Heart failure causes changes in skeletal muscle morphology and gene expression that are not explained by reduced activity. Circ Res 79:128–136.

Tatsuguchi M, Seok HY, Callis TE, et al. (2007). Expression of microRNAs is dynamically regulated during cardiomyocyte hypertrophy. J Mol Cell Cardiol 42(6):1137–1141. [Epub 2007 Apr 14.]

Thomas RD, Silverton NP, Burkinshaw L, et al. (1979). Potassium depletion and tissue loss in chronic heart disease. Lancet 2:9–11.

Timmerman LA, Clipstone NA, Ho SN, et al. (1996). Rapid shuttling of NF-AT in discrimination of Ca^{2+} signals and immunosuppression. Nature 383:837–840.

Uozumi H, Hiroi Y, Zou Y, et al. (2001). gp130 plays a critical role in pressure overload-induced cardiac hypertrophy. J Biol Chem 276:23115–23119.

van Rooij E, Sutherland LB, Qi X, et al. (2007). Control of stress-dependent cardiac growth and gene expression by a MicroRNA. Science 316:575–579.

Vescovo G, Serafini F, Tenderini P, et al. (1996). Specific changes in skeletal muscle myosin heavy chain composition in cardiac failure: differences compared with disuse atrophy as assessed on microbiopsies by high resolution electrophoresis. Heart 76:337–343.

Waddington CH (1942). The epigenotype. Endeavor 1:18–20.

Weber KT, Brilla CG (1991). Pathological hypertrophy and cardiac interstitium. Fibrosis and the renin-angiotensin-aldosterone system. Circulation 83:1849–1865.

Wollert KC, Taga T, Saito M, et al. (1996). Corticotrophin-1 activates a distinct form of cardiac muscle cell hypertrophy. Assembly of sarcomeric units in series via gp130/leukemia inhibitory factor receptor-dependent pathways. J Biol Chem 271:9535–9545.

Yamamoto K, Dang QN, Maeda Y, et al. (2001). Regulation of cardiac myocyte mechanotransduction by the cardiac cycle. Circulation 103:1459–1464.

Yang B, Lin H, Xiao J, et al. (2007). The muscle-specific microRNA miR-1 regulates cardiac arrhythmogenic potential by targeting GJA1 and KCNJ2. Nat Med 13:486–491.

Zhao Y, Ransom JF, Li A, et al. (2007). Dysregulation of cardiogenesis, cardiac conduction, and cell cycle in mice lacking miRNA-1-2. Cell 129:303–317.

CHAPTER 5

Cellular and Molecular Abnormalities in the Failing Heart

Arnold M. Katz • Marvin A. Konstam

Abnormalities in myocardial contraction and relaxation are found in virtually every patient with heart failure. These can be primary, where the underlying disease process involves the cardiac myocytes, but cellular and molecular changes in failing hearts are more commonly initiated when otherwise normal myocytes are subjected to abnormal neurohumoral signaling and various forms of chronic overloading. It is reasonable to ask what these abnormalities are and how they influence the clinical manifestations and course of heart failure, but unfortunately there are no simple answers to these questions. This is due in part to inconsistencies in the findings obtained from various animal models in which different stresses are used to cause heart failure; these include chronic pressure overload, myocardial infarction, and rapid incessant pacing. More recently, transgenic animal models have been used to define etiology, but inconsistencies remain because of species and other genetic differences, examination of tissue obtained at different stages of the syndrome, and variables such as diet and exercise. It is sometimes stated, for example, that transgenic mice in which a major protein has been knocked out or modified show no evidence of heart failure, but most of these studies describe caged mice, where the hearts are not stressed; one wonders how these animals would perform when faced with a hungry cat. Cellular and molecular data from human heart failure are also inconsistent, due partly to the many causes of this syndrome and effects of treatment. Furthermore, most tissue used in these clinical studies is obtained at the time of heart transplant, which of course represents end-stage disease. In spite of these daunting challenges, much valuable information has been obtained. The following attempt to summarize these data, while tenuous, provides clues as to what can go wrong in failing hearts, and so can help define guidelines for rational therapeutic approaches for this syndrome.

Two different mechanisms can depress ejection and impair filling in failing hearts (Table 5-1). The first comprises functional abnormalities that modify the behavior of otherwise normal proteins, membranes, and other structures responsible for such features of cardiac performance as excitation, excitation–contraction coupling, contraction, relaxation, and energy metabolism. These changes can be initiated when mediators of the neurohumoral response and other functional signals cause covalent posttranslational modifications such as protein phosphorylations, dephosphorylations, and acetylations (see Chapter 3), and by metabolic abnormalities like energy starvation, acidosis, and calcium overload. The second mechanism, which allows proliferative signals to change the composition, size, and shape of the heart, gives rise to various architectural phenotypes of cardiac hypertrophy, fibrosis, apoptosis, changes in myocyte structure, and molecular abnormalities such as reversion to the

TABLE 5-1

Two Mechanisms That Can Depress Ejection and Impair Filling in Failing Hearts

Functional Abnormalities: Changes in the Properties of Otherwise Normal Proteins, Membranes, and Other Structures
  Covalent posttranslational changes
    Phosphorylations
    Dephosphorylations
    Acetylations
  Metabolic abnormalities
    Energy starvation
    Acidosis
    Calcium overload

Proliferative Abnormalities: Changes in the Composition, Size, and Shape of the Heart
  Architectural changes
    Hypertrophy
    Remodeling
  Fibrosis
  Apoptosis
  Autophagy
  Changes in myocyte structure and composition
    Reversion to the fetal phenotype

fetal phenotype. The latter can be initiated by mediators of the neurohumoral response (see Chapters 3 and 4), chronic hemodynamic overloading (see Chapter 4), and familial cardiomyopathies (see subsequent text). In most patients with heart failure, functional and proliferative mechanisms play an important role in determining both the hemodynamic manifestations and clinical outcome.

OVERVIEW OF CONTRACTION AND RELAXATION IN THE NORMAL HEART

Cardiac contraction begins when energy-dependent interactions between the heart's contractile proteins are turned on by the passive, downhill flux of calcium into the cytosol and ends when this activator is actively transported out of the cytosol. *Excitation–contraction coupling*, the process that activates contraction in response to the signal generated by an action potential at the cell surface, triggers the delivery of calcium to high-affinity calcium-binding proteins that regulate the interactions between the contractile proteins. *Contraction* occurs when the latter transduce chemical energy released by ATP hydrolysis into the mechanical work that allows the cardiac myocytes to shorten and develop tension. *Relaxation*, which depends on calcium removal from the cytosol, is not simply a reversal of the processes involved in excitation–contraction coupling; instead, different structures activate excitation-contraction coupling and cause the heart to relax.

Cardiac Myocytes

Cardiac myocytes are arranged in a branched network in which specialized cell–cell junctions, called *intercalated discs*, provide mechanical linkages and allow free electrical communication between adjacent myocytes. Several types of cardiac myocyte are found in the adult human heart. These include the *working myocytes* of the atria and ventricles, *Purkinje fibers* in the atrioventricular (AV) bundle, bundle branches, and ventricular endocardium that are specialized for rapid conduction, and *nodal cells* in the SA and AV nodes that provide pacemaker activity and control atrioventricular conduction, respectively. Additional heterogeneity is seen at the molecular level; for example, working myocytes with different molecular phenotypes form a mosaic pattern in the walls of the heart (Sartore et al., 1981; Bouvagnet et al., 1984) that helps adapt form to function (Katz and Katz, 1989).

Almost half the volume of working cardiac myocytes is made up of the *contractile proteins*, which are organized in a regular array of cross-striated myofibrils (Fig. 5-1). Most of the remaining cell volume is occupied by *mitochondria* that generate the large amounts of high-energy phosphate required for contraction (Table 5-2). Two membrane systems regulate cardiac performance: the *plasma membrane*, which separates the cytosol from the surrounding extracellular space, and the intracellular membranes of the *sarcoplasmic reticulum*.

Myofibrils

The cross-striated pattern in working cardiac myocytes reflects the distribution of the contractile proteins in two types of filament: the more darkly staining *A-bands* made up of thick filaments and lighter *I-bands* that contain only thin filaments. Each I-band is bisected by a darkly staining *Z-line* which contains cytoskeletal proteins (see Chapter 4). The fundamental morphological unit of striated muscle, the

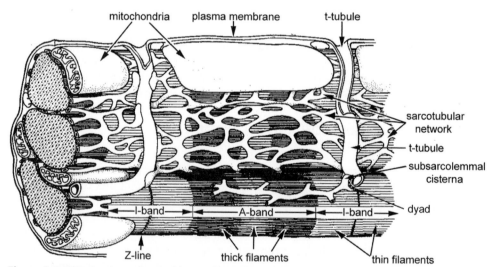

Figure 5-1: Ultrastructure of a working cardiac myocyte. Contractile proteins are arranged in a regular array of thick and thin filaments (seen in cross section at the left). The A-band is made up of thick filaments into which thin filaments extend from either side. The I-band contains only thin filaments that extend toward the center of the sarcomere from Z-lines that bisect each I-band. The functional unit of the contractile apparatus is the sarcomere, which lies between two Z-lines and contains one A-band and two half I-bands. The sarcoplasmic reticulum, an intracellular membrane system that surrounds the contractile proteins, consists of the sarcotubular network and subsarcolemmal cisternae. The latter form specialized composite structures with the transverse tubular system (t-tubules) called dyads. The t-tubular membrane is continuous with the sarcolemma, so that the lumen of the t-tubules contains extracellular fluid. Mitochondria are shown in the central sarcomere and in cross section at the left. From Katz AM (2006). *Physiology of the Heart*. 4th ed. Philadelphia, Lippincott Williams and Wilkins as modified from Katz AM, N Engl J Med (1975). 293:1184.

Morphology of a Working Myocardial Cell (Rat Left Ventricle)

Component	Percent of cell volume
Myofibrils	47
Mitochondria	36
Sarcoplasmic reticulum	3.5
Subsarcolemmal cisternae	0.35
Sarcotubular network	3.15
Nuclei	2
Other (mainly cytosol)	11.5

Modified from Page E (1978). Quantitative ultrastructural analysis in cardiac membrane physiology. Am J Physiol 63:C147–C158.

sarcomere, is the region between two Z-lines; each sarcomere therefore includes a central A-band and two adjacent half I-bands.

The thick filaments are made up of *myosin* and a number of cytoskeletal proteins, most important of which is *titin* (see Chapter 4). Other cytoskeletal proteins, including *myosin-binding protein C, M protein*, and *myomesin*, link the thick filaments in the center of the A-band where they provide lateral stability. *Cross-bridges* that project from the thick filaments represent the heads of myosin molecules that interact with the thin filaments. The latter are *actin* polymers that include *tropomyosin*, the three proteins of the *troponin complex*, and additional cytoskeletal proteins (see Chapter 4).

The lengths of the thick and thin filaments remain constant during contraction and relaxation, so that changes in sarcomere length are caused by variations in the extent of overlap between thick and thin filaments. In the resting heart the thin filaments extend almost to the center of the A-band (Fig. 5-2A), so that as

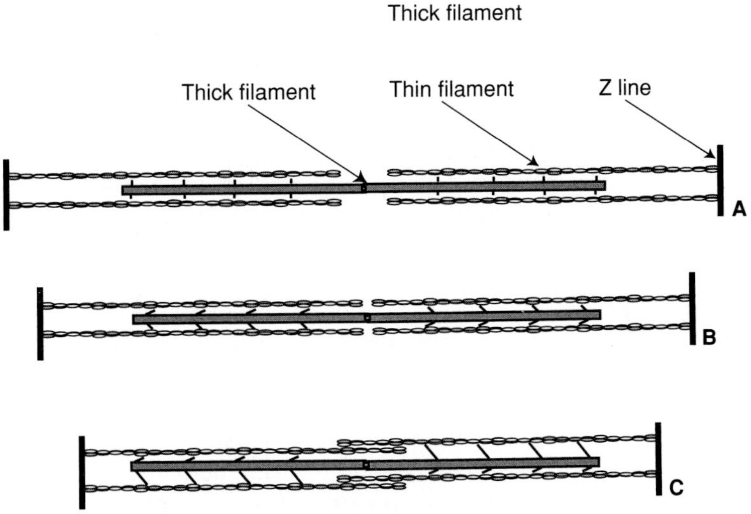

Thick filament

Figure 5-2: Schematic diagram of a sarcomere showing length-dependent changes in the overlap between thick and thin filaments. **A:** At the long sarcomere lengths in resting muscle, the ends of the thin filaments are pulled from the center of the A band. **B:** When the heart contracts, the thin filaments are drawn toward the center of the sarcomere. **C:** As the sarcomere shortens further, the thin filaments of adjacent I bands pass in the center of the A band (double overlap). From Katz AM (2006). *Physiology of the Heart*. 4th ed. Philadelphia, Lippincott Williams and Wilkins.

the heart contracts the thin filaments from either end of the sarcomere move toward the center of the A-bands (Fig. 5-2B). At short sarcomere lengths the thin filaments from each half of the sarcomere cross into the opposite half of the A-band, which causes double overlap (Fig. 5-2C).

Surface Membranes: The Plasma Membrane and Transverse Tubular System

The *plasma membrane (sarcolemma)*, which separates the intracellular and extra-cellular spaces, contains channels, exchangers, pumps, and other proteins that regulate cell composition and function, receptors and enzymes that participate in cell signaling, and adhesion molecules that link cells to each other and to the extracellular matrix. Many plasma membrane proteins are linked to the cytoskeleton and participate in cell signaling. Tubular invaginations, called *transverse tubules (t-tubules)*, extend from the surface membrane into the cell interior (Fig. 5-1). The t-tubules, which are open to the extracellular space and contain extracellular fluid, propagate action potentials rapidly into the cell and so play a key role in excitation–contraction coupling.

Internal Membranes: Nuclei, Mitochondria, and Sarcoplasmic Reticulum

Cardiac myocytes, like all eukaryotic cells, contain intracellular membrane-delimited organelles. These include the *nucleus*, which contains the cell's genetic material, and *mitochondria* that contain most of the oxidative enzymes that regenerate the ATP that provides the heart with energy. Mitochondria contain circular DNA that is characteristic of prokaryotes; this reflects the origin of these organelles as microorganisms that, hundreds of millions of years ago, crept into the cells of our progenitors where, in return for a nutrient-filled environment, these symbiotic invaders provide a generous supply of high-energy phosphate (Margulis, 1970). This origin explains why mitochondria in living cardiac myocytes are constantly changing shape by enlarging, contracting, branching, and fusing with one other.

Eukaryotes contain an internal membrane system, called the *endoplasmic reticulum*, that carries out protein synthesis and other functions. In cardiac myocytes, the major role of these internal membranes—called the *sarcoplasmic reticulum (SR)* or *sarcoendoplasmic reticulum (SERCA)*—is to take up, store, and release most of the calcium that activates contraction. The cardiac sarcoplasmic reticulum includes two specialized regions (Fig. 5-1): the *sarcotubular network*, which surrounds the myofilaments and pumps calcium from the cytosol into the interior of this membrane system, and flattened structures called *subsarcolemmal cisternae* that release calcium into the cytosol in response to plasma membrane depolarization. Cardiac myocytes contain *dyads* in which the subsarcolemmal cisternae and plasma membranes approach one another but do not fuse (Fig. 5-3); the narrow cytosolic space between these membranes contains electron-dense protein structures that are often called *feet* because they resemble the legs of a caterpillar (Franzini-Armstrong and Nunzi, 1983). The feet are a part of the sarcoplasmic reticulum *calcium release channels* that initiate contraction by allowing calcium to flow out of this intracellular membrane system into the cytosol. The calcium release channels, often called "ryanodine receptors" because they bind to this plant alkaloid, differ from the plasma membrane L-type calcium channels; the latter are also

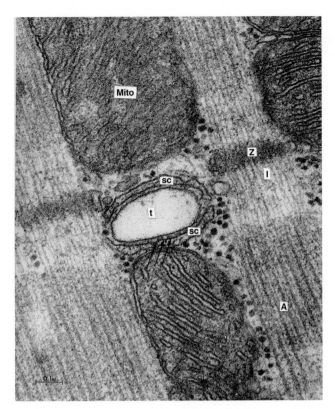

Figure 5-3: Cross section of dyad in rat ventricular muscle. The transverse tubular system (t), seen in cross section, lies between two subsarcolemmal cisternae (sc). Electron-dense "feet" (*arrows*) can be seen in the cytosol between the membranes of the t-tubule and subsarcolemmal cisterna. A, A-band; I, I-band; Mito, mitochondria; Z, Z-line. Scale = 0.1 μm. (Courtesy of Mrs. Judy Upshaw-Earley and Dr. Ernest Page. From Katz AM (2006). *Physiology of the Heart.* 4th ed. Philadelphia, Lippincott Williams and Wilkins.

called "dihydropyridine receptors" because they bind with high affinity to this class of calcium channel blocker.

Extracellular and Intracellular Calcium Cycles

In the middle of the 20th century, A.V. Hill (1949) noted that diffusion from the cell surface of large striated muscle myocytes is too slow to allow a chemical entering from outside the cell to activate their contractile machinery. This led Hill to postulate that excitation–contraction coupling depends on the release of an activator from within the myocytes or a process more rapid than diffusion. We now know that *both* postulates correctly describe activation of the adult human heart by calcium, the physiological activator. Unlike embryonic myocytes and smooth muscle, whose slow contractions can be activated by an *extracellular calcium cycle* in which calcium moves across the plasma membrane from the extracellular fluid into the cytosol, the larger more rapidly contracting myocytes in large striated muscles utilize an *intracellular calcium cycle* where much larger amounts of activator calcium are released from stores within the sarcoplasmic reticulum. In both, calcium enters the cytosol by passive diffusion through calcium-selective ion channels, but the channels are different. In the extracellular cycle, calcium enters the cell via L-type calcium channels in the plasma membrane in response to action potentials transmitted down the t-tubules, whereas in the intracellular cycle calcium release channels in the cardiac sarcoplasmic reticulum membrane admit a much larger amount of calcium into the cytosol in response to a calcium-mediated signal.

The heart relaxes when calcium is transported out of the cytosol by active "uphill" processes that utilize ion pumps and ion exchangers in both the plasma membrane and sarcoplasmic reticulum. ATP-dependent calcium pumps operate in both membranes, while a sodium/calcium exchanger in the plasma membrane uses energy provided by the sodium gradient across this membrane to lift calcium out of the cytosol into the extracellular space.

THE CONTRACTILE PROTEINS

The heart's contraction and relaxation depend on interactions among the six proteins listed in Table 5-3. These proteins interact with cytoskeletal proteins that support and organize the myofilaments, transmit tension to the surface of the myocytes, and participate in cell signaling (see Chapter 4).

Myosin

Myosin is one of a number of "motor proteins" that participate in cell motility, endocytosis, signal transduction, and sensory functions like hearing and vision. In the heart, myosin interacts with actin; the other motor proteins, *kinesins* and *dyneins*, interact with microtubules.

Cardiac myosin is a tadpole-shaped molecule made up of two heavy chains and four light chains (Fig. 5-4). In the "tail", two α-helical heavy chains are wound around each other in a coiled coil that provides rigidity to the thick filaments. The heavy chains contain an actin-activated ATPase that releases chemical energy used to power contraction; this enzyme is found in the paired "heads" which, along with the light chains, make up the cross-bridges that project from the thick filaments (Fig. 5-5). In the resting heart, where the thick and thin filaments are detached, the cross-bridges

TABLE 5-3

Contractile Proteins of the Heart

Protein	Location	Approximate molecular weight	Components	Salient biochemical properties
Myosin	Thick filament	500,000	Two heavy chains, four light chains	ATP hydrolysis interacts with actin
Actin	Thin filament	42,000	One	Activates myosin ATP ase, interacts with myosin
Tropomyosin	Thin filament	70,000	Two subunits	Modulates actin–myosin interactions
Troponin C	Thin filament	17,000	One, contains four E-F hand domains	Calcium binding
Troponin I	Thin filament	30,000	One	Inhibits actin–myosin interactions
Troponin T	Thin filament	38,000	One	Binds troponin complex to the thin filament

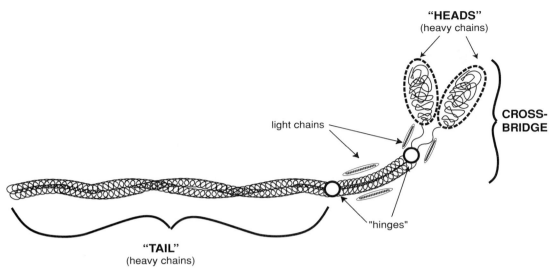

Figure 5-4: Myosin contains two heavy chains and four light chains. The "tail" of the elongated molecule is a coiled coil (two α-helical chains wound around each other) made up of the two heavy chains. The latter continue into the paired "heads" that, along with the light chains, form the cross-bridge. Myosin has two points of flexibility, or hinges: One lies below the heads, the other divides the tail into two unequal lengths. From Katz AM (2006). *Physiology of the Heart.* 4th ed. Philadelphia, Lippincott Williams and Wilkins.

are nearly perpendicular to the long axis of the muscle (Fig. 5-6). Following activation, the cross-bridges attach and detach from actin in a series of steps that, like the rowing of an oar, draws the thin filaments toward the center of the sarcomere. Although the lateral distance between the thick and thin filaments increases when the sarcomeres shorten, tension development and shortening velocity are only minimally affected by the change in lattice spacing because "hinges" in the myosin molecule (see Fig. 5-4) allow the cross-bridges to maintain contact with the thin filaments by extending the myosin heads from the thick filament.

Heavy Chains

Adult human atria and ventricles contain several myosin heavy chain isoforms (Table 5-4); additional isoforms are found in fetal and neonatal hearts. Human ventricles contain mainly the low ATPase β-myosin heavy chain along with a small amount (<10%) of a higher ATPase α-myosin heavy chain, while human atria contain two myosin heavy chain isoforms that differ from those in the ventricles. The

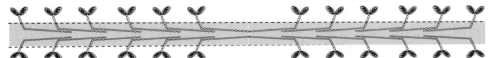

Figure 5-5: Myosin aggregates make up the thick filament whose "backbone", delineated by *dashed lines*, contains the tails of the myosin molecules along with cytoskeletal proteins including titin. The heads of the individual myosin molecules, whose polarities are opposite in the two halves of the filament (left and right), project from the long axis of the thick filament as the cross-bridges. The bare area in the center of the thick filament is devoid of cross-bridges because of the tail-to-tail organization of myosin. Modified from Katz AM (2006). *Physiology of the Heart.* 4th ed. Philadelphia, Lippincott Williams and Wilkins.

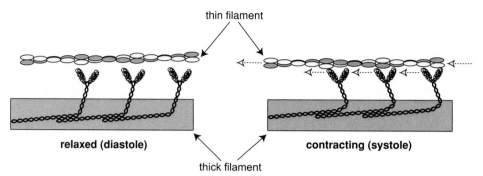

Figure 5-6: In resting muscle (**left**), the cross-bridges project almost at right angles to the longitudinal axis of the thick filament but do not interact with the thin filaments. During contraction (**right**), the cross-bridges interact with the thin filaments, which are drawn toward the center of the sarcomere. Modified from Katz AM 2006. *Physiology of the Heart*. 4th ed. 2006. Philadelphia, Lippincott Williams and Wilkins.

hypertrophic response to chronic overload is accompanied by an isoform shift that replaces the small amount of high ATPase (adult) isoform with the low ATPase (fetal) heavy chain. This isoform shift, which is part of the reversion to the fetal phenotype occurs in most overloaded and failing atria and ventricles where the lower myosin ATPase activity weakens the heart by slowing shortening velocity (Chapter 2).

Light Chains

Cardiac myosins contain two pairs of light chains, often referred to as *essential and regulatory light chains* (Table 5-4). These names refer to the fact that extraction of the essential light chains (also called LC_1, *ELC*, *MLC-1*, or *alkali-light chains*) inactivates myosin, whereas the regulatory light chains (also called LC_2, *RLC*, *MLC-2*, or *DTNB-* or *EDTA-light chains*) can be removed without abolishing myosin ATPase activity.

TABLE 5-4		
Cardiac Myosin Heavy and Light Chains		
HEAVY CHAINS		
Chamber	**Isoform**	
Atria	α (atrial)	High ATPase
	β (atrial)	Low ATPase
Ventricles	α (ventricular)	High ATPase
	β (ventricular)	Low ATPase
LIGHT CHAINS		
Chamber	**Isoform**	
Atria	LC_{1A}	Essential light chain
	LC_{2A}	Regulatory light chain
Ventricles	LC_{1V}	Essential light chain
	LC_{2V}	Regulatory light chain
	LC_{2V*}	Regulatory light chain

Five different light chain isoforms are found in human atrial and ventricular myosin. Two, LC_{1A} and LC_{1V}, are the essential light chains of atrial and ventricular myosin, respectively. The other three are regulatory light chains; two are found in the ventricles (LC_{2V} and LC_{2V*}) and one (LC_{2A}) in the atria. In chronically over-loaded ventricles, the atrial essential light chain LC_{1A} replaces some of the LC_{1V}. Because LC_{1A} is normally present in developing ventricles, this isoform shift is part of the reversion to the fetal phenotype. Myosin light chains are members of the family of *E-F hand calcium-binding proteins* that includes troponin C and calmodulin (see subsequent text). Human cardiac myosin light chains do not bind calcium but provide substrates for phosphorylations that regulate muscle-shortening velocity.

Actin

Actin, a highly conserved globular protein found in all eukaryotic cells, received its name because of its ability to activate myosin ATPase activity *in vitro*. Two isoforms are found in the human heart, *α-cardiac actin* and *α-skeletal actin*. Adult human ventricles contain mainly α-cardiac actin; α-skeletal actin, which is present in smaller amounts, is the fetal isoform. Actin can be stabilized *in vitro* as a monomer, called G-actin (G = globular), or as the filamentous F-actin polymer (F = fibrous). The latter, which makes up the backbone of the thin filaments (Fig. 5-7), is a macromolecular helix in which two chains of actin monomers are wound around one another like two strings of beads. Actomyosins reconstituted *in vitro* from purified actin and myosin can hydrolyze ATP and undergo physicochemical changes similar to those that occur during muscle contraction, but because they lack the regulatory proteins described in subsequent text, these two-protein actomyosins are not regulated by calcium.

Tropomyosin

Tropomyosin is a rigid elongated protein made up of two α-helical peptide chains, called *α-* and *β-tropomyosin*, that are linked by a single disulfide bond in dimers that can contain either or both isoforms. Although tropomyosin itself has no biological activity, when incorporated into the grooves between the two F-actin chains in the thin filament (Fig. 5-7), this protein regulates the interactions between myosin and actin.

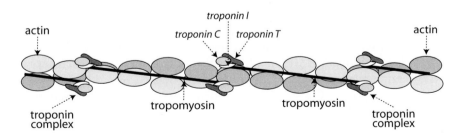

Figure 5-7: The thin filament. An F-actin polymer composed of two strands of G-actin monomers (*darkly and lightly shaded ovals*) wound around each other forms the backbone of the thin filaments. Tropomyosin (*dark lines*) lies in the grooves between the two strands of F-actin, where its ability to block the myosin-binding sites of actin is regulated by the three proteins of the troponin complex.

Figure 5-8: Cross section of the thin filament in resting muscle at the level of a troponin complex, showing relationships between actin, tropomyosin, and the three components of the troponin complex during diastole.

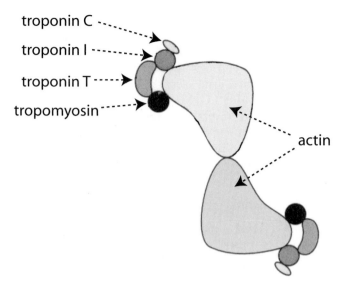

The Troponin Complex

The troponin complex includes three proteins (Table 5-3, Figs. 5-7 and 5-8) that, along with tropomyosin, regulate the interactions between the thick and thin filaments. *Troponin I* received its name because its most important effect is to inhibit actin–myosin interactions, *troponin T* binds the troponin complex to tropomyosin, and *troponin C* contains the calcium binding sites that participate in excitation–contraction coupling.

Troponin I

Changes in the strength of a labile bond linking troponin I to actin play a central role in regulating cardiac contraction. In the relaxed heart, where troponin C is not bound to calcium, troponin I binds tightly to actin and tropomyosin in a conformation that causes the latter to block the myosin-binding sites of actin. Calcium binding to troponin C loosens the bond linking troponin I to actin, which allows the latter to interact with the myosin cross-bridges. In this way, changes in the actin-binding affinity of troponin I that are initiated when calcium binds to troponin C provide a molecular switch that recognizes a rise in cytosolic calcium as a signal to initiate contraction.

Different troponin I isoforms are found in cardiac, fast skeletal, and slow skeletal muscles; a fourth troponin I isoform has been identified in developing muscle. Cardiac troponin I contains several sites for regulatory phosphorylations. One, which is catalyzed by protein kinase A (cyclic AMP-dependent protein kinase), reduces the calcium sensitivity of troponin C; this posttranslational response accelerates relaxation during sympathetic stimulation by favoring dissociation of activator calcium from the contractile proteins. Calcium/calmodulin-dependent protein kinase (CAM kinase) and protein kinase C also catalyze cardiac troponin I phosphorylations, but these reduce contractility by inhibiting interactions between the thick and thin filaments.

Troponin T

Troponin T, the largest of the three troponin components, mediates allosteric interactions between the proteins of the thin filament that influence the calcium sensitivity of tension development. In failing hearts, cardiac troponin T isoform shifts result from alternate splicing of the gene that encodes this protein. These isoform shifts modify both myocardial contractility and the calcium sensitivity of the contractile process (see subsequent text).

Troponin C and Other E-F Hand Proteins

Troponin C is one of a family of *E-F hand proteins* that includes the myosin light chains and calmodulin. All of these intracellular calcium-binding proteins contain peptide chains of ~30 amino acids in which two α-helical regions, designated E and F, are separated by a short nonhelical sequence. The term E-F hand reflects the fact that these α-helices resemble the extended index finger and thumb of a right hand which includes several oxygen-containing amino acids that form an anionic "pocket" that tightly binds calcium ions (Fig. 5-9). Most calcium-binding proteins contain two or four E-F hand regions, but amino acid substitutions in the calcium binding regions of some members of this family often cause the proteins to lose their ability to bind calcium with high affinity.

Three different mechanisms can allow E-F hand proteins to mediate the calcium-induced signal that activates muscle contraction. In the heart and mammalian skeletal muscle, troponin C located on the thin filament causes a rearrangement of the regulatory proteins when it binds activator calcium (see below). In a few other muscles, such as the scallop adductor, contraction is activated when calcium binds to an E-F hand myosin light chain instead of troponin C. In vascular smooth muscle, calcium binds to calmodulin, a soluble E-F hand protein, rather than an E-F hand protein in the myofilaments; the resulting calcium/calmodulin complex activates a *myosin light chain kinase (MLCK)* that initiates contraction by phosphorylating a smooth muscle myosin light chain. The ability of the latter, which is an E-F hand protein that has lost the ability to bind calcium, to stimulate contraction when it is phosphorylated in response to a calcium-mediated signal illustrates how various members of a single protein family can perform similar functions but in different ways.

Troponin C contains four E-F hand amino acid sequences. Some of these sequences bind only calcium and so are designated *calcium-specific sites*, while others, called *calcium-magnesium sites*, also bind magnesium. Because the ionized magnesium concentration in most cells is much higher than that of calcium, the calcium-magnesium sites remain occupied by magnesium and cannot mediate signaling by small changes in cytosolic calcium. For this reason, only the calcium-specific sites participate in excitation–contraction coupling by recognizing a rise in cytosolic calcium concentration as a signal to activate contraction. In human cardiac troponin C, only one of the four E-F hand sites serves as the physiological calcium receptor.

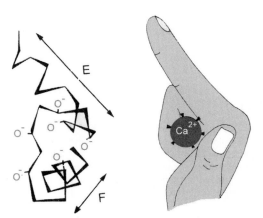

Figure 5-9: Structure of an E-F hand protein (**left**) showing two α-helical regions (E and F) separated by a nonhelical loop. This structure, which orients six oxygen atoms (O^-) to form a high-affinity calcium-binding peptide, is called an "E-F hand" because it resembles a right hand (**right**). From Katz AM (2006). *Physiology of the Heart.* 4th ed. Philadelphia, Lippincott Williams and Wilkins.

Calmodulin, which like troponin C contains four E-F hands, responds to a rise in cytosolic calcium by forming a calcium/calmodulin complex that exposes a hydrophobic surface on the calmodulin molecule. Interactions of this surface with the hydrophobic domains of several proteins, including members of a family of calcium-dependent protein kinases called *calcium/calmodulin kinases* (*CAM kinases*) participate in cell signaling by catalyzing protein phosphorylations (see Chapter 4).

Actomyosin

Actomyosins reconstituted *in vitro* from various combinations of the proteins described in Table 5-3 provide useful models of contraction. In the early 1940s, A. Szent-Györgyi found that ATP causes actomyosin threads made up of F-actin and myosin to shorten and, if a load is attached, to perform work. He also found that high concentrations of ATP could dissolve these threads, which demonstrated that ATP has two effects on actomyosin—the ability to energize the interactions between actin and myosin that cause muscle contraction and a relaxing effect that dissociates actin and myosin. Both of these effects occur in the living heart. During systole, ATP hydrolysis by the catalytic site of myosin provides energy for contraction, whereas ATP helps dissociate the thick and thin filaments during diastole by inhibiting interactions between the myosin cross-bridges and actin. Loss of the latter effect, which occurs only at very low ATP concentrations, causes rigor mortis in skeletal muscle and ischemic contracture in the heart (see below).

Regulation by Calcium

Calcium binding to troponin C regulates the properties of actomyosin by initiating a series of cooperative interactions among the proteins of the thin filament that, by shifting the position of tropomyosin in the grooves of the thin filament, exposes reactive sites on actin (Fig. 5-10). In the relaxed heart, where troponin C is not bound to calcium, tropomyosin lies toward the outside of the grooves of the double-stranded F-actin polymer where it prevents active sites on actin from inter-

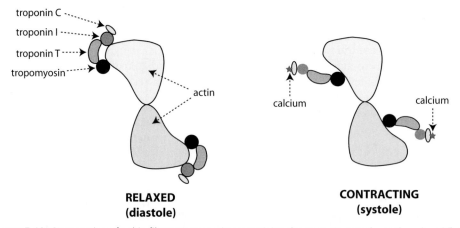

RELAXED
(diastole)

CONTRACTING
(systole)

Figure 5-10: Cross section of a thin filament at a region containing the troponin complex in the relaxed (**left**) and contracting heart (**right**). During diastole the troponin complex holds the tropomyosin molecules toward the periphery of the groove between adjacent actin strands, which prevents active sites on actin from interacting with the myosin cross-bridges. During systole, calcium binding to troponin C weakens the bond linking troponin I to actin; this alters the conformation of the regulatory proteins so as to shift tropomyosin deeper into the groove between the strands of actin, which allows actin to interact with the myosin cross-bridges.

acting with the myosin cross-bridges. Binding of calcium to troponin C weakens the bond connecting troponin I to actin, which by shifting tropomyosin from its blocking position, allows actin to interact with myosin. The heart relaxes when dissociation of calcium from troponin C returns tropomyosin to its inhibitory position.

In addition to providing the on–off switch that allows a rise of cytosolic calcium to initiate contraction, tropomyosin and the troponin complex modulate the intensity of the contractile process. Some of these effects are modified by troponin I and troponin T phosphorylation (see previous discussion) and an allosteric effect that reduces the calcium binding affinity of troponin C when protons bind to troponin I in the acidotic heart. The length–tension relationship and Starling's law of the heart are due largely to length-dependent allosteric effects that modify the interactions among the myofibrillar proteins (see Chapter 2). Isoform shifts involving these proteins modify cardiac performance and efficiency in hypertrophied and failing hearts (see below).

EXCITATION–CONTRACTION COUPLING

Excitation–contraction coupling utilizes two external membrane systems, the plasma membrane and t-tubules, along with the internal membranes of the sarcoplasmic reticulum, to deliver calcium to the contractile proteins (Table 5-5). The

TABLE 5-5

Membrane Structures That Participate in Cardiac Excitation–Contraction Coupling and Relaxation

Structure	Excitation–contraction coupling	Relaxation
Plasma Membrane		
Sarcolemma		
Na channel	Depolarization of cell surface	
	Open plasma membrane Ca channels	
Ca channel	Action potential plateau	
	Open intracellular Ca release channels	
Ca pump (PMCA)		Ca efflux
Na/Ca exchanger	Ca influx	Ca efflux
Na pump		Establish Na gradient
Transverse tubule		
Na channel	Propagate action potential into cell	
Ca channel	Open intracellular Ca release channels	
Sarcoplasmic Reticulum		
Subsarcolemmal cisternae		
Ca release channel	Ca release for binding to troponin C	
Calsequestrin	Ca storage, regulation	
Sarcotubular network		
Ca pump (SERCA2a)		Ca efflux

electrochemical gradient that drives calcium across the plasma membrane from the extracellular fluid into the cytosol is due primarily to a ~10,000-fold concentration gradient, augmented by the electronegativity within resting cardiac myocytes; calcium also enters the cytosol from the sarcoplasmic reticulum by passive diffusion. Both calcium influx and efflux across the plasma membrane are accompanied by depolarizing currents, but calcium fluxes into and out of the sarcoplasmic reticulum do not influence transmembrane potential because these internal membranes contain anion channels that allow chloride and phosphate ions to neutralize the charge carried by the positively charged calcium ions (see below).

In mammalian skeletal muscles, the amount of calcium released from the sarcoplasmic reticulum is generally sufficient to bind to virtually all of the troponin C, so that active state is normally at its maximum. However, the lower content of sarcoplasmic reticulum in adult mammalian cardiac myocytes provides only enough calcium under basal conditions to bind ~40% of the troponin C; this allows the intensity of the contractile response to be regulated by interventions that vary calcium release from the sarcoplasmic reticulum, the calcium affinity of troponin C, or both.

THE EXTRACELLULAR CALCIUM CYCLE

Calcium Influx across the Plasma Membrane

Calcium influx through L-type calcium channels provides the major source of this activator in smooth muscles and the embryonic heart, where contractions are weak and tension develops slowly. In adult working cardiac myocytes, however, calcium derived from the extracellular space provides only enough of the activator to bind to ~5% of the troponin C; the other ~95% is released from intracellular stores. Calcium that enters cells from the extracellular fluid does, however, play a key role in excitation–contraction coupling by triggering the release of the much larger amount of calcium from the sarcoplasmic reticulum (see below). Because some of the calcium derived from the extracellular fluid is taken up and stored by these internal membranes, where it is added to the calcium released in *subsequent* contractions, the amount of calcium that enters the heart via the extracellular calcium cycle is a major determinant of myocardial contractility.

Calcium Efflux across the Plasma Membrane

The calcium that enters the cytosol through the L-type calcium channels during each action potential must, at any steady state, be pumped out of the cell during diastole. Two mechanisms effect this uphill transport: a plasma membrane calcium pump and a sodium/calcium (Na/Ca) exchanger; the latter has a greater capacity than the plasma membrane calcium pump and so is responsible for most of this calcium efflux.

The Plasma Membrane Calcium Pump ATPase

The *plasma membrane calcium pump ATPase (PMCA)* is one of a family of *P-type ion pumps* that couple energy derived from ATP hydrolysis to active cation transport (Fig. 5-11); other members of this family include the sarcoplasmic reticulum calcium pump, the sodium pump, and proton pumps. Binding of calcium to a transport site on the cytosolic side of the membrane directly stimulates the pump. Increased intracellular calcium can also increase pump turnover indirectly, when the

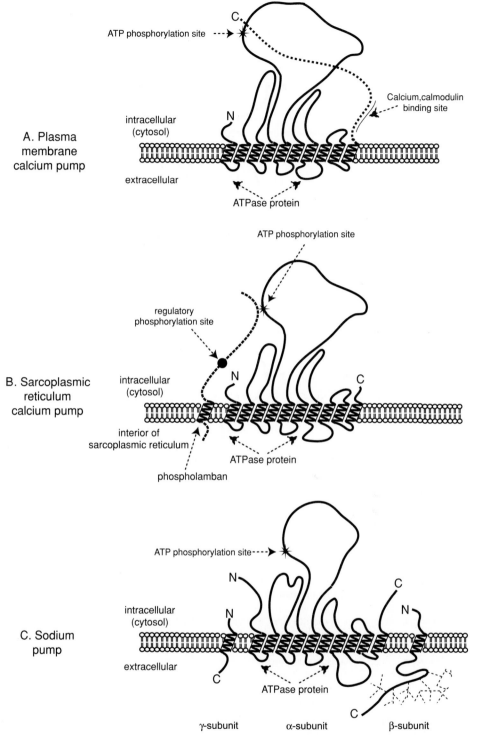

Figure 5-11: Three P-type ion pump proteins. The plasma membrane calcium pump (**A**), sarcoplasmic reticulum calcium pump (**B**), and the α-subunit of the sodium pump (**C**) all contain ten membrane-spanning α-helices and a large cytosolic domain that includes an ATPase site that provides the energy for active transport. The ions that are transported bind to several membrane-spanning α-helices. In the plasma membrane calcium pump, a portion of the C-terminal peptide chain provides a regulatory site that binds the calcium/calmodulin complex. Phospholamban, which regulates calcium transport into the sarcoplasmic reticulum, is homologous to the C-terminal portion of the plasma membrane calcium pump. The sodium pump contains three subunits: The larger α-subunit binds sodium, potassium, ATP and cardiac glycosides. A glycosylated β-subunit and a small γ-subunit regulate pump activity. Modified from Katz AM (2006). *Physiology of the Heart.* 4th ed. Philadelphia, Lippincott Williams and Wilkins.

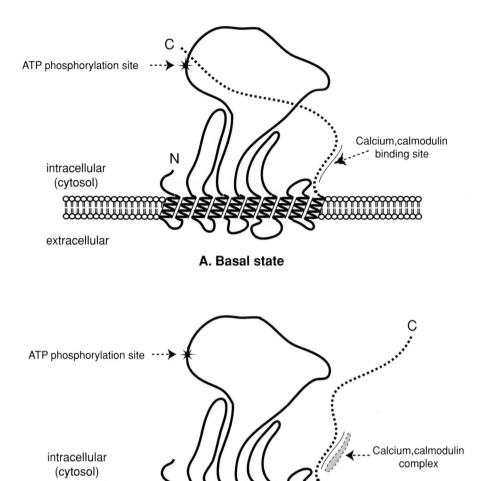

Figure 5-12: Regulation of the plasma membrane calcium pump by the calcium/calmodulin complex. **A:** In the basal state, where low cytosolic calcium concentration precludes formation of the calcium/calmodulin complex, a portion of the C-terminal peptide chain interacts with an intracellular regulatory site to inhibit calcium transport. **B:** Binding of the calcium/calmodulin complex to the C-terminal peptide inhibits calcium efflux by abolishing its inhibitory effect on the pump. From Katz AM (2006). *Physiology of the Heart.* 4th ed. Philadelphia, Lippincott Williams and Wilkins.

C-terminal region of the pump binds to the calcium/calmodulin complex (Fig. 5-12). This response helps cardiac myocytes avoid calcium overload by recognizing increased cytosolic calcium concentration as a signal to increase calcium efflux from these cells.

The Sodium/Calcium Exchanger

The most important protein that removes calcium from cardiac myocytes is the *sodium/calcium (Na/Ca) exchanger (NCX)*, an antiport that uses the sodium gradient across the plasma membrane to energize uphill calcium transport. The discovery of this exchanger has an interesting history. In the 1940s, the strength of cardiac contraction was found not to change when extracellular calcium and sodium concentrations were varied at a constant ratio, which indicated that contractility is regulated by a mechanism that is sensitive to the ratio between extracellular calcium and sodium (Wilbrandt and Koller, 1948). These and other findings suggested that calcium and sodium compete for binding to an exchanger that can transport either ion in either direction across the plasma membrane (Lüttgau and Niedergerke, 1958). According to this hypothesis, binding of extracellular calcium to the exchanger causes the heart to contract more strongly by increasing calcium influx, whereas increasing extracellular sodium weakens contraction by causing the exchanger to transport sodium, rather than calcium, into the cell. At the same time, calcium efflux was postulated to be determined by the relative concentrations of sodium and calcium that are available for binding to the intracellular side of the exchanger. The importance of Na/Ca exchange was established by Reuter and Seitz (1968), who found that the exchanger accounts for ~80% of the calcium efflux from the myocardium.

Discovery of Na/Ca exchange provided the key to understanding the positive inotropic effect of cardiac glycosides, which in the 1950s had been discovered to inhibit the sodium pump (Schätzmann, 1953). These drugs are now known to increase contractility when the increased intracellular sodium that results from sodium pump inhibition favors sodium efflux and so reduces calcium efflux by the exchanger. By retaining calcium within the myocytes, this response increases the amount of calcium available for release during excitation–contraction coupling (Repke, 1964).

The Na/Ca exchanger is an intrinsic membrane protein that includes nine membrane-spanning α-helices and a large cytosolic domain, called the *f-loop* (Fig. 5-13). The membrane-spanning helices, along with intervening amino acid sequences, mediate cation transport across the plasma membrane. The intracellular f-loop contains phosphorylation and other regulatory sites that alter the turnover of the exchanger in response to protein kinase-mediated phosphorylations, an allosteric effect of ATP, and changing intracellular concentrations of sodium and calcium (see below).

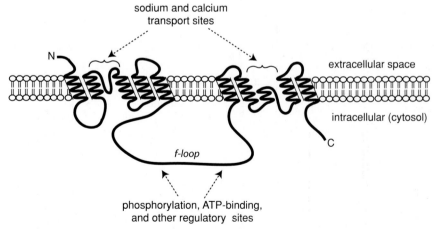

Figure 5-13: The sodium/calcium exchanger contains nine membrane-spanning α-helices organized in two groups that are linked by a large intracellular peptide chain. The sodium and calcium transport sites include regions of both groups of membrane-spanning helices along with hydrophobic amino acids that lie in the plane of the bilayer. The intracellular peptide chain includes a large f-loop that contains sites that allow the exchanger to be regulated by an allosteric effect of ATP, phosphorylations, and changes in cytosolic sodium and calcium concentrations. From Katz AM (2006). *Physiology of the Heart*. 4th ed. Philadelphia, Lippincott Williams and Wilkins.

A simple way to understand Na/Ca exchange is to view this antiport as a negatively charged carrier that, after binding either three sodium ions or one calcium ion within and outside the cell, moves the bound cations in opposite directions across the membrane (Fig. 5-14). The driving force for calcium efflux is the normal sodium gradient across the plasma membrane, so that the ultimate source of the energy for Na/Ca exchange is the ATP used by the sodium pump to establish the sodium gradient (see below).

The Na/Ca exchanger is *electrogenic* because, by transporting three sodium ions in exchange for one calcium ion, it generates an ionic current. This current, defined by the flux of positive charge, flows in the same direction as the sodium flux and is opposite to the movement of calcium (Fig. 5-14A); this can be remembered by the statement "current follows sodium." Although the currents generated by the exchanger are small, contributing only a few millivolts to membrane potential, they can be very important clinically. This is especially true in calcium-overloaded hearts, where increased calcium efflux generates a depolarizing current that can cause afterdepolarizations, torsades de pointes, and ventricular fibrillation (see below).

Although Na/Ca exchange does not require ATP hydrolysis, turnover of the exchanger is stimulated by an allosteric effect of ATP. This is one example of the general ability of ATP to accelerate ion fluxes by exchangers, channels, and pumps (see below). A corollary to this effect is that Na/Ca exchange is inhibited when ATP concentration falls in energy-starved failing hearts, which can exacerbate calcium overload. The exchanger is activated when it is phosphorylated by protein kinases A and C, and by calcium/calmodulin-dependent protein kinase (CAM kinase). In addition, elevated intracellular calcium increases the turnover of the exchanger by a regulatory effect that, like activation by CAM kinase, helps prevent calcium overload.

Figure 5-14: Overview of Na/Ca exchange. **A:** The exchanger can be viewed as a carrier (R) that can transport three Na$^+$ in either direction across the plasma membrane in exchange for a single Ca^{2+}. The directions of these fluxes are determined largely by cytosolic calcium concentration. This exchange generates an ionic current (*dotted line*) in which calcium efflux is accompanied by a depolarizing current and calcium influx by a repolarizing current; in both cases, current follows sodium. **B:** The exchanger can be represented as a well in which two buckets move in opposite directions; one bucket contains a single divalent calcium ion, the other three sodium ions. Modified from Katz AM (2006). *Physiology of the Heart*. 4th ed. Philadelphia, Lippincott Williams and Wilkins.

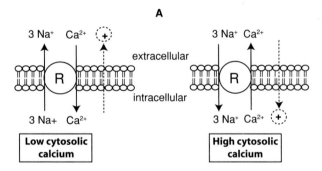

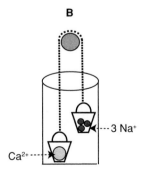

The Sodium Pump

The sodium pump (also called the *sodium-potassium ATPase* or *Na-K-ATPase* because its ability to hydrolyze ATP is increased when sodium and potassium are present together) exchanges the small amount of sodium that enters the cytosol during each action potential for the potassium that leaves the cell during repolarization. Because both sodium efflux and potassium influx are uphill processes, the sodium pump requires energy, which is derived from ATP hydrolysis. The energy cost of sodium pump activity is very high; for example, in nonmotile tissues like the kidneys the sodium pump accounts for 20% to 30% of the ATP consumed under basal conditions.

The electrochemical gradients established by the sodium pump are essential for cardiac excitability because they provide the driving force for the depolarizing sodium currents that activate atrial and ventricular myocytes and Purkinje cells, the repolarizing potassium currents that return membrane potential to its resting level at the end of systole, and the potassium concentration gradient across the plasma membrane that determines resting potential. The sodium gradient also energizes calcium efflux by the Na/Ca exchanger (see previous discussion), proton efflux by the Na/H exchanger (see below), and active transport of several substrates and metabolites across the plasma membrane.

The sodium pump includes three subunits (Fig. 5-15). The largest, the α-subunit, is a P-type ion pump ATPase (see Fig. 5-11) whose intracellular domain contains a phosphorylation site that uses chemical energy derived from ATP hydrolysis to perform osmotic work, along with several regulatory sites. The extracellular side of the α-subunit also contains the sites that transport potassium into the cell, while the sites that transport sodium out of the cell are on the cytosolic side. Cardiac glycosides inhibit the sodium pump when they bind to a site on the extracellular side of the α-subunit (see below); interactions of this site with the potassium-binding site explains why increased extracellular potassium reduces the sensitivity of the sodium pump to inhibition by cardiac glycosides, and why hypokalemia potentiates the response to these drugs. The smaller β-subunit, which is essential for normal transport activity, is a glycoprotein that includes a single membrane-spanning domain; the γ-subunit, like the β-subunit, regulates interactions between sodium, potassium, and the sodium pump.

The sodium pump is electrogenic because it transports three sodium ions out of the cell in exchange for two potassium ions that enter the cytosol (Fig. 5-16). The movement of positive charge by the sodium pump, like that by the Na/Ca exchanger (Fig. 5-14), is in the same direction as the flux of sodium ions, which provides another example where current follows sodium. The contribution of this repolarizing current to membrane potential is small, usually <10 mV. Under some circumstances this current can be of functional importance; for example, in injured cells where resting potential is reduced and sodium "leak" into the cell is increased, the outward current generated by the sodium pump helps maintain intracellular electronegativity. The arrhythmogenic effects of sodium pump inhibition, which are seen in patients given high doses of cardiac glycosides, are due in part to reduction of this repolarizing current, but a more important cause of arrhythmias following sodium pump inhibition is slowed conduction that results from resting depolarization. The latter occurs when reduced potassium efflux decreases intracellular potassium concentration and so reduces the electrochemical gradient responsible for maintaining resting potential.

The *cardiac glycosides*, which were the first class of drugs found to be useful in treating heart failure (see Chapter 1), have four major actions, all due to sodium

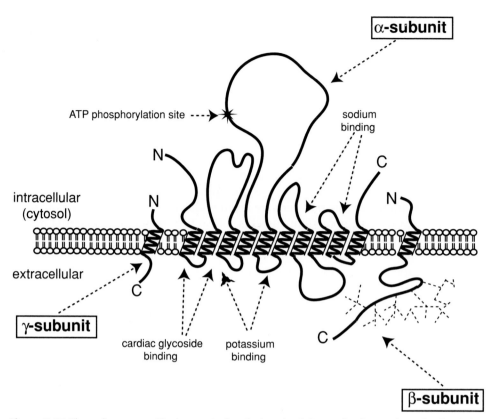

Figure 5-15: The sodium pump. The large cytoplasmic domain of the α-subunit contains a site that, when phosphorylated by ATP, provides the energy needed for active ion transport. The extracellular portions of several membrane-spanning α-helices bind potassium and cardiac glycosides, while sodium binds to membrane-spanning helices from the intracellular side of the membrane. Several sites on the intracellular domain of the α-subunit, along with the β- and γ-subunits, regulate sodium pump activity. Modified from Katz AM (2006). *Physiology of the Heart*. 4th ed. Philadelphia, Lippincott Williams and Wilkins.

pump inhibition. Their ability to increase myocardial contractility, which is traditionally viewed as the desired effect, occurs when sodium pump inhibition increases intracellular sodium concentration near a region of the plasma membrane that is rich in the Na/Ca exchanger. Because the higher sodium concentration at the cytosolic side of the membrane inhibits calcium efflux via the Na/Ca exchanger, less calcium leaves the cell, which, by increasing intracellular calcium stores, explains the positive inotropic effect. The second action, resting membrane depolarization caused by a fall in intracellular potassium concentration, is responsible for many of the arrhythmogenic effects of these drugs; this depolarizing effect is increased by the

Figure 5-16: Overview of ion transport by the sodium pump. Because three sodium ions are exchanged for two potassium ions, the pump generates an ionic current that follows sodium. From Katz AM (2006). *Physiology of the Heart*. 4th ed. Philadelphia, Lippincott Williams and Wilkins.

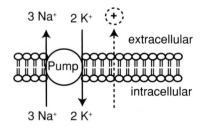

third action, reduction of the small repolarizing current generated by the sodium pump. However, a fourth mechanism now appears to account for many of the beneficial effects of the cardiac glycosides in heart failure. This consists of counterregulatory responses that are initiated when sodium pump inhibition in the brain stem increases vagal tone and reduces sympathetic activity. Together, these central reflexes decrease heart rate, contractility, and peripheral resistance and so have an energy-sparing effect that benefits the failing heart. Interactions between cardiac glycosides and potassium at extracellular sites on the pump, as noted in the previous discussion, explain why hyperkalemia, which displaces these drugs from their extracellular binding site, reduces their potency, as well as the dangerous potentiation of the cardiac glycoside effects by low serum potassium levels.

Several protein kinases regulate the sodium pump; for example, phosphorylation by protein kinase-A allows sympathetic activation to stimulate sodium transport. Pump activity is also regulated by acylation of the α-subunit and glycosylation of the β-subunit, and stimulated by an allosteric effect of high ATP concentration. Sodium pump activity is decreased in failing hearts by both isoform shifts and reduced concentration of this protein in the plasma membrane.

The Sodium/Hydrogen Exchanger

Because energy production is accompanied by the generation of protons, mechanisms are needed to prevent intracellular acidosis, which has several deleterious effects on the heart. The latter include inhibition of enzymes involved in energy production, a negative inotropic effect caused when protons compete with calcium for binding to the troponin complex, and inhibition of calcium fluxes that relax the heart. The normal intracellular pH is about 7.2, which is more alkaline than would be expected if protons were distributed according to their electrochemical gradient. This intracellular alkalinity is maintained by a symport, the sodium/bicarbonate transporter, and three antiports: a chloride/bicarbonate exchanger, a chloride/hydroxyl exchanger, and, most important, the *sodium/hydrogen (Na/H) exchanger (NHE)*.

Sodium/hydrogen exchangers use energy derived from the sodium gradient across the plasma membrane to transport protons uphill out of the cell; because the stoichiometry between proton efflux and sodium influx is 1:1, this exchange is electrically neutral. Na/H exchangers are members of a large and ancient superfamily of transporters found in both prokaryotes and eukaryotes; NHE1, the major isoform in the heart, is a glycoprotein that contains twelve membrane-spanning α-helices, an N-terminal portion that participates in the ion exchange reaction, and a large intracellular C-terminal domain that includes several regulatory sites (Fig. 5-17). Intracellular acidosis stimulates the Na/H exchanger in two ways: a direct response to increased proton concentration and an indirect effect that occurs when the protons bind to an intracellular pH sensor that increases the turnover of the antiport. Both increase intracellular sodium because increased proton efflux is coupled to increased sodium influx; this response increases contractility by reducing calcium efflux by the Na/Ca exchanger. NHE1 is activated by an allosteric effect of ATP and regulated by the calcium/calmodulin complex; other protein kinases phosphorylate the exchanger in response to agonist-binding to G protein–coupled receptors, receptor tyrosine kinases, and integrins. Linkage of the NHE1 to the actin cytoskeleton through a cytoskeletal "organizer" called *ezrin*, one of a family of ezrin-radixin-moesin (ERM) proteins that connect membrane proteins and the cytoskeleton, allows the

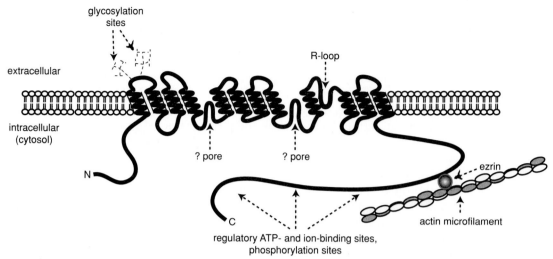

Figure 5-17: The sodium/hydrogen exchanger contains 12 membrane-spanning α-helices and a glycosylated extracellular region between the first and second helices. The N-terminal region, including the adjacent membrane-spanning helices, participates in ion transport, while the large intracellular C-terminal peptide chain contains phosphorylation sites that, along with ion-binding, ATP-binding, and calcium/calmodulin-binding sites, regulate the exchanger. Turnover of the exchanger is accelerated in the acidotic heart when protons bind to its intracellular surface. Ezrin, a cytoskeletal organizer that links the exchanger to actin microfilaments, allows the exchanger to participate in signal transduction. From Katz AM (2006). *Physiology of the Heart.* 4th ed. Philadelphia, Lippincott Williams and Wilkins.

exchanger to participate in the proliferative signaling systems that mediate the hypertrophic response to overload. The complexity of this control attests to the importance of the Na/H exchanger, which in addition to regulating intracellular pH, participates in signals that regulate both cell growth and cell death.

Impaired oxidative phosphorylation increases the susceptibility of failing hearts to intracellular acidosis by accelerating anaerobic glycolysis. The latter increases lactate production, which releases protons that are extruded by the NHE1 in exchange for sodium. Because the latter decreases calcium efflux by the Na/Ca exchanger, the net effect can be a vicious cycle where increasing calcium overload worsens energy starvation both by increasing energy utilization and further inhibiting oxidative phosphorylation (see below).

THE INTRACELLULAR CALCIUM CYCLE

Calcium Release from the Sarcoplasmic Reticulum

Action potentials initiate calcium release from the sarcoplasmic reticulum by a mechanism called "calcium-triggered calcium release," where the small amount of calcium that enters the cytosol from the extracellular fluid via the L-type calcium channels releases a much larger amount of activator calcium from within the sarcoplasmic reticulum (Fabiato, 1983). This is analogous to the firing mechanism of a flintlock musket, where the small charge exploded when the flint strikes the primer pan—like calcium entry through the L-type calcium channels—ignites the larger amount of powder within the barrel of the musket, which is analogous to the larger quantity of calcium released through calcium release channels from within the sarcoplasmic reticulum.

Calcium Release Channels

The electron-dense "feet" between the plasma membrane and subsarcolemmal cisternae (Fig. 5-3) are the intracellular calcium release channels. These membrane proteins, which are imbedded in the subsarcolemmal cisternae (Fig. 5-18), include four subunits, each of which contains a large cytosolic domain (the foot) and at least four α-helical membrane-spanning segments. The calcium release channels in the heart are opened when binding of the trigger calcium causes the foot to rotate so as to align a central pore within the plane of the membrane with radial channels in each of the four cytosolic subunits, and close when the central pore is disconnected from the radial channels. These channels are grouped in functional clusters that include plasma membrane L-type calcium channels, the Na/Ca exchanger, and the sodium pump (Stern et al., 1999; Franzini-Armstrong et al., 1999). Calcium is released from

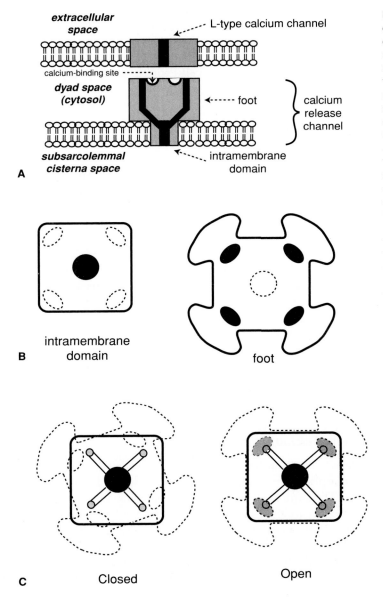

Figure 5-18: Schematic representation of the dyad. **A:** View through the plane of the bilayer showing the plasma membrane (above) and subsarcolemmal cisternal membrane (below). The former contains L-type calcium channels that deliver calcium to binding sites on the sarcoplasmic reticulum calcium release channels. The latter are made up of an intramembrane domain and a large "foot" that projects into the cytosolic space. *Dark areas* represent the pores through which calcium crosses the membrane when these channels are open. **B:** The intramembrane domain of the intracellular calcium release channel as seen from within the subsarcolemmal cisterna (**left**) and from the cytosolic space within the dyad (**right**). The intramembrane domain contains a central pore that, in the open channel, is connected to radial channels within each of the four cytoplasmic domains of the foot. **C:** Depiction of the rotation that opens the channel. In the closed state, the four radial channels do not connect with the central pore. The channel opens when the radial channels become aligned with the central pore. From Katz AM. *Physiology of the Heart*. 4th ed. Philadelphia, Lippincott Williams and Wilkins.

these clusters in small packages, which causes localized areas of increased calcium concentration, called "calcium sparks" (Wang et al., 2004).

Cardiac calcium release channels are highly regulated. Phosphorylation by calcium/calmodulin kinase provides a protective mechanism by which high cytosolic calcium concentration can inhibit channel opening in situations of calcium overload. During sympathetic stimulation, on the other hand, phosphorylation by protein kinase A increases calcium release, which contributes to the inotropic response to exercise. Interactions among the four subunits of the cardiac calcium release channels are regulated by a protein, called *FKBP12* or *calstabin2*, that facilitates channel opening by coordinating the gating of the four intracellular subunits. A number of additional proteins in the subsarcolemmal cisternae also regulate these channels (see below).

Inositol trisphosphate (InsP$_3$)-gated calcium channels in the sarcoplasmic reticulum are related to the calcium-gated calcium release channels but are smaller and open and close more slowly than the latter. InsP$_3$-gated calcium channels play a major role in delivering the calcium that activates smooth muscle contraction, and the small number of InsP$_3$-gated calcium channels in adult hearts may also regulate resting tension. These channels also participate in proliferative signaling, so that they can help regulate protein synthesis, cell growth, and apoptosis (see Chapter 4).

Calcium Uptake by the Sarcoplasmic Reticulum

Understanding of the role of the sarcoplasmic reticulum in muscle relaxation began to emerge in the 1950s, when supernatants obtained after low speed centrifugation of muscle minces were found to relax actomyosins *in vitro*. This effect, which requires ATP and can be abolished by calcium, was initially believed to be caused by a "soluble relaxing factor" (Gergely, 1959). However, Hasselbach and Makinose (1961) and Ebashi and Lipmann (1962) discovered independently that the relaxing effect occurs when tiny membrane vesicles in homogenized muscle minces (called microsomes) derived from the sarcoplasmic reticulum use energy from ATP hydrolysis to pump calcium into their interior. The concurrent discovery that actin–myosin interactions are activated under physiological conditions by micromolar concentrations of ionized calcium (Weber and Winicur, 1961) made it clear that muscles relax when calcium is taken up by the sarcoplasmic reticulum. Within a few years it was possible to show that the cardiac contractile proteins are also regulated by calcium (Katz et al., 1966) and that the cardiac sarcoplasmic reticulum contains a calcium pump that has both sufficient capacity and calcium affinity to relax the heart (Katz and Repke, 1967; Harigaya and Schwartz, 1969).

The Sarcoplasmic Reticulum Calcium Pump

The activator calcium released from intracellular stores is returned to this internal membrane system by the sarcoplasmic reticulum calcium pump, which is one of the P-type ion pumps (Fig. 5-11). The cardiac isoform, SERCA2a, forms a densely packed array in the membranes of the sarcotubular network (Fig. 5-19). Like the plasma membrane calcium pump, SERCA2a includes a large intracellular domain that contains a calcium-transport site, an ATP phosphorylation site, and several regulatory sites (Fig. 5-20). Unlike the sodium pump, which pumps sodium and potassium in opposite directions, the calcium pump does not exchange calcium for a counter ion. However, the

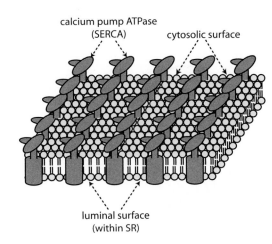

calcium pump ATPase
(SERCA)

cytosolic surface

luminal surface
(within SR)

Figure 5-19: Three-dimensional depiction of the membrane of the sarcotubular network; the cytosolic surface is above and the lumen below. Calcium pump ATPase molecules are packed into the bilayer with most of their mass projecting into the cytosol. Modified from Katz AM (2006). *Physiology of the Heart.* 4th ed. Philadelphia, Lippincott Williams and Wilkins.

fluxes of positively charged calcium ions into and out of the sarcoplasmic reticulum do not generate electrical currents because this internal membrane contains nonspecific anion channels that allow negatively charged chloride and phosphate anions to accompany the calcium ions, which neutralizes any charge movement (Beil et al., 1977).

The key regulator of calcium pump activity is the level of cytosolic calcium because binding of cytosolic calcium is a prerequisite for pump turnover. Elevated cytosolic calcium also stimulates calcium transport indirectly by forming a calcium/calmodulin complex that activates a CAM kinase that phosphorylates a regulatory site on the pump. An allosteric effect of the normally high concentration of cytosolic ATP in the heart stimulates the calcium pump, which is one reason why energy starvation, by attenuating this regulatory effect, slows relaxation in failing hearts. Also important in energy-starved hearts is the effect of increased ADP concentration, along with a smaller decrease in ATP concentration, to reduce the free energy that is made available by ATP hydrolysis ($-\Delta G$); the major consequence is slowing of calcium uptake into the sarcoplasmic reticulum (Tian and Ingwall, 1996), which contributes to both the negative lusitropic and inotropic effects of energy starvation (see below).

Phospholamban

Phospholamban, a small membrane protein that contains a single α-helical membrane-spanning segment, regulates the calcium pump of the cardiac sarcoplasmic reticulum (Fig. 5-20). In the dephospho-form (Fig. 20A), phospholamban slows relaxation by reducing the calcium sensitivity of SERCA2a. This effect also decreases contractility because reduced calcium uptake into the sarcoplasmic reticulum allows more of this activator to be transported out of the cytosol into the extracellular space, which reduces intracellular calcium stores. These inhibitory effects are reversed when phospholamban is phosphorylated by protein kinase A (Fig. 20B), which by accelerating relaxation and increasing contractility, is an important component of the heart's response to sympathetic stimulation. Phosphorylation of phospholamban by calcium/calmodulin kinase, which also stimulates calcium uptake into the sarcoplasmic reticulum, helps protect the heart in situations of calcium overload.

Comparison of the stimulation of sarcoplasmic reticulum calcium transport by phospholamban with that of the calcium/calmodulin-binding domain of the plasma

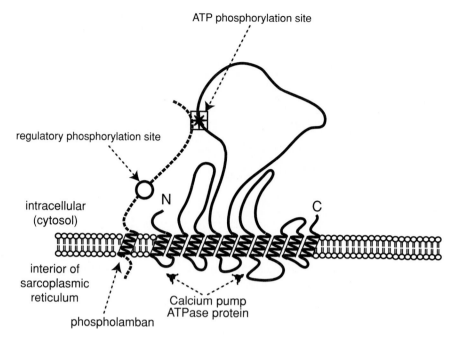

A. Basal State

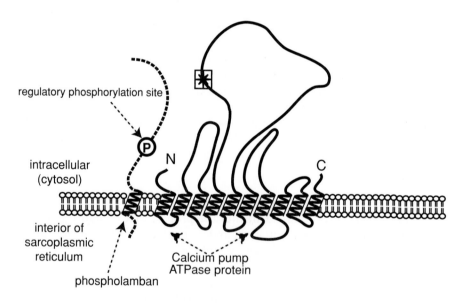

B. Activated State

Figure 5-20: Regulation of the cardiac sarcoplasmic reticulum calcium pump by phospholamban. **A:** In the basal state phospholamban inhibits calcium transport when it interacts with the phosphorylation site of the intracellular regulatory domain. **B:** Phosphorylation of phospholamban accelerates calcium transport by reversing this inhibitory effect. Modified from Katz AM (2006). *Physiology of the Heart*. 4th ed. Philadelphia, Lippincott Williams and Wilkins.

membrane calcium pump (Figs. 5-12 and 5-20) illustrates how homologous structures in different systems can generate similar responses. Although the inhibitory action of the calcium/calmodulin-binding domain of the plasma membrane calcium pump resembles that of phospholamban, in the former this regulatory peptide is part of the pump protein whereas phospholamban is a separate protein. Homologies between these two peptide chains suggest that a regulatory peptide in the ancestral calcium pump evolved in two ways: In the plasma membrane calcium pump it remained attached to the pump molecule where it responds to a calcium-activated signal, whereas the homologous region in SERCA2a became a separate protein that mediates a signal initiated by cyclic AMP.

Calcium-Binding and Regulatory Proteins of the Subsarcolemmal Cisternae

Much of the calcium stored within the sarcoplasmic reticulum is associated with calcium-binding proteins in the subsarcolemmal cisternae. Most important of the latter is *calsequestrin*, each molecule of which contains between 18 and 50 calcium-binding sites. Other calcium-binding proteins present in smaller amounts include a *histidine-rich calcium-binding protein, sarcalumenin*, and *calreticulin*. Sequestration of calcium by these proteins maintains a low calcium concentration within the sarcoplasmic reticulum, which is important because high intraluminal calcium inhibits the calcium pump. Additional proteins, *triadin* and *junctin*, interact with calsequestrin to regulate the opening of the calcium release channels. Most of these proteins, including triadin, junctin, calsequestrin, sarcalumenin, and the histidine-rich calcium-binding protein, along with the calcium release channels themselves, participate in proliferative signaling and are regulated by a variety of protein kinases.

Abnormalities in the calcium release channels and associated proteins in the subsarcolemmal cisternae cause a clinical syndrome, called *catecholaminergic polymorphic ventricular tachycardia*, that is characterized by dangerous ventricular arrhythmias. The underlying abnormality, a calcium leak from the sarcoplasmic reticulum into the cytosol, generates a depolarizing current across the plasma membrane when the excess calcium is transported out of the cell by the Na/Ca exchanger. These abnormalities can also be accompanied by cardiomyopathies.

Mitochondria

Mitochondrial calcium uptake and release play little or no role in normal cardiac excitation–contraction coupling because of the low calcium affinity and slow turnover of mitochondrial calcium transport. In energy-starved hearts, however, calcium overload causes the mitochondria to accumulate calcium. Although this helps protect the myocardium from the detrimental effects of calcium overload, the ability of mitochondrial calcium uptake to buffer calcium is limited. More important, calcium accumulation by mitochondria worsens energy starvation by uncoupling oxidative phosphorylation.

SUMMARY OF THE INTRACELLULAR AND EXTRACELLULAR CALCIUM CYCLES

The extracellular and intracellular calcium cycles (Fig. 5-21) involve five pools, or compartments: the *extracellular space, sarcoplasmic reticulum, cytosol, contractile proteins*, and *mitochondria* (Fig. 5-21A). The major calcium fluxes in the adult

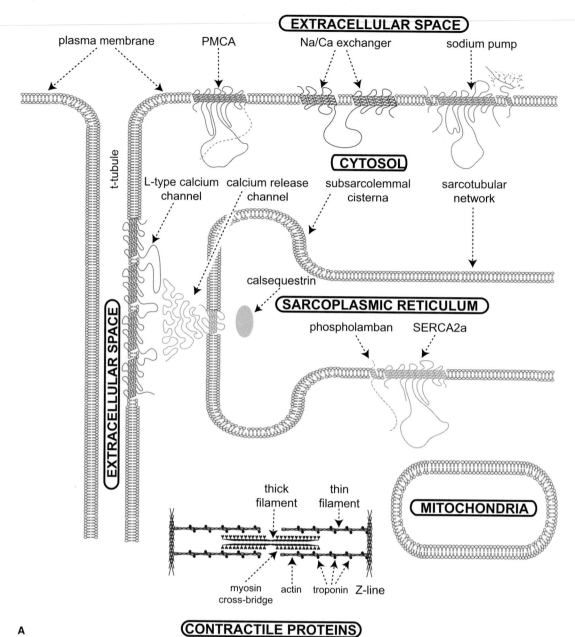

Figure 5-21: Key structures (**A**) and calcium fluxes (**B**) that control cardiac excitation–contraction coupling and relaxation. In **A**, Calcium pools are in bold capital letters. In **B**, the thickness of the arrows indicates the magnitude of the calcium fluxes, while their vertical orientations describe their energetics: *downward arrows* represent passive calcium fluxes; *upward arrows* represent energy-dependent active calcium transport. Most of the calcium that enters the cell from the extracellular fluid via L-type calcium channels (*arrow A*) triggers calcium release from the sarcoplasmic reticulum; only a small portion directly activates the contractile proteins (*arrow A1*). Calcium is actively transported out of the cytosol into the extracellular fluid by the plasma membrane calcium pump ATPase (PMCA; *arrow B1*) and the Na/Ca exchanger (*arrow B2*). The sodium that enters the cell in exchange for calcium (*dashed line*) is pumped out of the cytosol by the sodium pump. Two calcium fluxes are regulated by the sarcoplasmic reticulum: calcium efflux from the subsarcolemmal cisternae via calcium release channels (*arrow C*) and calcium uptake into the sarcotubular network by the calcium pump ATPase (*arrow D*). Calcium diffuses within the sarcoplasmic reticulum from the sarcotubular network to the subsarcolemmal cisternae (*arrow G*), where it forms a complex with calsequestrin and other calcium-binding proteins. Calcium binding to (*arrow E*) and dissociation from (*arrow F*) high-affinity calcium-binding sites of troponin C activate and inhibit the interactions of the contractile proteins. Calcium movements into and out of mitochondria (*arrow H*) buffer cytosolic calcium concentration. The extracellular calcium cycle is shown by *arrows A, B1,* and *B2*, while the intracellular cycle involves *arrows C, E, F, D,* and *G*. From Katz AM (2006). *Physiology of the Heart.* 4th ed. Philadelphia, Lippincott Williams and Wilkins. (continued)

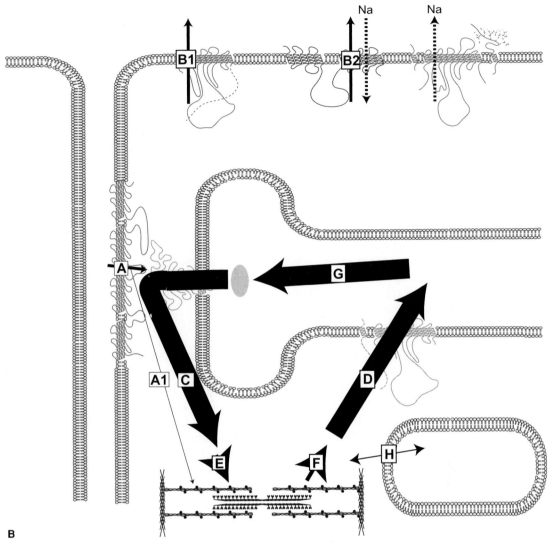

Figure 5-21: (Continued)

mammalian heart are shown in Fig. 5-21B, where upward arrows represent active fluxes and downward arrows passive fluxes; the thickness of each arrow is roughly proportional to the amount of the calcium flux. In the extracellular calcium cycle, calcium influx across the plasma membrane is mediated by voltage-gated L-type calcium channels (arrow A), while active calcium efflux is effected by the plasma membrane calcium pump (arrow B1) and Na/Ca exchanger (arrow B2). The most important function of the calcium that enters the cytosol from the extracellular space is to open calcium release channels in the sarcoplasmic reticulum (calcium-triggered calcium release); only a small fraction binds directly to the contractile proteins (arrow A1). In the intracellular calcium cycle, the calcium fluxes out of (arrow C), into (arrow D), and within (arrow G) the sarcoplasmic reticulum are much greater than those of the extracellular calcium cycle (arrows A, B1, and B2). The contractile proteins are activated when calcium binds to troponin C (arrow E), while the heart relaxes when lowering of cytosolic calcium concentration causes the activator to dissociate from the high-affinity E-F hand calcium binding sites on this protein (arrow F). The limited ability of mitochondria to buffer high cytosolic calcium levels is shown by the double arrow H.

ARRHYTHMIAS AND SUDDEN DEATH

Sudden death, along with progressive deterioration of the failing heart, has emerged as a major determinant of long-term prognosis in heart failure. Many arrhythmias result from architectural changes in the walls of the heart, notably enlargement and fibrosis, which slow conduction and disorganize the spread of the wave of depolarization. Variations in conduction velocity that depend on abnormalities in fiber orientation, called *anisotropy*, are an important cause of arrhythmias in patients whose heart failure is due to ischemic heart disease but do not appear to be important in nonischemic dilated cardiomyopathies. The likelihood of a lethal arrhythmia in these patients is also increased by changes in the channel proteins that are responsible for the heart's electrical activity.

Cardiac action potentials, which last several hundred milliseconds, result from the orchestrated opening and closing of ion-selective channels in the plasma membrane. These vary in different regions of the heart. The action potentials in the His-Purkinje system include five phases (Fig. 5-22): a rapid upstroke (phase 0), early transient repolarization (phase 1), a plateau (phase 2), delayed repolarization (phase 3), and a resting phase (phase 4). Action potentials in the working cells of the ventricles resemble those of Purkinje cells but are slightly smaller, while atrial action potentials are much briefer. The initial inward current in all of these cells, which is carried by sodium, develops rapidly and lasts only a short time, and so is often referred to as a *fast inward current*. Action potentials in the SA and AV nodes are of lower amplitude and lack a plateau because they depend on the opening of lower-conductance calcium channels. Their lower amplitude and slower rate of depolarization cause these action potentials to conduct slowly.

Resting membrane depolarization establishes a substrate for lethal arrhythmias by inactivating sodium channel opening in the atria, His-Purkinje system, and ventricles. The resulting decrease in the rate of rise and amplitude of the action potential slows the velocity of impulse conduction, which tends to disorganize conduction and favor the appearance of reentrant arrhythmias. Resting potential is proportional to the electrochemical gradient for potassium across the plasma membrane (K_i/K_o) because these membranes are selectively permeable to potassium during diastole. For this reason, sodium pump inhibition caused by energy starvation, which decreases intracellular potassium concentration, contributes to the likelihood of sudden cardiac death in patients with heart failure (see below). Cardiac glycosides, which also reduce resting membrane potential by inhibiting the sodium pump, have a similar effect. Depolarizing currents generated by premature systoles, which can reach excitable regions of the heart before the sodium channels have had time to reactivate fully from a prior depolarization, are dangerous because of their ability to generate small, slowly rising action potentials that can initiate reentry.

Sodium Channels

The major sodium channel in human hearts is encoded by the gene SCN5A. Mutations in this gene can cause both gain-in-function and loss-of-function abnormalities that are responsible for long QT syndromes and an electrocardiographic abnormality called the *Brugada syndrome*, respectively; both are substrates for lethal arrhythmias.

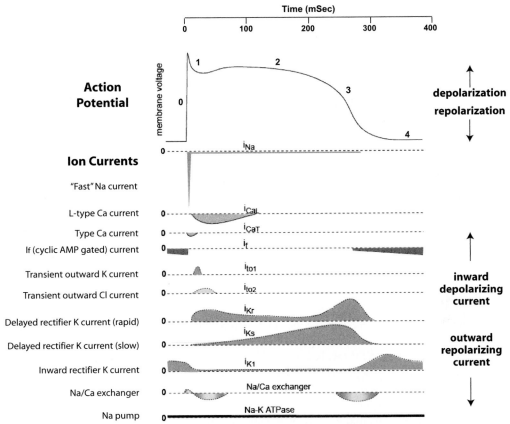

Figure 5-22: Ion currents responsible for the Purkinje fiber action potential. **Upper** tracing: voltage changes during the action potential. **Lower** tracings: Membrane currents; inward currents are downward, outward currents are upward. Depolarizing currents include i_{Na}, i_{CaL}, i_{CaT}, and i_f; both i_{CaT}, and i_f participate in pacemaker activity. Repolarizing currents include three outward potassium currents (i_{to1}, i_{Kr}, and i_{Ks}) and an outward chloride current (i_{to2}), while resting potential is maintained by the inward rectifier i_{K1}. Currents generated by the Na/Ca exchanger and Na pump are shown below. Modified from Katz AM (2006). *Physiology of the Heart.* 4th ed. Philadelphia, Lippincott Williams and Wilkins.

Smaller amounts of neuronal and skeletal muscle sodium channel isoforms have also been described in the heart, but the clinical importance of changes in these channels in failing hearts is not yet clear.

Calcium Channels

Two types of calcium channel are found in the human heart: These are L- and T-type calcium channels whose names reflect the slower inactivation of L-type calcium channels than T-type channels (L, long-lasting; T, transient). L-type calcium currents in the working cells of the atria and ventricles carry the inward calcium flux that contributes to the action potential plateau and opens sarcoplasmic reticulum calcium release channels (see previous discussion). T-type calcium channels also generate inward currents, but these are too small either to play an important role in depolarization of the atria, ventricles, and His-Purkinje system or to participate in excitation–contraction coupling. Calcium flux through T-type channels may contribute to resting tension in working cardiac myocytes, and these calcium channels participate in SA node pacemaker activity. In many cell types, including the developing heart, T-type calcium channels play a role in proliferative signaling, but the significance of an increase in the content of these channels in hypertrophied hearts is not clear.

Potassium Channels

Cardiac myocytes contain several types of potassium channel; some are responsible for maintaining resting potential, while others repolarize the heart after the passage of an action potential has depolarized its cells.

Potassium currents commonly exhibit a property called *rectification*, which means that opening of these channels is influenced by membrane potential. Potassium currents can be rectified in two ways. *Outward rectification*, which occurs when depolarization *increases* the flow of repolarizing current, tends to restore membrane potential to its resting level. *Inward rectification* occurs when depolarization *decreases* repolarizing current, so that inward rectifier potassium currents tend to maintain the membrane of an activated cell in a depolarized state. Outward and inward rectification are now known to reflect the properties of structurally different potassium channels.

There are several types of inward rectifier channels in the heart. One, which carries a current called i_{K_1}, is open during diastole and so is a major determinant of resting potential. Another class of inward rectifier channels, called $i_{K,ATP}$, is inhibited by the normally high levels of cytosolic ATP so that, like a contented house cat asleep before the hearth, $i_{K,ATP}$ channels spend most of their life in a dormant state. Opening of $i_{K,ATP}$ channels when ATP levels fall and ADP levels rise in energy-starved failing hearts increases resting depolarization, which by reducing excitability, has an energy-sparing effect. Acetylcholine-gated inward rectifier channels in the SA node, called $i_{K,Ach}$, slow the heart in response to vagal stimulation, adenosine, and other purines by hyperpolarizing these pacemaker cells. Vagal stimulation also opens $i_{K,Ach}$ channels in the atria; this response, which shortens the action potential, is largely responsible for the negative inotropic response of the atria to parasympathetic stimulation.

Transient repolarization (phase 1) is caused by an outward rectifying potassium current called i_{to1} which, along with a brief outward chloride current called i_{to2}, shortens action potential duration by accelerating the cycling of the channels that open later during the action potential. Activation of i_{to1} channels by protein kinase. A catalyzed phosphorylation helps shorten the action potential during exercise, when sympathetic stimulation increases heart rate. Conversely, decreased expression of the genes that encode the i_{to1} channels in patients with heart failure prolongs both the action potential and the open state of the L-type calcium channels, and delays the onset of the potassium currents that end the cardiac action potential; both of these effects favor the appearance of arrhythmias (see below).

Two delayed outward rectifier potassium channels repolarize the ventricles and His-Purkinje cells: one, called i_{Kr}, carries an outward current that initiates repolarization early during the action potential plateau; the other, called i_{Ks}, opens later and generates more sustained repolarizing currents. Slowed cycling of both of these channels prolongs the action potential, which tends to disorganize repolarization and so favors reentrant arrhythmias.

Other Ion Currents

The Na/Ca exchanger, which generates a depolarizing current when it exchanges one calcium ion for three sodium ions (see previous discussion), plays an important role in causing sudden death in patients with heart failure. This current, which accompanies calcium efflux from the heart's cytosol at the beginning of diastole, is especially dangerous because it can initiate afterdepolarizations at the end of the action potential, during the vulnerable period when the ventricles are most susceptible to fibrillation. Reversion to the fetal phenotype, which increases dependence on the extracellular calcium cycle in failing hearts, increases this depolarizing current (see below). Calcium overload further exacerbates the dangerous situation caused by the inward current generated by the Na/Ca exchanger and is one reason for the arrhythmogenic effects of inotropic agents, notably those that increase cellular cyclic AMP levels (see Chapter 7).

The sodium pump generates an outward current when it transports three sodium ions out of the cell in exchange for two potassium ions (see previous discussion), but the effects of this current, which stabilizes membrane potential, are normally small.

Gap Junctions

Intercalated discs contain large nonspecific channels that are a major determinant of internal electrical resistance. Closure of these channels, which are made up of proteins called *connexins* that are organized in the gap junctions, increases internal resistance, which, by slowing conduction, provides a substrate for reentrant arrhythmias. Phosphorylation of connexins by protein kinases A and C and MAP kinases speeds impulse conduction by favoring the open state of these channels, whereas tyrosine phosphorylation generally slows conduction by closing these channels. Other gap junction phosphorylations regulate intracellular resistance by modifying the assembly and disassembly of connexin subunits. Acidosis and calcium overload close gap junctions in failing hearts, and so are arrhythmogenic. Isoform shifts involving connexins can also modify internal resistance.

FUNCTIONAL ABNORMALITIES IN HEART FAILURE

Until the end of the 1980s, it was generally accepted that reduced myocardial contractility represented the central problem in heart failure. This led to the seemingly logical conclusion that this syndrome should be treated by inotropic drugs—and that the more powerful they were, the better would be the clinical outcome. At about the same time, recognition of the adverse effects of increased afterload (see Chapter 2) provided a rationale for the use of vasodilators. It is now clear, however, that most drugs that increase contractility, even though they lead to short-term improvement, worsen long-term prognosis (see Chapter 7). Furthermore, even though vasodilators generally cause short-term hemodynamic improvement, clinical trials showed that most do not improve long-term survival, and several shorten life expectancy. By the end of the 1990s, therefore, it had become clear that impaired pump performance, while important in causing symptoms in patients with heart failure (see Chapter 2), is not the only determinant of long-term prognosis.

Posttranslational Modifications

The most important functional mechanisms that depress the hemodynamic performance of failing hearts are covalent posttranslational changes initiated by the neurohumoral response and metabolic abnormalities caused by energy starvation (Table 5-1). Phosphorylations and other posttranslational changes can modify most of the proteins discussed in this chapter. High circulating norepinephrine levels activate protein kinase A and, along with other extracellular messengers such as angiotensin II, increase protein kinase C activity. Most protein kinase A–catalyzed phosphorylations increase myocardial contractility, whereas protein kinase C phosphorylations generally depress cardiac performance. Examples of the latter include phosphorylation of myosin regulatory light chains, which reduces the calcium sensitivity of the contractile proteins, and phosphorylation of troponin I and troponin T, which slows cross-bridge turnover. Some protein kinase C activators, however, increase myocardial contractility. Additional post-translational phosphorylations are catalyzed by *p21-activated protein kinase* and *Rho-dependent protein kinase*, while *protein phosphatase 2A* catalyzes protein dephosphorylation. The overall effect of the changes in the thin filaments in human heart failure has been reported to be a 19% increase in maximal shortening velocity and a 27% decrease in maximum force development (Noguchi et al., 2004). However, these are approximations in part because the extent of the reduction in contractile performance in failing hearts is highly dependent on heart rate, increasing markedly as the heart beats more rapidly.

Many of the membrane proteins that participate in the excitation–contraction coupling and relaxation undergo functional modifications in animal models of heart failure, but the findings in different studies are often inconsistent and data from failing human hearts are limited. There is general agreement that phosphorylation of phospholamban is decreased in failing hearts, an effect that would impair relaxation and depress myocardial contractility. On the other hand, increased phosphorylation of intracellular calcium release channels by calcium/calmodulin kinase, along with calcium overload, has been suggested to increase the leakiness of these channels so as to favor the appearance of arrhythmias when the excess calcium leaves the myocardium by way of the Na/Ca exchanger. Some reports, however, describe impaired coupling of calcium entry through plasma membrane L-type calcium channels to calcium-triggered calcium release from the sarcoplasmic reticulum. Because of conflicting data, it is not now possible to define a general role of these and other functional abnormalities in the pathophysiology of clinical heart failure.

Energy Starvation

Suggestions that failing hearts might be in an energy-starved state go back to the 19th century, but it is only recently that analytic tools like NMR spectroscopy were able to show conclusively that ATP and phosphocreatine levels are significantly reduced in overloaded and failing hearts. Energy starvation is especially marked in the subendocardial regions of the left ventricle, because of a combination of high wall stress and low perfusion. In malignant hypertension and end-stage aortic stenosis, energy starvation can become so severe as to cause subendocardial necrosis.

Energy starvation impairs relaxation more than it does contraction in part because the active transport mechanisms that relax the heart are intrinsically slower than those that deliver this activator into the cytosol to initiate systole. For example, the velocity of calcium uptake by a single sarcoplasmic reticulum calcium pump at 37°C is ~30 ions per second, which is 25,000 times slower than the ~750,000 ions per second for the downhill calcium flux through a single intracellular calcium release channel. Even though the sarcoplasmic reticulum contains almost 200 times more SERCA2a than intracellular calcium release channels, the maximum rate of calcium uptake into the sarcoplasmic reticulum during diastole by the densely packed calcium pump molecules (see Fig. 5-19) cannot compensate for the much greater rate at which calcium diffuses into the cytosol during systole. These flux rates, which illustrate the well-known precept that it is easier to get into trouble than out of trouble, help in understanding the greater impact of energy starvation on relaxation than contraction.

Causes of Energy Starvation

Energy starvation in the failing heart results from an imbalance between energy consumption, which is generally increased, and energy production, which is usually decreased. In systolic (low EF) heart failure, energy utilization is increased when dilation of the ventricle and thinning of its walls increase systolic wall stress and reduce cardiac efficiency. Cardiac energy demands are also increased in elderly patients who have diastolic heart failure (heart failure with normal EF) when left ventricular afterload is increased by arterial hypertension and decreased aortic compliance, both of which are common causes of this syndrome. High levels of pressure–volume work in most forms of valvular and congenital heart disease also increase cardiac energy expenditure, while ischemic heart disease, which reduces the number of normally perfused ventricular myocytes, adds to the work that must be done by each of the remaining myocardial cells.

Cardiac hypertrophy exacerbates energy starvation in part because the greater number of working sarcomeres in the enlarged cells increases energy demand. At the same time, energy supply in hypertrophied hearts is reduced by structural abnormalities that impair diffusion of substrates, notably oxygen. These include a decrease in capillary density relative to ventricular mass, which, by increasing intercapillary spacing, adds to the distance that oxygen must diffuse to working cardiac myocytes (Shipley et al., 1938). The greater diameter of the hypertrophied cardiac myocytes also impairs energy production by causing the core of the enlarged fibers to become hypoxic.

A number of metabolic changes can impair energy production in failing hearts (Fig. 5-23), but the tight coupling between various pathways makes it difficult to isolate and evaluate the importance of specific abnormalities. Impaired mitochondrial function is especially detrimental because of the heart's dependence on ATP regeneration by oxidative phosphorylation. The limited ability of glycolysis to supply the energy needs of the heart makes it impossible for anaerobic pathways to provide enough ATP for the contractile machinery when mitochondrial energy production is impaired.

Abnormalities that have been implicated in decreasing oxidative phosphorylation in failing hearts include cellular hypoxia (see previous discussion) and reduced activities of both the respiratory chain and ATP synthase caused by calcium overload. Decreased synthesis of oxidative enzymes, notably mitochondrial creatine phosphokinase, slows the phosphocreatine shuttle, which transfers high-energy phosphates from the mitochondria, where they are regenerated, to cytosolic energy-utilizing systems such as the myofibrillar proteins and ion pumps. Another consequence of impaired mitochondrial function is release of reactive oxygen species that damage cells, and cytochromes that induce apoptosis (see Chapter 4). Mitochondrial dysfunction also reduces fatty acid oxidation, which leads to lipid accumulation that can contribute to necrosis by damaging membranes.

Figure 5-23: Some metabolic abnormalities in failing hearts. The major change in substrate utilization is a decrease in fatty acid oxidation; increased glycolysis partly compensates for this abnormality in early heart failure. Oxidative phosphorylation is impaired by reduced delivery of oxygen to working cardiac myocytes, decreased respiratory chain and ATP synthase activities, and uncoupling of oxidation and ATP regeneration. Energy transfer by the phosphocreatine shuttle is reduced when phosphocreatine and creatine kinase levels fall; consequences include a minor fall in cytosolic ATP and a more marked increase in cytosolic ADP; together these decrease the free energy of ATP hydrolysis, which is proportional to the ratio between ATP and ADP concentrations.

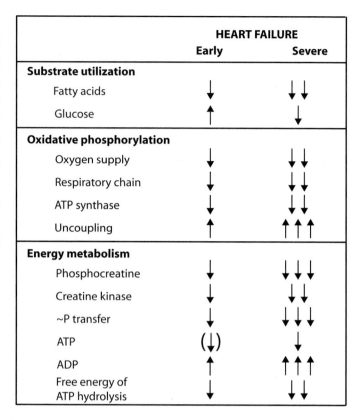

Consequences of Energy Starvation

High-energy phosphate content falls slightly in severe heart failure, but levels of ATP do not become low enough to deprive the substrate-binding sites of the contractile proteins, ion pumps, and other energy-consuming systems of their energy source. This is because normal cytosolic ATP concentration is 5 to 10 mM, whereas most substrate-binding sites are saturated at ATP concentrations below 1 μM. For this reason, lack of substrate for energy-consuming reactions occurs only in dying hearts, where ATP concentration reaches levels low enough to deplete high-affinity sites of this substrate. More important is attenuation of the allosteric effects of ATP, which are seen at high ATP concentrations and do not require hydrolysis of the nucleotide (Table 5-6). These allosteric effects allow a modest fall in ATP concentration to increase diastolic stiffness and depress myocardial contractility because attenuation of these effects inhibits dissociation of actin and myosin and slows ion pumps, Na/Ca exchange, and downhill calcium fluxes through calcium channels. Reduction in the allosteric effect of ATP also slows the sodium pump, which by increasing cytosolic sodium, impairs relaxation by reducing calcium efflux via the Na/Ca exchanger. Sodium pump inhibition also decreases resting membrane potential, which inactivates sodium channel opening and so provides a substrate for reentrant arrhythmias (see previous discussion).

The most important consequence of ATP depletion in energy-starved hearts appears to be a decrease in the free energy available from ATP hydrolysis ($-\Delta G$), which is proportional to the ATP/ADP ratio. Even a slight fall in ATP concentration,

Effects of Diminished Allosteric Effects of ATP on Myocardial Contraction and Relaxation

Process	Immediate consequence	Mechanical effect
Plasma membrane L-type Ca channels	Reduced Ca influx into cytosol → less Ca release from sarcoplasmic reticulum	Negative inotropic
Plasma membrane Ca pump	Reduced Ca efflux from cytosol → increased intracellular Ca	Negative lusitropic
Na/Ca exchanger	Reduced Ca efflux from cytosol → increased intracellular Ca	Negative lusitropic
Plasma membrane Na pump	Reduced Na efflux into cytosol → increased intracellular Na → decreased Ca efflux by Na/Ca exchange → increased intracellular Ca	Negative lusitropic
Sarcoplasmic reticulum Ca release channels	Reduced Ca release during systole → less Ca for binding to contractile proteins	Negative inotropic
Sarcoplasmic reticulum Ca pump	Reduced Ca uptake during diastole → less Ca removed from contractile proteins	Negative lusitropic
Actin–myosin interactions	Reduced dissociation of thick and thin filaments → decreased diastolic compliance	Negative lusitropic

because of the disproportional increase in ADP concentration, which is normally very low, can reduce $-\Delta G$ to levels that slow the sarcoplasmic reticulum calcium pump (see previous discussion). The resulting increase in cytosolic calcium is among the most detrimental consequences of energy starvation because it accelerates energy-consuming interactions between the contractile proteins during diastole. These and other problems caused by increased cytosolic calcium can initiate a number of vicious cycles that can lead to myocyte necrosis and literally destroy the myocardium (Fig. 5-24). These mechanisms explain why heart failure, by causing energy demand to exceed energy supply, can lead to the release of cardiac myocyte proteins, notably troponin T and I, into the blood of these patients.

Acidosis

Impaired oxidative phosphorylation accelerates glycolysis (see previous discussion), which increases lactate formation, and releases inorganic phosphate as the result of ATP hydrolysis. Because lactate and phosphate are weak acids that liberate hydrogen ions at the neutral cytosolic pH, both acidify the energy-starved cardiac myocytes. Although some of these protons are absorbed when phosphocreatine hydrolysis releases creatine, which is a weak base, the net effect is to reduce intracellular pH.

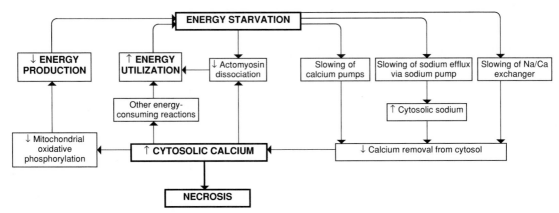

Figure 5-24: Energy starvation contributes to several vicious cycles that can cause cardiac myocyte necrosis by increasing energy utilization and decreasing energy production. Reduced turnover of the calcium pumps of the sarcoplasmic reticulum and plasma membrane, the Na/Ca exchanger, and the sodium pump impair calcium removal from the cytosol. The resulting increase in cytosolic calcium inhibits actomyosin dissociation, which in addition to impairing relaxation, increases energy utilization and so worsens the energy starvation. Aerobic energy production is also inhibited when cytosolic calcium is taken up by the mitochondria, which uncouples oxidative phosphorylation. The resulting increase in cytosolic calcium amplifies these vicious cycles and can lead to necrosis of the energy-starved cells. From Katz AM (2006). *Physiology of the Heart*. 4th ed. Philadelphia, Lippincott Williams and Wilkins.

Acidosis interferes with many of the reactions involved in excitation–contraction coupling, contraction, and relaxation because protons compete with calcium for binding sites on troponin and calcium channels, pumps, and exchangers. Acidosis also slows energy production because it inhibits key glycolytic enzymes. The ability of acidosis to inhibit the opening of voltage-gated ion channels and to close gap junctions in the intercalated disc also provides a substrate for reentrant arrhythmias and sudden death.

PROLIFERATIVE ABNORMALITIES

Functional abnormalities that modify the behavior of otherwise normal proteins are not the only causes of the impaired cardiac performance and poor prognosis in patients with heart failure. Additional maladaptive changes occur when altered proliferative signaling changes the architecture and cellular and molecular composition of failing hearts (Table 5-7). The clinical importance of the latter became apparent in the 1990s when long-term clinical trials showed that inotropic agents and most vasodilators, in spite of their ability to alleviate the hemodynamic abnormalities in patients with heart failure, worsen long-term prognosis. Neurohumoral blockers, on the other hand, generally improve long-term survival (see Chapter 6), in most cases by reversing, at least temporarily, the maladaptive proliferative responses that lead to progressive dilatation (remodeling). As described below, proliferative responses can be both beneficial and deleterious, often at the same time!

Myofibrillar Proteins

Thick Filaments

The first molecular change to be described in failing human hearts was increased expression of the slow (β) myosin heavy chain isoform. This isoform shift, which is

---

TABLE 5-7

Some Molecular Alterations in Hypertrophied and Failing Hearts[‡]

A. CONTRACTILE AND CYTOSKELETAL PROTEINS

Protein	Heart Failure
Myosin heavy chain	Isoform shift[*]
Myosin light chains	Isoform shift[*]
Actin	Isoform shift[*]
Troponin I	No change
Troponin T	Isoform shift[*]
Troponin C	No change
Tropomyosin	No change
Titin	Isoform shift[§]

B. SARCOPLASMIC RETICULUM PROTEINS

Protein	Heart Failure
Calcium pump ATPase (SERCA)	Decreased content[*]
Phospholamban	Decreased content[*]
Calcium release channel (ryanodine receptor)	No change or decreased content

C. PLASMA MEMBRANE PROTEINS

Protein	Heart Failure
Transient outward potassium channels (i_{to})	Decreased current
Delayed rectifier potassium channels (i_{Kr})	Decreased current
Delayed rectifier potassium channels (i_{Ks})	Decreased current
Inward rectifying potassium channels (i_{K1})	Decreased current
L-type calcium channels	Normal
Na/Ca exchanger	Increased content[*]
Sodium pump	Decreased content, isoform shift[*]
β_1-Adrenergic receptor	Decreased content
β_1-Adrenergic receptor kinase	Increased content
$G_{\alpha i}$	Increased content

[‡]These abnormalities are not found in all models of heart failure.
[*]Reversion to the fetal phenotype.
[§]Appear to differ in systolic and diastolic heart failure.

now recognized to be part of the reversion to the fetal phenotype in pathological hypertrophy, both reduces myocardial contractility and has an energy-sparing effect. In exercise-induced physiological hypertrophy (the athlete's heart), however, cardiac enlargement is associated with the *opposite* response: greater expression of the fast (α) myosin heavy chain isoform, which increases contractility (Scheuer and Buttrick, 1987). The extent of the myosin heavy chain isoform shift in pathological hypertrophy depends on the severity, duration, and even the nature of the overload; for example, overexpression of the slow β-isoform is less in chronic volume overload than in chronic pressure overload (Calderone et al., 1995). Replacement of substantial amounts of the ventricular isoform of the essential myosin light chain with the atrial isoform, unlike the myosin heavy chain isoform shift, increases contractility in pathological hypertrophy by accelerating the interactions between myosin and actin.

Thin Filaments

Chronic overload and heart failure are accompanied by isoform shifts in troponin T and actin, but tropomyosin, troponin I, and troponin C isoform shifts do not appear to occur. The troponin T isoform shifts, which result from changes in alternative splicing, increase the content of a fetal isoform that slows cross-bridge turnover. In some heart failure models, small amounts of α-cardiac actin, the normal isoform, is replaced with α-skeletal actin, the fetal isoform, but the functional consequences of this change are not clear.

The Cytoskeleton

Isoform shifts in several cytoskeletal proteins, including titin, α-actinin, myosin-binding protein C, microtubules, and fibronectin have been found in overloaded and failing hearts. Changes in titin, which is an important determinant of diastolic compliance, appear to be clinically significant because different titin isoforms have been found to be expressed preferentially in systolic and diastolic heart failure: the less stiff N2BA isoform is increased in dilated hearts whereas more of the stiffer N2B is found in diastolic heart failure (van Heerebeck et al., 2006). Participation of cytoskeletal proteins in proliferative signaling (see Chapter 4) suggests that these changes may have additional effects on the structure and composition of diseased hearts.

Membrane Proteins

Gap Junctions

Slowed conduction caused by increased internal resistance can play an important role in causing arrhythmias in patients with heart failure (see previous discussion). As already noted, gap junctions in energy-starved myocytes are closed by acidosis and increased cytosolic calcium; internal resistance can also be increased in severe heart failure when stress-activated c-Jun down-regulates the expression of connexin. Gap junction structure in overloaded hearts can also be modified when proliferative signals are generated by cytoskeletal responses to abnormal cell deformation.

Plasma Membrane Ion Channels

Action potential prolongation and resting depolarization in patients with heart failure increase the likelihood of reentrant arrhythmias. A major cause of action potential prolongation in hypertrophied and failing hearts is reduced expression of the potassium channels that carry i_{to}, which is a major determinant of the rate of cycling of the ion channels that open and close later during the cardiac action potential. By decreasing early repolarization, attenuation of the transient outward current increases the heterogeneity of repolarization by delaying the onset and decreasing the amplitudes of the delayed rectifier currents i_{Kr} and i_{Ks} (Fig. 5-25). (Reported decreases in the expression of i_{Kr} and i_{Ks} would also prolong action potential duration.) An additional consequence of the reduction of i_{to} is an increase in i_{CaL} that, by increasing calcium influx during the plateau, increases energy expanditure, which worsens energy starvation and adds to the arrhythmogenic current generated when the Na/Ca exchanger removes this calcium from the cell. The content of L-type plasma membrane calcium channels does not appear to change in failing hearts.

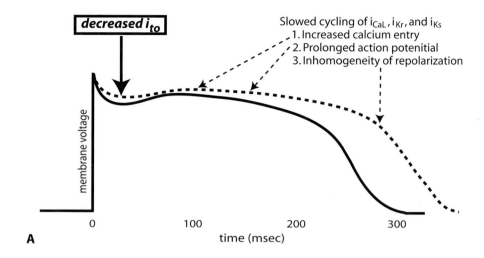

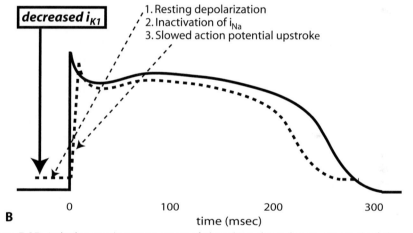

Figure 5-25: Arrhythmogenic consequences of altered ion channel expression in the failing ventricle. **A:** Decreased expression of the potassium channels responsible for the transient outward current i_{to} slows the cycling of L-type calcium channels and the delayed rectifier potassium channels that repolarize the heart. Prolongation of the open state of i_{CaL} increases calcium entry, which contributes to calcium overload and increases the inward current generated when this calcium leaves the cell via the Na/Ca exchanger. Slowed cycling of i_{Kr} and i_{Ks} prolongs the action potential, which by increasing the heterogeneity of repolarization, favors the appearance of reentrant arrhythmias. **B:** Decreased expression of the inward rectifying i_{K1} channels reduces resting potential, which, by inactivating sodium channel opening and slowing the action potential upstroke, increases the susceptibility to reentrant arrhythmias. Normal action potentials are depicted by *solid lines.*

Reduced density of the inward rectifying potassium channels that carry i_{K1} decreases resting potential, which inactivates sodium channels (Fig. 5-25). The resulting decrease in the rate of rise and amplitude of the action potential increases the susceptibility of failing hearts to reentrant arrhythmias by slowing conduction velocity. Reduced $i_{K.ATP}$ channel opening caused by energy starvation is also arrhythmogenic. Evidence for greater heterogeneity of potassium channel expression in different regions of hypertrophied and failing hearts would add to these arrhythmogenic effects.

The Sodium/Calcium Exchanger

The most important cause of sudden death in patients with heart failure is probably an increase in the inward current generated by the Na/Ca exchanger when it transports calcium from the cytosol into the extracellular fluid (see previous discussion). This change, which is associated with greater reliance on the extracellular calcium cycle, is part of the reversion to the fetal phenotype (see Chapter 4). The arrhythmogenic currents are maximal during the vulnerable period at the end of the action potential, when even small depolarizing currents can initiate afterdepolarizations, triggered activity, torsades de pointes, and ventricular fibrillation.

Calcium efflux via the exchanger in failing hearts is increased further by energy starvation and inotropic agents, both of which amplify this dangerous current by elevating cytosolic calcium. This mechanism is probably a major cause for the increased mortality associated with the use of inotropic drugs, like β-adrenergic agonists and phosphodiesterase inhibitors, that increase calcium influx into the cytosol through L-type channels.

Sarcoplasmic Reticulum

Reduced expression of the calcium pump ATPase (SERCA2a) slows relaxation in hypertrophied and failing hearts by decreasing the rate of calcium uptake into the sarcoplasmic reticulum, and depresses contractility by reducing intracellular calcium stores (Table 5-7). Both of these effects appear to be partially offset by a decrease in phospholamban phosphorylation, which would reduce the normal inhibitory effect of this regulatory protein on calcium uptake. The decreased content of the calcium pump ATPase is an example of reversion to the fetal phenotype because the sarcoplasmic reticulum is poorly developed in embryonic hearts, which depend mainly on the extracellular calcium cycle (see previous discussion). The density of the intracellular calcium release channels appears either not to change or to be slightly reduced in heart failure.

FAMILIAL CARDIOMYOPATHIES

In 1990, the report of myosin heavy chain mutations in familial hypertrophic cardiomyopathies (Geisterfer-Lowrance et al., 1990) opened a new era in understanding the pathophysiology of heart failure. Since then, hundreds of mutations affecting genes that encode dozens of proteins have been found to cause both hypertrophic (HCM) and dilated (DCM) cardiomyopathies (Table 5-8). It now appears that 20% to 50% of patients with dilated cardiomyopathies have familial disease and that about half of what appear to be sporadic cases of childhood onset cardiac hypertrophy are due to genetic abnormalities. Molecular studies of the human cardiomyopathies have shown that even a small change in genotype, such as a single missense mutation or a small deletion, can lead to severe disease. However, the view that analysis of gene abnormalities can predict who will have these diseases has been shown not to be correct because not all individuals who carry a specific gene abnormality will exhibit the typical phenotype; in fact, some may have few if any cardiac abnormalities (see below).

The typical histological phenotype in HCM is loss of the parallel orientation of the hypertrophied myofibrils within and among adjacent myocytes, called "myofibrillar disarray." This pattern, which leads to heterogeneities in mechanical performance and regional variations in contractility, reduces cardiac efficiency. The histology of DCM, on the other hand, is characterized by myocyte degeneration and

TABLE 5-8

Some Molecular Causes of Human Familial Cardiomyopathies

	Hypertrophic	Dilated
Myofibrillar Proteins		
β-Myosin heavy chain	X	X
α-Myosin heavy chain	X	X
Regulatory myosin light chain	X	
Essential myosin light chain	X	
Troponin T	X	X
Troponin I	X	X
Troponin C	X	X
α-Tropomyosin	X	X
Cardiac α-actin	X	X
Cytoskeletal Proteins		
Sarcomere related		
Myosin-binding protein C	X	X
Cardiac LIM proteins	X	X
T-cap	X	X
Titin	X	X
Myosin light chain kinase	X	
Z-line-related		
α-Actinin		X
Cypher/ZASP		X
Vinculin		X
Desmin		X
Metavinculin		X
Calsarcin 1 (myozenin 2)	X	
Dystrophin related		
Sarcoglycans (α, β, γ, δ)[§]		X
Dystrophin[§]		X
Dystrobrevin[§]		X
Syntrophin[§]		X
Caveolin-3[§]		X
Desmosome related		
Desmin (see above)		
Plakoglobin		X
Desmoplakin[§]		X
Desmoglein-2[§]		X
Desmocollin-2[§]		X
Plakophilin-2[§]		X
Nuclear		
Emerin		X
Lamin A/C		X
Membrane Proteins		
Calcium release channel (ryanodine receptor)[§]	X	X
Phospholamban		X
Sodium channel (i_{Na})		X
ATP-regulated potassium channel ($i_{K,ATP}$)		X

(continued)

TABLE 5-8

Some Molecular Causes of Human Familial Cardiomyopathies (Continued)

	Hypertrophic	Dilated
Metabolic Proteins		
AMP-activated protein kinase*	×	
Lysosome-associated membrane protein-2* (Danon's Disease)	×	×
α-Galactosidase A (Fabry's Disease)*	×	
α-1,4 Glucosidase (Pompe's Disease)*	×	
Polysaccharide metabolism (Hurler, Hunter, and Morquio syndromes)	×	
Carnitine transporter (carnitine deficiency)	×	
Tafazzin [phospholipid acyltransferase] (Barth syndrome)	×	×
Frataxin [heme synthesis] (Friedreich's ataxia)	×	
Acyl-CoA deficiency	×	
Mitochondrial DNA [point mutations]	×	×
Other Proteins		
Tyrosine phosphatase SHP-2 (Noonan syndrome)	×	
Dystrophia myotonica protein kinase (Myotonic dystrophy)	×	
Nkx2.5 [homeobox]	×	

*Glycogen storage disease.
§Associated with arrhythmogenic right ventricular dysplasia.

fibrosis. These differences may be due in part to the functional consequences of different mutations. For example, the sarcomeric mutations that cause HCM are usually accompanied by changes in the interactions between the myosin cross-bridges and actin that increase force generation and shortening velocity, whereas both tend to be reduced in DCM. Recent additions to the diseases listed in Table 5-8, however, weaken this generalization, so that the mechanistic links between abnormal cardiac architecture and specific mutations remain obscure. It is possible that specific local stress abnormalities caused by different mutations, by activating proliferative signaling pathways that determine whether sarcomeres are added in series or in parallel, play a central role in determining the appearance of these phenotypes.

Both HCM and DCM, like other types of heart failure, are commonly associated with lethal arrhythmias. In many cases these are caused by the mechanisms described previously. Patients with HCM in whom myocyte mass is increased by mutations that cause intracellular glycogen accumulation often exhibit pre-excitation (Wolff-Parkinson-White syndrome) because glycogen-filled myocytes can short-circuit atrioventricular conduction when they cross the central fibrous body, a connective tissue insulator that normally separates the atria and ventricles. The association of atrioventricular conduction abnormalities in DCM, notably those with lamin A/C mutations, is not well understood.

As already noted, the genomics of cardiovascular disease once seemed to be straightforward; a single mutation, which can be defined as a DNA abnormality found in <1% of the population, leads to a phenotypic abnormality that causes a clinical syndrome. Early data also suggested that hypertrophic cardiomyopathies could be attributed to contractile protein mutations and dilated cardiomyopathies to cytoskeletal protein abnormalities, but it is now clear that this generalization is not correct (see previous discussion). Although it came as no surprise that different mutations in a single gene could lead to variations in the severity of these clinical syndromes, the finding that mutations in closely related regions of a single protein could cause the phenotypically distinct syndromes of HCM and DCM was unexpected. During the past few years, new information has made the link between genotype and phenotype increasingly tenuous, notably the fact that not all carriers of mutations known to cause familial diseases exhibit the typical phenotypes, and some remain free of obvious disease (Cambien and Tiret, 2007).

There are several reasons for variations in the severity of the clinical syndrome caused by a specific mutation. Factors that influence these variations, called "penetrance," include the patient's age (the clinical manifestations of genetic diseases frequently increase as patients get older), environmental factors such as the ability of high salt intake to increase the likelihood that a susceptible individual will develop hypertension, and effects of therapy, for example β-blockers can slow the progression of dilated cardiomyopathies. Penetrance is also determined by the way that a mutation modifies the structure into which the abnormal protein is incorporated. For example, the consequences of a *dominant negative* effect, where function is impaired disproportionally by incorporation of an abnormal protein into a cellular structure, can differ from those caused by *haploinsufficiency*, in which the mutation reduces the amount of the protein available for assembly into the structure. More recently, other genetic features in affected individuals have been found to influence the clinical severity of the disease caused by a given mutation. These include the presence of *single nucleotide polymorphisms* (*SNPs*) in the abnormal gene, which are defined as the appearance of different nucleotides at a given point in the genome in a significant fraction of a population, and runs of linked polymorphisms, called *haplotypes*, in the same or other genes. This is especially clear in the "channelopathies"; for example, the severity of the clinical syndrome caused by a given sodium channel (SCN5A) mutation can be profoundly modified by SNPs (Poelzing et al., 2006) and haplotype variations (Bezzina et al., 2006) that, by themselves, are of no obvious clinical significance. Epigenetic mechanisms (see Chapter 4) can also allow carriers of an abnormal gene that usually causes a mild cardiomyopathy to exhibit atypical or severe abnormalities, and vice versa.

SOME THERAPEUTIC IMPLICATIONS

Until the late 1980s, treatment of patients with heart failure sought to correct the hemodynamic abnormalities; diuretics were given to reduce preload, vasodilators to reduce afterload, and inotropes to increase contractility. However, clinical trials carried out over the past 20 years have shown that although these strategies generally improve symptoms, many vasodilators and virtually all inotropes worsen prognosis (see Chapter 6). In the case of the vasodilators, functional effects on the peripheral circulation that reduce afterload account for an immediate hemodynamic benefit but do not explain why most direct-acting arteriolar vasodilators fail to improve long-term survival. Some vasodilators do have significant survival benefits; these include nitrates, ACE inhibitors, and angiotensin II receptor blockers, all of which are neurohumoral blockers which inhibit the maladaptive proliferative signaling pathways that lead to progressive dilatation (remodeling). Similarly, the long-term beneficial effect of β-blockers, which because of their negative inotropic effect had been almost universally viewed as contraindicated in these patients, appear to be due to their ability to inhibit remodeling as well as to reduce the energy demands of the heart, while spironolactone and other aldosterone antagonists, which also improve long-term prognosis, inhibit maladaptive hypertrophy as well as reducing fibrosis. Even cardiac resynchronization therapy, which was introduced to minimize electrical heterogeneities in the left ventricles of patients with end-stage heart failure, has been found to inhibit remodeling. These findings highlight the clinical importance of maladaptive proliferative signaling in determining the long-term prognosis in heart failure.

BIBLIOGRAPHY

General

Bugaisky L, Gupta M, Gupta MG, et al. (1992). Cellular and molecular mechanisms of hypertrophy In: *The Heart and Cardiovascular System*. 2nd ed. Fozzard H, Haber E, Katz A, et al., eds. 1621–1640. New York, Raven Press.

Collucci WS (2005). *Atlas of Heart Failure. Cardiac Function and Dysfunction*. 4th ed. Philadelphia, Current Med.

Katz AM (2006). *Physiology of the Heart*. 4th ed. Philadelphia, Lippincott Williams and Wilkins.

Langer GA, ed. (1997). *The Myocardium*. San Diego, Academic Press.

Mann DL, ed. (2004). *Heart Failure: A Companion to Braunwald's Heart Disease*. Philadelphia, Saunders.

Opie LH (2006). *Heart Physiology. From Cell to Circulation*. 4th ed. Philadelphia, Lippincott Williams & Wilkins.

Page E, Fozzard HA, Solaro RJ, eds. (2002). *Handbook of Physiology*, Section 2: The Cardiovascular System, Vol. I. *The Heart*. New York, Oxford.

Sipido KR, Eisner D (2005). Something old, something new: changing views on the cellular mechanisms of heart failure. Cardiovasc Res 68:167–174.

Excitation–Contraction Coupling, Contraction, Relaxation, and the Cytoskeleton

Beard NA, Laver DR, Dulhunty AF (2004). Calsequestrin and the calcium release channel of skeletal and cardiac muscle. Prog Biophys Mol Biol 85:3369.

Bers DM (2001). *Excitation-Contraction Coupling and Cardiac Contractile Force*. Dordrecht, Kluwer.

Bodi I, Mikala G, Koch SE, et al. (2005). The L-type calcium channel in the heart: the beat goes on. J Clin Invest 115:3306–3317.

Bretscher A, Edwards K, Fehon RG (2002). ERM proteins and merlin: integrators at the cell cortex. Nat Rev Mol Cell Biol 3:586–599.

Cingolani HE, Ennis IL (2007). Sodium-hydrogen exchanger, cardiac overload, and myocardial hypertrophy. Circulation 115:1090–1100.

Fill M, Copello JA (2002). Ryanodine calcium receptor calcium release channels. Physiol Rev 82:893–922.

Granzier HL, Labeit S (2004). The giant protein titin. A major player in myocardial mechanics, signaling and disease. Circ Res 94:284–295.

Kaplan JH (2002). Biochemistry of Na,K-ATPase. Annu Rev Biochem 71:511–535.

Karmayzn M, Gan XT, Humphreys RA, et al. (1999). The myocardial Na^+/H^+ exchange. Structure, regulation, and its role in disease. Circ Res 85:777–786.

Kretsinger RH (1979). The informational role of calcium in the cytosol. Adv Cyclic Nucl Res 11:1–26.

Lehnart SE, Wehrens XHT, Kushnir A, et al. (2004). Cardiac ryanodine receptor function and regulation in heart disease. Ann N Y Acad Sci 1015:144–159.

Levi AJ, Boyett MR, Lee CO (1994). The cellular actions of digitalis glycosides on the heart. Prog Biophy Molec Biol 62:1–54.

MacLennan DH, Kranias EG (2003). Phospholamban: a crucial regulator of cardiac contractility. Nat Rev Mol Cell Biol 4:566–577.

Maier LS, Bers DM (2007). Role of Ca(2+)/calmodulin-dependent protein kinase (CaMK) in excitation-contraction coupling in the heart. Cardiovasc Res 73:631–640.

Mermall V, Post PL, Mooseker MS (1998). Unconventional myosins in cell movement, membrane traffic, and signal transduction. Science 279:527–533.

Palmer BM (2005). Thick filament proteins and performance in human heart failure. Heart Fail Rev. 10:187–197.

Pitt GS, Dun W, Boyden PA (2006). Remodeled calcium channels. J Mol Cell Cardiol 41:373–388.

Putney LK, Denker SP, Barber DL (2002). The changing face of the Na^+/H^+ exchanger, NHE1: structure, regulation, and cellular actions. Annu Rev Pharmacol Toxicol 42:527–552.

Rossi D, Sorrentino V 2002. Molecular genetics of ryanodine receptors Ca^{2+}-release channels. Cell Calcium 32:307–319.

Schillinger W, Fiolet JW, Schlotthauer K, et al. (2003). Relevance of Na^+–Ca^{2+} exchange in heart failure. Cardiovasc Res 57:921–933.

Solaro RJ (2005). Remote control of A-band cardiac thin filaments by the I-Z-I protein network of cardiac sarcomeres. Trends Cardiovasc Med 15:148–152.

Solaro RJ, Rarick HM (1998). Troponin and tropomyosin. Proteins that switch on and tune in the activity of cardiac myofilaments. Circ Res 83:471–480.

Tardiff JC (2005). Sarcomeric proteins and familial hypertrophic cardiomyopathy: linking mutations in structural proteins to complex cardiac phenotypes. Heart Failure Rev 10:237–248.

Therien AG, Pu HX, Karlish SJ, et al. (2001). Molecular and functional studies of the gamma subunit of the sodium pump. J Bioenerg Biomembr 33:407–414.

VanBuren P, Okada Y (2005). Thin filament remodeling in failing myocardium. Heart Failure Rev 10:199–209.

Wang SQ, Wei C, Zhao G, et al. (2004). Imaging microdomain Ca^{2+} in muscle cells. Circ Res 94:1011–1022.

Yano M, Ikeda Y, Matsuzuki M (2005). Altered intracellular Ca^{2+} handling in heart failure. J Clin Invest 1154:556–564.

Arrhythmias

Akar FG, Tomaselli GF (2005). Conduction abnormalities in nonischemic dilated cardiomyopathy: basic mechanisms and arrhythmic consequences. Trends Cardiovasc Med 15:259–264.

George CH, Jundi H, Thomas NL, et al. (2007). Ryanodine receptors and ventricular arrhythmias: emerging trends in mutations, mechanisms and therapies. J Mol Cell Cardiol 42:34–50.

Haufe V, Chamberland C, Dumaine R (2007). The promiscuous nature of the cardiac sodium current. J Mol Cell Cardiol 42:469–477.

Hille B (2001). *Ionic Channels of Excitable Membranes*. 3rd ed. Sunderland MA, Sinauaer.

Kontula K, Laitinen PJ, Lehtonen A, et al. (2005). Catecholaminergic polymorphic ventricular tachycardia: recent mechanistic insights. Cardiovasc Res. 15:379–387.

Lampe PD, Lau AF (2000). Regulation of gap junctions by phosphorylation of connexins. Arch Biochem Biophys 384:205–215.

Nerbonne JM (2000). Molecular basis of functional voltage-gated K^+ channel diversity in the mammalian myocardium. J Physiol (Lond) 525:285–298.

Pogwizd SM, Bers DM (2004). Cellular basis of triggered arrhythmias in heart failure. Trends Cardiovasc Med 14:61–66.

Saffitz JE, Kléber AG (2004). Effects of mechanical forces and mediators of hypertrophy on remodeling of gap junctions in the heart. Circ. Res 94:585–591.

Yu H, McKinnon D, Dixon JE, et al. (1999). Transient outward current, i_{to1}, is altered in cardiac memory. Circulation 99:1898–1905.

Energy Starvation

Barger PM, Kelly DP (1999). Fatty acid utilization in the hypertrophied and failing heart: Molecular regulatory mechanisms. Am J Med Sci 318:36–42.

Giordano FJ (2005). Oxygen, oxidative stress, hypoxia, and heart failure. J Clin Invest 115:500–508.

Huss JM, Kelly DP (2005). Mitochondrial energy metabolism in heart failure: a question of balance. J Clin Invest 115:547–555.

Ingwall JS (2002). *ATP and the Heart*. Norwall MA, Kluwer.

Ingwall JS, Weiss RG (2004). Is the failing heart energy starved? On using chemical energy to support cardiac function. Circ Res 95:135–145.

Kane GC, Liu X-K, Yamada S, et al. (2005). Cardiac K_{ATP} channels in health and disease. J Mol Cell Cardiol 38:937–943.

Neubauer S (2007). The failing heart — An engine out of fuel. N Engl J Med 356:1140–1151.

Stanley WS, Chandler MP (2002). Energy metabolism in the normal and failing heart: Potential for therapeutic interventions. Heart Failure Rev 7:115–130.

Proliferative Signaling

Akazawa H, Komuro I (2003). Roles of cardiac transcription factors in cardiac hypertrophy. Circ Res 92:1079–1088.

Calderone A, Takahashi N, Izzo NJ Jr, et al. (1995). Pressure- and volume-induced left ventricular hypertrophies are associated with distinct myocyte phenotypes and differential induction of peptide growth factor mRNAs. Circulation 92:2385–2390.

de Tombe PP, Solaro RJ (2000). Integration of cardiac myofilament activity and regulation with pathways signaling hypertrophy and failure. Ann Biomed Eng 28:991–1001.

Dorn GW II, Force T (2005). Protein kinase cascades in the regulation of cardiac hypertrophy. J Clin Invest 115:527–537.

Foo RS-Y, Mani K, Kitsis RN (2005). Death begets failure in the heart. J Clin Invest 115:565–571.

Frey N, Katus HA, Olson EN, et al. (2004). Hypertrophy of the heart. A new therapeutic target. Circulation 109:1580–1589.

Hoshijima M, Chien KR (2002). Mixed signals in heart failure: cancer rules. J Clin Invest 1098:849–855.

Lips DJ, deWindta LJ, van Kraaij DJW, et al. (2003). Molecular determinants of myocardial hypertrophy and failure: alternative pathways for beneficial and maladaptive hypertrophy. Europ Heart J 24:883–896.

McKinsey TA, Olson EN (2005). Toward transcriptional therapies of the failing heart: chemical screens to modulate genes. J Clin Invest 115:538–546.

Molkentin JD (2006). Dichotomy of Ca^{2+} in the heart: contraction versus intracellular signaling. J Clin Invest 116:623–626.

Selvetella G, Hirsch E, Notte A, et al. (2004). Adaptive and maladaptive hypertrophic pathways: points of convergence and divergence Cardiovasc Res 63:373–380.

Familial Cardiomyopathies

Arad M, Seidman JG, Seidman CE (2002). Phenotypic diversity in hypertrophic cardiomyopathy. Hum Mol Genet 11:2499–2506.

Arad M, Maron BJ, Gorham JM, et al. (2005). Glycogen storage diseases presenting as hypertrophic cardiomyopathy. N Engl J Med 352:362–372.

Ashrafian H, Watkins H (2007). Reviews of translational medicine and genomics in cardiovascular disease: new disease taxonomy and therapeutic implications. J Am Coll Cardiol 49:1251–1264.

Burkett EL, Hershberger RE (2005). Clinical and genetic issues in familial dilated cardiomyopathy. J Am Coll Cardiol 45:969–981.

Casademont J, Miro O (2002). Electron transport chain defects in heart failure. Heart Failure Rev 7:131–139.

Chang A, Potter JD (2005). Sarcomeric protein mutations in dilated cardiomyopathy. Heart Failure Rev 10:225–235.

Colan SD, Lipshultz SE, Lowe AM, et al. (2007). Epidemiology and cause-specific outcome of hypertrophic cardiomyopathy in children: findings from the Pediatric Cardiomyopathy Registry. Circulation 115:773–781.

Gomes AV, Potter JD (2004). Molecular and cellular aspects of troponin cardiomyopathies. Ann N Y Acad Sci 1015:214–224.

Ho CY, Seidman CE (2006). A contemporary approach to hypertrophic cardiomyopathy. Circulation 113:e858–e862.

Kamisago M, Schmitt JP, McNamara D, et al. (2006). Sarcomere protein gene mutations and inherited heart disease: a beta-cardiac myosin heavy chain mutation causing endocardial fibroelastosis and heart failure. Novartis Found Symp 274:176–189.

Keller DI, Carrier L, Schwartz K (2002). Genetics of familial cardiomyopathies and arrhythmias. Swiss Med Weekly 132:401–407.

Morita H, Rehm HL, Menesses A, McDonough B, Roberts AE, Kucherlapati R, Towbin JA, Seidman JG, Seidman CE (2008), Shared genetic causes of cardiac hypertrophy in children and adults. New Engl J Med 358:1899–1908.

Sabatine MS, Seidman JG, Seidman CE (2006). Cardiovascular genomics. Circulation 113:e450–e455.

Taylor MR, Bristow MR (2006). Alterations in myocardial gene expression as a basis for cardiomyopathies and heart failure. Novartis Found Symp 274:73–89.

REFERENCES

Beil FU, von Chak D, Hasselbach W, et al. (1977). Competition between oxalate and phosphate during active calcium accumulation by sarcoplasmic vesicles. Z Naturforsch 32:281–287.

Bezzina CR, Shimizu W, Yang P, et al. (2006). Common sodium channel promoter haplotype in Asian subjects underlies variability in cardiac conduction. Circulation 113:338–344.

Bouvagnet P, Leger J, Dechesne C, et al. (1984). Fiber types and myosin types in human atrial and ventricular myosin. An anatomical description. Circ Res 55:794–804.

Calderone A, Takahashi N, Izzo NJ Jr, et al. (1995). Pressure- and volume-induced left ventricular hypertrophies are associated with distinct myocyte phenotypes and differential induction of peptide growth factor mRNAs. Circulation 92:2385–2390.

Cambien F, Tiret L (2007). Genetics of cardiovascular diseases: from single mutations to the whole genome. Circulation 116:1714–1724.

Ebashi S, Lipmann F (1962). Adenosine triphosphate-linked concentration of calcium ions in a particulate fraction of rabbit muscle. J Cell Biol 14:389–400.

Fabiato A (1983). Calcium-induced release of calcium from the cardiac sarcoplasmic reticulum. Am J Physiol 245:C1–C14.

Franzini-Armstrong C, Nunzi G (1983). Junctional feet and particles in the triads of a fast-twitch muscle fibre. J Muscle Res Cell Motil 4:233–252.

Franzini-Armstrong C, Protasi F, Ramesh V (1999). Shape, size, and distribution of Ca(2+) release units and couplons in skeletal and cardiac muscles. Biophys J 77:1528–1539.

Furukawa T, Kurokawa J (2006). Potassium channel remodeling in cardiac hypertrophy. J Mol Cell Cardiol 41:753–761.

Geisterfer-Lowrance AAT, Kass S, Tanigawa G, et al. (1990). A molecular basis for familial hypertrophic cardiomyopathy: a beta cardiac myosin heavy chain gene missense mutation. Cell 62:999–1006.

Gergely J (1959). The relaxing factor of muscle. Ann N Y Acad Sci 81:490–504.

Harigaya S, Schwartz A (1969). Rate of calcium binding and uptake in normal and failing human cardiac muscle. Circ Res 25:781–794.

Hasselbach W, Makinose M (1961). Die calciumpumpe der "ershlaffungsgrana" des muskels und ihre abhangigkeit von der ATP-spaltung. Biochem Z 333:518–528.

Hill AV (1949). The abrupt transition from rest to activity in muscle. Proc Roy Soc B 136:399–420.

Katz AM (2002). Ernest Henry Starling, his predecessors, and the "Law of the Heart." Circulation 106:2986–2992.

Katz AM, Repke DI (1967). Quantitative aspects of dog cardiac microsomal calcium binding and calcium uptake. Circulation Res 21:153–162.

Katz AM, Katz PB (1989). Homogeneity out of heterogeneity. Circulation 79:712–717.

Katz AM, Repke DI, Cohen B (1966). Control of the activity of highly purified cardiac actomyosin by Ca^{++}, Na^+ and K^+. Circulation Res 19:1062–1070.

Kobayashi T, Solaro RJ (2005). Calcium, thin filaments, and the integrative biology of cardiac contractility. Annu Rev Physiol 676:39–67.

Lüttgau HC, Niedergerke R (1958). The antagonism between Ca and Na ions on the frog's heart. J Physiol (Lond) 143:486–505.

Margulis L (1970). *Origin of Eukaryotic Cells*. New Haven, CT Yale Univ Press.

Noguchi T, Hunlich M, Camp PC, et al. (2004). Thin-filament-based modulation of contractile performance in human heart failure. Circulation 110:982–987.

Page E (1978). Quantitative ultrastructural analysis in cardiac membrane physiology. Am J Physiol 63:C147–C158.

Poelzing S, Forleo C, Samodell M, et al. (2006). SCN5A polymorphism restores trafficking of a Brugada syndrome mutation on a separate gene. Circulation 114:368–376.

Repke K (1964). Über den biochemischen Wirkungsmodus von Digitalis. Klin Wochschr 41:156–165.

Reuter H, Seitz N (1968). The dependence of calcium efflux from cardiac muscle on temperature and external ion composition. J Physiol (London) 195:451–470.

Sartore S, Gorza L, Pierobon Bormioli S, et al. (1981). Myosin types and fiber types in cardiac muscle. I: Ventricular myocardium. J Cell Biol 88:226–233.

Schätzmann HJ (1953). Herzglykoside als hemmstoffe für den aktiven Kalium-und Natriumtransport durch die Erythrocytenmembran. Helv physiol Acta 11:346–354.

Scheuer J, Buttrick P (1987). The cardiac hypertrophic responses to pathologic and physiologic loads. Circulation 75(1 Pt 2):I63–I68.

Shipley RA, Shipley LJ, Wearn JT (1938). The capillary supply in normal and hypertrophied hearts of rabbits. J Exp Med 65:29–42.

Stern M, Song L-S, Cheng H, et al. (1999). Local control models of cardiac excitation-contraction coupling. A possible role for allosteric interactions between ryanodine receptors. J Gen Physiol 113:469–489.

Tian R, Ingwall JS (1996). Energetic basis for reduced contractile reserve in isolated rat hearts. Am J Physiol 270(4 Pt 2):H1207–H1216.

van Heerebeck L, Borbély A, Niessen HWM, et al. (2006). Myocardial structure and function differ in systolic and diastolic heart failure. Circulation 113:1966–1973.

Wang SQ, Wei C, Zhao G, et al. (2004). Imaging microdomain Ca^{2+} in muscle cells. Circ Res 94:1011–1022.

Weber A, Winicur S (1961). The role of calcium in the superprecipitation of actomyosin. J Biol Chem 236:3198–3202.

Wilbrandt W, Koller H (1948). Die Calcium-Wirkung am Froschherzen als Funktion des Ionengleichgewichts zwischen Zellmembran und Umgebung. Helv Physiol Acta 6:208–221.

CHAPTER 6

Therapeutic Options for Patients with, or at Risk for, Heart Failure

Marvin A. Konstam • Arnold M. Katz

These final two chapters are devoted to the management of patients with heart failure and to those who are at risk for developing this condition. The present chapter first lays the groundwork for this discussion by describing the recent evolution of thinking related to heart failure treatment and by articulating treatment goals. It is then organized according to treatment or management modality, describing the conceptual basis for each modality and summarizing the data that provide a basis and guidance for its use. The following chapter focuses on approaches to managing specific patient groups, drawing on the various modalities previously covered. It is organized according to categories of patients, determined by symptom status and mode of presentation and divided into broad anatomic/cardiac functional categories based on the presence or absence of left ventricular (LV) remodeling with dilation. In aggregate, these chapters are intended to provide the reader with both an understanding of the basis for various management approaches and a practical guide to approaching the management of specific categories of patients.

EVOLVING CONCEPTS IN THE TREATMENT OF HEART FAILURE

The past two decades have seen a revolution in thinking regarding an approach to therapy for patients with heart failure and those at risk for this condition (Fig. 6-1). These changes can be traced to three parallel developments in the field. The first is improved sophistication in the design and conduct of cardiovascular clinical trials, with an increasing affinity by clinicians and clinical investigators for evidence-based medicine. The second is the discovery that some treatments (e.g., inotropic agents) with an intuitive attractiveness regarding treating this population failed to effect long-term clinical benefits, whereas other agents (e.g., angiotensin-converting enzyme [ACE] inhibitors and beta-adrenergic receptor blockers [beta blockers]) with less or absent intuitive attractiveness provided us with our first evidence of improvement in the natural history of these patients. The third is a shifting paradigm of the pathophysiology of heart failure, with interdependent systemic (neurohormonal) and cardiovascular (structural remodeling and functional modification) components.

It would be logical to infer that the second factor, based on clinical trial evidence, has been driven by the third, based on mechanistic insight. However, clinical trial evidence has contributed importantly to shifts in the mechanistic paradigm, often providing unexpected results and requiring rethinking basic evidence or disparaging a popular concept in favor of a less-popular one. One prominent example was the observation that treatment with the mixed inotrope-vasodilator milrinone was associated with an excess mortality, compared with placebo.[1] A second was observed survival

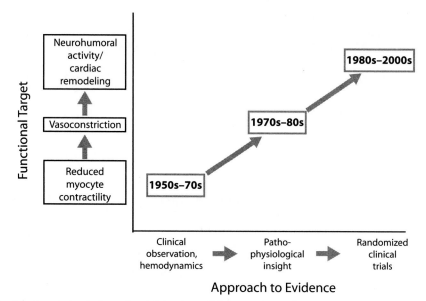

Approach to Evidence

Figure 6-1: Progression in focus for defining heart failure treatment, from 1950s to today.

benefit with beta blocker treatment in a series of clinical trials[2,3,4] transforming a minority view regarding the deleterious effect of adrenergic excess into a broadly accepted component of the heart failure paradigm.

During the 1970s and early 1980s clinicians viewed heart failure as a uniformly fatal condition, varying only moderately in the pace of progressive cardiac functional and symptomatic deterioration, for which mere palliation was medically feasible, with prescription of digoxin, diuretics, and bed rest (see Chapter 1). We now have therapies that are well documented to prolong survival, improve symptom status and health-related quality of life, and arrest or reverse the progression of adverse cardiac remodeling and dysfunction (Fig. 6-2). Complete normalization of LV volumes and ejection fraction (EF) is a frequent observation during treatment with ACE inhibitors and beta blockers in patients with dilated cardiomyopathy.

Three characteristics of the pathophysiology of heart failure are worthy of mention and re-emphasis as an introduction to these chapters on therapeutics in heart failure: neurohormonal activation (see Chapter 3), ventricular remodeling (see Chapters 4 and 5), and heart failure as a cardiovascular-renal syndrome.

Figure 6-2: Drugs and devices and the year they were first definitively demonstrated to have a beneficial effect on clinical outcomes in at least some subsets of patients with chronic heart failure, generally with reduced LV ejection fraction (LV dilation). (No such data are available for diuretics, although all clinical trials were performed using background diuretic treatment.) ACE, angiotensin-converting enzyme; Aldo, aldosterone; ARB, angiotensin receptor blocker; CRT, cardiac resynchronization therapy; ICD, implantable cardioverter-defibrillator; VAD, ventricular assist device.

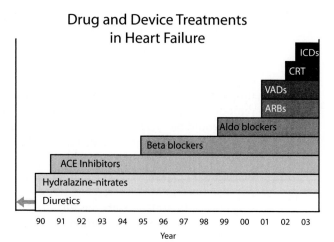

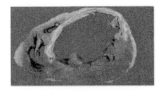

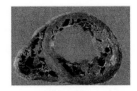

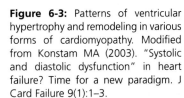

Figure 6-3: Patterns of ventricular hypertrophy and remodeling in various forms of cardiomyopathy. Modified from Konstam MA (2003). "Systolic and diastolic dysfunction" in heart failure? Time for a new paradigm. J Card Failure 9(1):1–3.

**Ischemic
Cardiomyopathy**

**Dilated
Cardiomyopathy**

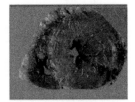

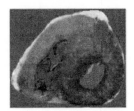

**Hypertensive
Cardiomyopathy**

**Hypertrophic
Cardiomyopathy**

The term *ventricular remodeling* most commonly applies to a restructuring of cardiac architecture, which may result in LV dilatation and transformation from an ellipsoidal to a spherical configuration[5,6,7,8] (Fig. 6-3). Histologically, these findings are associated with myocyte hypertrophy and increases in interstitial collagen. The myocardium within pathologically remodeled ventricles displays various functional changes in calcium handling, receptor signaling, metabolism, contraction, and relaxation (see Chapter 5). Increased interstitial collagen is associated with increased myocardial stiffness. Many of the drugs demonstrated to improve clinical outcomes in patients with heart failure have also been found to slow or reverse the progression of pathologic remodeling (Table 6-1). These findings support both a central role of

TABLE 6-1		
Comparison of Left Ventricular Remodeling and Survival Effects for Various Drug Classes		
	Remodeling effects	**Survival effects**
Established Therapy		
ACEI	Benefit	Benefit
ARB	Benefit	Benefit
Aldo blockers	Benefit to neutral	Benefit
β-blockers	Benefit	Benefit
Other Therapy		
Vasopeptidase-I	Benefit (ACEI-neutral)	Benefit (ACEI-neutral)
Endothelin-1-B	Neutral	Neutral
TNFα-B	Neutral to adverse	Neutral to adverse
Ibopamine	Adverse	Adverse
Vasopressin-B	Neutral	Neutral

Comparison of effects of various drug classes on parameters of left ventricular remodeling and on survival. ACE-I, angiotensin converting enzyme inhibitor; ARB, angiotensin receptor blocker; Aldo, aldosterone; I, inhibitor; TNFα, tumor necrosis factor – alpha;

Figure 6-4: Approximate magnitude of relative risk reduction in mortality demonstrated in clinical trials with the drug classes shown. Each subsequent drug class was investigated using background therapy that included the class(es) of drugs previously shown to convey outcome benefit. ACEI, ACE (angiotensin-converting enzyme) inhibitor; ARB, angiotensin receptor blocker; Aldo, aldosterone.

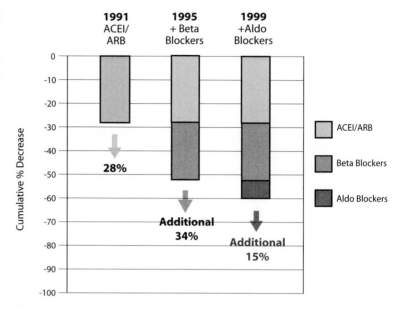

ventricular remodeling in driving the natural history of heart failure and the likelihood that clinical benefit from these drug classes is driven, at least in part, through modulation of ventricular remodeling and prevention of myocardial cell death.

Activation of neurohormonal systems, particularly the renin–angiotensin–aldosterone axis and the adrenergic nervous system,[9] is closely linked to observed therapeutic advances in heart failure (see Chapter 3) (Fig. 6-4). Most of the drugs documented to improve the natural history of this condition—ACE inhibitors, angiotensin receptor blockers (ARBs), aldosterone receptor blockers, and beta blockers—act through interference of these systems. Activation of these systems contributes to the cellular and interstitial changes that drive ventricular remodeling.

There is increasing recognition of the contribution of renal and vascular factors in the pathogenesis and clinical expression of heart failure. Investigators and clinicians are turning to the terms *cardiorenal syndrome* and *cardiovascular-renal syndrome* in reference to the complex interactions among these three organs/organ systems. The same factors—e.g., neurohormones, hypertension, diabetes, lipid derangement—that contribute to cardiac disease also promote vascular and renal pathology. Both endothelial dysfunction[10] and excessive arterial stiffness[11] contribute to the syndrome of heart failure through impaired reactive vasodilation and inability to handle an intravascular volume load. Conversely, heart failure promotes endothelial dysfunction.[12,13] Impaired renal sodium handling and increased renin production promote the progression and clinical expression of heart failure. Conversely, heart failure impairs renal function and sodium excretion and promotes renin production.[14] Thus, cardiac, vascular, and renal pathology and functional impairment conspire in a complex series of vicious cycles. It is likely that direct renal and/or vascular effects of agents such as ACE inhibitors, ARBs, and nitrates contribute importantly to their observed benefits in patients with heart failure. Renal impairment limits the efficacy of diuretics, and diuretics may worsen renal function. Investigational strategies are increasingly focusing on the renal and vascular contributions to the heart failure syndrome.

We can now look back at the therapeutic advances that have occurred in treating patients with heart failure and observe a logic to evidence-based clinical practice, which fits well with current constructs for the pathophysiology of this condition. But this unified image evolved in a nonlinear and often counterintuitive fashion, driven by disappointing and unexpected clinical trial findings at least as much as by trial results that fit neatly with underlying basic hypotheses. Regardless of the path that has brought us to our present understanding, clinicians now possess the therapeutic tools to improve the lives of patients with heart failure and of those at risk for this condition. Although the present mechanistic paradigms—including ventricular remodeling and neurohormonal activation—will undoubtedly evolve in the coming years, they form a solid basis for moving forward along a pathway to future clinical advances through the conduct of well-designed clinical trials.

TREATMENT GOALS

Arguably, the clinician has only two goals in managing patients: prolonging survival and maximizing health-related quality of life. We use the latter term broadly to encompass all factors that influence both symptom profile and functional status. For example, symptoms, such as dyspnea, light-headedness, or edema, and functional impairment, such as inability to climb stairs, sleep comfortably, or engage in sexual activity, all detract from health-related quality of life. Appropriate treatment goals, therefore, include eliminating or minimizing all of the aforementioned factors, each of which detracts from the patient's satisfaction with life.

Much debate centers on the relative value of these two goals in managing patients with heart failure. Although the relative desirability of living longer versus feeling better (or being more functional) varies from patient to patient, generally, the worse a patient's health-related quality of life, the greater importance he or she places on treatments that will improve symptoms or functional status, relative to those that may prolong life.[15] In examining clinical trial results, regulatory decision making, and guideline recommendations, it appears that greater weight is placed on treatments that prolong survival over those that improve health-related quality of life. This apparent preference is likely driven more by the broad methodological consensus and consistency of findings from study to study for determining treatment effect on survival as much as by a bias toward the desirability for optimizing survival over health-related quality of life. In contrast, the goal of achieving convincing symptom or functional status improvement has been more elusive, with disagreement on the optimal instruments and timing of measurement and with inconsistency of findings from study to study.

Preventing hospitalization is a frequently mentioned goal in managing patients with heart failure. It is an endpoint that has been successfully incorporated into clinical trials (most commonly structured as time to death or initial cause-specific hospitalization) and contributes to the basis for regulatory approval of several widely used drugs. Since hospital utilization represents the principal driver for the high health care cost associated with heart failure, use of this endpoint may be rationalized because of its implication for health care economics. However, for the purpose of this discussion, it is best to focus on goals related to the needs of the individual patient. Need for hospitalization may be considered a marker for disease severity or disease progression. As such, the hospitalization event may be viewed as a surrogate (see subsequent text), its inferred value based on the view that greater or more rapid disease severity or progression (indicated by the need for hospitalization) will ultimately lead to a greater likelihood for early death or to worsening of health-related quality of life. A more straightforward rationale for accepting the goal of preventing heart failure–related hospitalizations is that these events are direct indicators of a worsening quality of life. A patient's appearance in an emergency department and a willingness to be hospitalized may imply intolerability of, or greater concern over, symptoms or deterioration of functional status. Certainly, the need to be in a hospital is a direct detractor of a patient's ability to function optimally in life. So the treatment goal of preventing hospitalizations can be viewed most simply as part of the clinician's efforts to help the patient to feel better or optimize health-related quality of life.

Surrogate Endpoints

All treatment goals other than prolonging survival and maximizing health-related quality of life may be viewed as surrogate markers, or intermediate targets in patient management. If one understands enough about a disease process and what drives its impact on survival, symptoms, and functional status, one can incorporate goals that have no direct consequence to the patient but, if achieved, will secondarily reduce the adverse consequences.[16] To draw an analogy to golf, using a surrogate endpoint is like lining up a putt by identifying a near-field target that the golfer calculates as lying along the correct pathway between the ball position and the hole. There is no reward for reaching the intermediate target. However, if the golfer has calculated correctly, then hitting the surrogate target will improve the likelihood of the ball finding the hole.

Reductions in blood pressure and low density lipoprotein (LDL) cholesterol represent two broadly accepted surrogate treatment targets for the prevention of cardiovascular disease, since in each case, the abnormality correlates strongly with subsequent adverse clinical outcome. Furthermore, treatment-related improvement in the abnormality (i.e., reducing blood pressure or reducing LDL cholesterol) has been uniformly observed to be associated with reduced subsequent incidence of adverse cardiovascular events. Unfortunately, in heart failure, there are no universally accepted surrogates.

Measures of ventricular remodeling, such as LV volume, have been advocated as surrogate treatment targets,[7] given the strong association of these markers with subsequent morbidity and mortality (Table 6-1). Furthermore, most classes of drugs—e.g., ACE inhibitors, ARBs, and beta blockers—that have been shown to reduce morbidity and mortality also improve measures of LV dilation or slow their progression. Reversal or slowing of LV remodeling may be viewed as a means to an end, because a drug that achieves this effect is likely to improve clinical outcomes. Nevertheless, therapeutic impact on measures of LV volume or mass has not yet been shown to be predictive of a benefit on morbidity and mortality with sufficient reliability to be accepted as a standard for regulatory approval or for widespread application by clinicians.

Assays for several natriuretic peptides and their derivatives—e.g., B-type natriuretic peptide and N-terminal pro-B-type natriuretic peptide—have been found useful in diagnosing, grading, and judging treatment effect in patients with heart failure. These measures correlate with both severity of LV dysfunction and subsequent morbidity.[17,18] They are effective in distinguishing acute heart failure exacerbation from alternative causes of dyspnea[19,20] and have been suggested as adjunctive tools to clinical assessment in gauging response to treatment. As with measures of LV remodeling, therapeutic impact on levels of the natriuretic peptides have not been sufficiently reliably linked to treatment effect on clinical outcomes to warrant acceptance of these measures as a clinical or regulatory standard.

TREATMENT OF UNDERLYING CONDITIONS

Management of the patient with heart failure must always entail considering and addressing etiologic and exacerbating factors. Potentially remediable causes include coronary occlusive disease, hypertension, valvular heart disease, congenital heart disease, pericardial disease, toxins—including alcohol and cocaine—infection, collagen-vascular and vasculitic diseases, infiltrative processes, endocrine and metabolic disorders, and obstructive sleep apnea (see also Chapter 2). Detailed discussion of treatment approaches to each of these disorders is beyond the scope of this book. However, several of these etiologic factors deserve special attention.

Coronary Occlusive Disease

Ischemic heart disease represents a major etiologic factor responsible for heart failure in the developed world. Its diagnosis should be considered in all patients. Ischemic heart disease may manifest itself as heart failure for one or more of several reasons. First, energy starvation caused by ongoing ischemia adversely impacts both diastolic and systolic myocardial function (See Chapter 5). Its potential impact in driving manifestations of heart failure should particularly be considered in patients with angina or angina-equivalent symptoms and in those with episodic or purely exertional symptoms. However, even in patients with signs and symptoms that appear more stable and without symptoms referable to angina, recurrent ischemia, associated with myocardial "hibernation"[21,22] and/or "stunning,"[23] may be contributing to myocardial dysfunction. Second, patients may manifest chronic heart failure due to loss of myocardium, secondary to prior infarction. Most often, cardiac dysfunction results not only from the infarction itself but also from the progressive reactive hypertrophy and fibrosis in noninfarcted zones, contributing to left ventricular dilation. Pathologically hypertrophied myocardium manifests abnormal calcium handling, increased stiffness, and functional abnormalities during both systole and diastole (See Chapter 5). The latter processes may be slowed or at least partially reversed through pharmacologic therapy (see subsequent text). Third, ischemic heart disease may result in mitral valve dysfunction, because of (a) infarction involving the papillary muscle apparatus or adjacent myocardium, (b) recurrent ischemia of these same tissues, or (c) functional impairment related to left ventricular remodeling and dilation.

The diagnostic evaluation of patients with heart failure must include an approach that provides confidence that there is, or is not, a contributing element of ischemic heart disease. The aggressiveness with which this diagnosis is pursued is influenced by (a) the presence or absence of anginal symptoms; (b) telltale evidence of prior infarction by electrocardiography, echocardiography, and/or magnetic resonance imaging; and (c) the presence and extent of risk factors for coronary artery disease. Some clinicians feel that every patient with heart failure, in the absence of advanced age or substantial comorbidity, should undergo coronary angiography to confirm or exclude significant coronary artery disease. However, increased sophistication of noninvasive imaging techniques has substantially diminished the need for this approach. Current diagnostic options include tests for inducible ischemia—e.g., radionuclide myocardial perfusion imaging and stress echocardiography—and less-invasive methods to image the major epicardial coronary arteries—e.g., computerized tomographic angiography. Where results of such investigations yield a low probability of obstructive coronary disease, coupled with a low pretest probability, based on the previously discussed factors, the need for invasive coronary angiography is obviated. On the other hand, if significant doubt remains following clinical evaluation and noninvasive testing, cardiac catheterization should be performed.

The diagnosis of coronary artery disease, as by coronary angiography, is not necessarily sufficient to drive appropriate therapeutic decision making. Rather, functional and/or myocardial perfusion imaging often adds essential information by delineating myocardial zones that are or are not viable and viable zones that are or are not subject to active ischemia.[24,25] Such information is critical in determining whether or not to proceed with coronary revascularization and, if so, which areas to revascularize.

The importance of the diagnosis of ischemic heart disease is driven by its impact on treatment decision making. Percutaneous or surgical revascularization should be strongly considered for patients with prior myocardial infarction and either clinical or imaging evidence of spontaneous or inducible myocardial ischemia. The rationale for revascularization is strengthened where (a) extensive—particularly three-vessel—obstructive coronary artery disease is present, (b) substantial amounts of viable myocardium are supplied by arteries with significant obstructive disease, and (c) the disease is relatively focal—that is, arteries distal to discrete obstruction are not diffusely diseased. The following specific recommendation is made in the Heart Failure Society of America heart failure guideline[26]:

> It is recommended that coronary revascularization be performed in patients with heart failure and suitable coronary anatomy for relief of refractory angina or acute coronary syndrome. (Strength of Evidence = B)
>
> Coronary revascularization with coronary artery bypass or percutaneous coronary intervention as appropriate should be considered in patients with heart failure and suitable coronary anatomy who have demonstrable evidence of myocardial viability in areas of significant obstructive coronary artery disease or the presence of inducible ischemia. (Strength of Evidence = C)

Despite the pathophysiological rationale, to date no randomized controlled trial has demonstrated the value of coronary revascularization in patients with heart failure. Instead, evidence supporting a value to revascularization in this setting is derived from observational analyses comparing outcomes in apparently comparable cohorts who have or have not undergone surgical revascularization.[25] Such analyses have demonstrated that viable myocardial areas undergoing revascularization manifest improvement in systolic function over time, with associated augmentation of global left ventricular EF, and patients with substantial areas of viable myocardium undergoing surgical revascularization manifest better survival than similar patients not undergoing these procedures. Such observational analyses do not carry the same weight as randomized, controlled clinical trial findings because of potential bias in treatment selection. One randomized controlled trial[27] failed to demonstrate improved survival associated with percutaneous revascularization of a stenosed or occluded coronary artery responsible for myocardial infarction, beyond the time usually associated with an opportunity for myocardial salvage. However, this finding does not negate the potential for improved outcomes from revascularizing areas of viable myocardium supplied by stenosed coronary arteries. In the absence of randomized controlled data, the combination of a pathophysiological rationale and existing observational analyses supports strong consideration of revascularization in this setting.

Aside from, and in addition to, percutaneous or surgical revascularization, the diagnosis of significant coronary artery disease influences medical treatment. ACE inhibitors, ARBs, beta blockers, and/or aldosterone blockers are warranted in many patients with heart failure, regardless of the presence or absence of ischemic heart disease. But beyond these treatments, if active ischemia is considered to be contributing to clinical heart failure, greater consideration should be given to drugs that may directly diminish ischemia, such as nitrates and calcium channel blockers, even though randomized clinical trial evidence for an improvement in outcomes from such treatments is sparse or absent. The presence of coronary disease also provides a rationale for use of antiplatelet treatment in patients with heart failure.

Hypertension

Population-based analyses have identified hypertension as the most important attributable risk for the development of heart failure among previously healthy individuals.[28] A history of hypertension is present in most patients with heart failure, with little difference between patients with and without LV dilation and reduced EF.[29] Blood pressure elevation directly provokes heart failure signs and symptoms by increasing LV afterload (see Chapter 2) and so is a critical factor in triggering and potentiating acute exacerbations of heart failure. Long-standing hypertension promotes pathologic myocyte hypertrophy, driving abnormalities in contraction, relaxation, and compliance. Hypertension is an important risk factor for coronary artery disease, a major cause of heart failure. Furthermore, hypertensive vascular disease contributes to the heart failure syndrome by increasing vascular resistance and impedance, reducing vascular capacitance, and impairing endothelial function. For all of these reasons, management of hypertension is an essential element of strategies designed to prevent heart failure and to treat patients with both acute and chronic heart failure. Treatments directed at correcting hypertension have been shown to reduce the risk for development of heart failure.[30,31]

For patients hospitalized with acute heart failure exacerbation, there is growing evidence for an association between higher blood pressure at time of admission and better short-term prognosis.[32,33] However, this finding almost certainly reflects variations in the underlying physiology among patients with higher versus lower blood pressures in this setting and the poor prognostic implication of cardiac dysfunction severe enough to drive blood pressure down. These findings should not detract from recognizing the importance of aggressive antihypertensive treatment, particularly in the setting of acute decompensated heart failure.

In the acute setting, vasodilators with little or no cardiac effects are ideal choices, because acute heart failure is characterized by vasoconstriction, and caution must be exerted in administering drugs that reduce cardiac contractility in the setting of severe hemodynamic derangement. Nitrates offer substantial value, directly reducing venous pressure as well as arterial blood pressure.[34] By relieving pulmonary edema, diuretics may reduce an acute adrenergic stimulus to vasoconstriction, although excessive diuresis may provoke neurohormonal activation. ACE inhibitors or ARBs may be initiated and incorporated into the chronic regimen, as long as renal function permits. As the patient returns to a more compensated state, strong consideration should be given to the gradual initiation of beta adrenergic blockade.

In the chronic setting, control of hypertension is a major avenue toward preventing heart failure. In patients who have not manifested heart failure, the principal goal should be to decrease systolic and diastolic pressure by whatever means necessary to reach therapeutic targets, without inducing unacceptable adverse effects. A general approach to hypertension management is provided elsewhere[35] and may include sodium restriction, a diuretic, ACE inhibitor, ARB, beta blocker, calcium channel blocker, aldosterone receptor blocker, and/or alpha adrenergic blocker.

Large trials of patients with hypertension have not identified substantial differences among the various drug choices in preventing major adverse cardiovascular events.[36] Alpha adrenergic blockers[37,38] and perhaps calcium channel blockers,[36] have been associated with more heart failure–related events (or less prevention of heart failure–related events) than other drugs achieving the same degree of blood pressure lowering. In the case of calcium channel blockers, this point is not a major consideration for patients without clinical heart failure or cardiac dysfunction, because calcium channel blockers are at least as beneficial as other agents in preventing all-cause cardiovascular events in hypertensive populations without heart failure. In some studies, ARBs have been associated with a greater reduction in LV mass among hypertensive patients with LV hypertrophy,[39] a finding that might translate into relative benefits on clinical outcomes in at least some patient subsets. In other trials targeting patients with atherosclerosis, other coronary risk factors, or patients with diabetic nephropathy, ACE inhibitors[40] or ARBs[41] have reduced the frequency of subsequent heart failure events, lending credence to the attractiveness of these choices in managing hypertension, even in the absence of overt heart failure.

In patients with clinical heart failure or reduced LVEF, agents with demonstrated benefit on long-term clinical outcomes—ACE inhibitors, ARBs, beta blockers, and, in at least some populations, aldosterone blockers—represent important elements of an antihypertensive treatment regimen. Nitrates may be useful adjuncts. Although they are less potent than other drug classes in lowering blood pressure, they have important adjunctive benefits, including reduction in venous pressure and providing a source of vascular nitric oxide. The combination of hydralazine and isosorbide dinitrate has shown benefit in improving clinical outcomes and symptoms, with findings most clear-cut in African Americans.[42] The possible rationale for this combination is discussed in detail in subsequent text, but the combination remains an important consideration for aiding blood pressure control in the hypertensive patient with heart failure. Diuretics should be used wherever there is evidence of, or a propensity toward, volume overload. Sodium restriction represents a major constituent of treatment for all patients with heart failure, particularly those with hypertension.

Once the combination of agents, selected from those mentioned previously (together with dietary sodium restriction), has reached its target or maximal tolerated dose, but without achieving optimal blood pressure control, additional drug treatment should be initiated. Despite concern regarding the negative inotropic effect of agents such as diltiazem and verapamil, calcium channel blockers represent an important additional treatment option. Adverse effects are more likely related to reflex neurohormonal activation than to negative inotropy. For the heart failure patient with persistent hypertension being treated with appropriate neurohormonal blockers and diuretics, the potential added value of these agents—particularly longer-acting agents and newer dihydropyridine agents, such as amlodipine—in reducing blood pressure far outweighs any theoretical risk.

Although there is general consensus that hypertension should be treated more aggressively in the setting of present or prior heart failure, the appropriate blood pressure target in treating hypertensive patients with heart failure remains controversial. There is no evidence for a J-shaped curve, that is a blood pressure below which risk increases with further blood pressure reduction, as had once been believed. Rather, population-based studies suggest that the hypertensive risk is linear over a broad range of blood pressure.[43] The Heart Failure Society of America (HFSA) 2006 Comprehensive Heart Failure Guideline[44] recommends a target of <130/80. It further states:

> In hypertensive patients with evidence for LV dysfunction, particularly when the LV dysfunction is associated with signs and symptoms of heart failure and preserved LV chamber dimension and EF, therapy should be aimed at blood pressure reduction to the lowest levels that can be achieved without side effects. Most guidelines agree that a systolic pressure <130 or even lower may be optimal.

Valvular Disease

As recently as 50 years ago, rheumatic heart disease was responsible for heart failure in a large proportion of patients with this syndrome (see Chapter 1), with congenital aortic valve disease, syphilitic aortitis, and endocarditis also representing significant contributing causes. Currently, in the developed world, with the near disappearance of acute rheumatic fever, early surgical intervention for congenital heart disease, and appropriate antibiotic and surgical treatments for endocarditis, valvular heart disease contributes only a small proportion of cases of heart failure. Rheumatic heart disease continues to contribute importantly to the development of heart failure in regions of Asia and Africa.[45]

Obstruction to mitral inflow, most commonly due to rheumatic mitral stenosis, but occasionally due to atrial myxoma and rarely due to congenital mitral valve or subvalvular pathology, directly impedes forward flow and raises pulmonary venous pressure, causing the heart failure syndrome in the absence of myocardial disease. Unlike for other valvular lesions that can cause progressive myocardial deterioration, medical treatment of rheumatic mitral stenosis is a reasonable option, as long as symptoms can be controlled and pulmonary hypertension is absent to mild.

Medical treatment includes maintenance of sinus rhythm, where possible, heart rate reduction, with beta blockers, calcium channel blockers and/or digoxin (the latter to show ventricular response in atrial fibrillation), to maximize diastolic filling time, appropriate fluid management with sodium restriction and diuretics, endocarditis prophylaxis, and anticoagulation for those with more than mild stenosis and those with atrial fibrillation. However, where symptoms of dyspnea and/or functional impairment persist despite medical treatment, surgical or percutaneous intervention is warranted to relieve the obstruction to flow. Furthermore, delay in correction of obstruction in the presence of significant pulmonary hypertension can lead to pulmonary vascular obstructive disease, which may not correct following valve replacement or repair. Therefore patients must be carefully monitored during medical therapy for mitral stenosis, clinically and using echocardiography and

Doppler imaging, for evidence of worsening symptoms and increasing pulmonary artery pressures. Intervention for rheumatic mitral stenosis may take the form of valve replacement, surgical mitral commissurotomy, or transcatheter valvuloplasty.

There are numerous causes for mitral regurgitation, including rheumatic, ischemic (due to papillary muscle dysfunction), myxomatous, infectious (endocarditis), and congenital (e.g., cleft mitral valve, related to endocardial cushion deformity). Mitral regurgitation may also be functional, related to LV dilation due to ischemic or idiopathic dilated cardiomyopathy. Because in the presence of a leaky mitral valve, the left ventricle partially ejects directly into the left atrium, mitral regurgitation may provoke the heart failure syndrome in the absence of LV pathology and dysfunction. Consideration can be given to delaying surgical correction as long as symptoms are readily managed medically and there is little or no evidence of LV dilation or systolic dysfunction, although in the setting of moderate to severe mitral regurgitation, an LVEF <60% may indicate a significant degree of ventricular remodeling and/or diminished myocardial systolic function. Medical therapy includes diuretics and vasodilators. Strong consideration should be given to the use of ACE inhibitors or ARBs. Although there are no clear-cut data documenting improved outcomes with these classes of agents, it seems reasonable to extrapolate from findings in other forms of dilated cardiomyopathy to infer that these agents may slow the progression of LV dilation and remodeling in patients with primary mitral valvular regurgitation.

A joint guideline committee of the American Heart Association and American College of Cardiology provides recommendations regarding indications for surgical correction of valvular disease.[46] In asymptomatic patients with chronic severe mitral regurgitation, indications for surgical repair or replacement include LVEF ≤60%, LV end-systolic dimension ≥40 mm, new-onset atrial fibrillation or pulmonary arterial hypertension (systolic pressure >50 mm Hg at rest or 60 mm Hg during exercise). For symptomatic patients, repair or replacement is indicated in the absence of severe LV dysfunction (LVEF <30%) and/or dilation (LV end-systolic dimension >55 mm). Surgical correction is controversial in patients with mitral regurgitation and severe LV dysfunction and/or dilation. These findings increase the risk of surgery, and clear-cut evidence for outcome benefit is lacking. There is active investigation underway exploring nonsurgical, catheter-based approaches to mitral valve repair.

Aortic stenosis, with its three principal causes—congenital bicuspid valve, rheumatic disease, and degenerative sclerocalcific disease—is a progressive condition that requires surgical repair once any symptoms appear. Clinical evaluation entails quantifying the hemodynamic lesion and exploring alternative explanations for symptoms. Any reasonable assumption that symptoms of heart failure, angina, or syncope are caused by aortic stenosis should prompt early surgical intervention. Early attempts at percutaneous balloon aortic valvular disease uniformly met with restenosis within months, relegating this procedure to one of palliation under circumstances where surgery is felt to be inadvisable. Otherwise, definitive treatment entails surgical aortic valve replacement. For patients with bicuspid aortic valves, evidence exists to suggest that statin treatment may delay progression of degenerative calcific stenosis. However, firm recommendations regarding this treatment await more definitive evidence based on randomized controlled trials.

Numerous causes may lead to aortic regurgitation, including valvular (e.g., congenital, infectious, rheumatic) and supravalvular (aortic root: e.g., cystic medial necrosis, aortic dissection, infectious or autoimmune aortitis) causes. The danger in aortic regurgitation resides in progressive myocardial damage and remodeling that result from the chronic volume overload. Signs and symptoms of heart failure denote a failing left ventricle. For these reasons, although symptoms may be managed with diuretics and vasodilators, they indicate a need for surgical repair or valve replacement. Similarly, in patients with aortic regurgitation, LV dimensions and function should be monitored, as with serial (at least yearly) echocardiograms to screen for early signs of remodeling and dysfunction. A decrease in EF to ≤50% or an increase in LV end-diastolic dimension to >75 mm or in LV end-systolic dimension to >55 mm in a patient with aortic regurgitation is considered an indication for surgical intervention, regardless of signs and symptoms of heart failure.[46]

NONPHARMACOLOGIC, NONDEVICE MODALITIES IN HEART FAILURE

Although most of the attention regarding management of patients with heart failure or ventricular remodeling and dysfunction has been directed toward the outcome benefits that may be achieved through drug and device prescription, a number of nondrug, nondevice interventions should be emphasized during initial treatment and at every subsequent patient visit. These include diet, exercise, toxic substance avoidance, heart rate and rhythm management, and careful monitoring for early signs and symptoms of physiologic or clinical worsening, particularly in terms of fluid status.

Patient Education and Counseling

Patient education and counseling represent major pillars of any management plan for patients with, or at risk for, heart failure. Noncompliance to medication and dietary prescription represent important, often unrecognized, obstacles to patient management. Inability or unwillingness of patients and their caregivers to recognize and respond to weight gain and early symptoms of clinical worsening represent major causes of emergency department visits and urgent hospitalizations.

Successful care plans must include regular education efforts directed toward both patients and caregivers to overcome these sources of treatment failure.[47] Key components of an educational initiative are (a) an understanding of the patient's condition at an individually appropriate level, (b) emphasis on adherence to medication and dietary prescription, (c) avoidance of toxic substances, and (d) awareness of the early signs of clinical worsening and appropriate response. These points should be reinforced at every visit and as part of a disease management effort. Clinicians should be aware of materials that can be provided to patients and caregivers to facilitate these efforts (see http://www.hfsa.org/hf_modules.asp).

In addition, all patients presenting with heart failure should be advised to strongly consider advance directives, contemplating emergency treatment options that the patient does or does not wish delivered under various clinical circumstances, and assigning a health care proxy to make critical decisions in the event that the patient is unable to make them.[48] During early stages of illness, these directives are best kept general, conveying a sense of the patient's viewpoint on the desire for aggressive treatment to prolong life, versus a focus on patient comfort. They provide guidance for the health care proxy in making specific decisions at a later time. For patients with more advanced symptoms and short life expectancy, the directives may be amended to provide greater specificity regarding which measures a patient does or does not desire. In seeking advance directives, care must be exercised to minimize discomfort in the patient and caregiver, particularly in addressing issues for which they are unprepared. Whenever possible, the clinician should approach these issues in a relaxed, patient manner, allowing the patient and caregiver to approach them if and when they are comfortable doing so. The optimal outcome is having the patient receive the type of management that he or she desires, and providing comfort to caregivers that the patient's desires were respected, rather than their being forced to make urgent critical decisions arbitrarily.

The subsequent sections detail several elements of an extrapharmacologic treatment plan, which should be incorporated into the educational content.

Diet

The most important element of dietary management in patients with heart failure is sodium restriction. The degree of sodium restriction should match to the individual patient's propensity to retain fluid. Dietary sodium restriction is as important as any other element in a clinical management plan for the patient with heart failure prone to fluid retention, the single most prevalent cause for clinical worsening and hospitalization among patients with heart failure. Since most diuretics work by reducing renal tubular sodium reabsorption, dietary sodium intake directly negates their action. In addition to the impact on fluid balance per se, dietary sodium restriction represents an important element of antihypertensive treatment, particularly among patients whose hypertension is difficult to manage.

There is often a striking degree of ignorance and noncompliance to sodium restriction among patients with heart failure. A number of factors are to blame; these include widespread emphasis on a heart-healthy diet (generally low cholesterol and low saturated fat diet), with inadequate attention to sodium intake, even in the hospital setting. Physicians are typically more focused on medication adjustment and procedural considerations, to the detriment of attention to diet. Nurse educators and disease management interventions can help focus the patient and the caregiver on dietary prescription.

The Heart Failure Society of America 2006 Comprehensive Heart Failure Guideline[49] recommends limiting dietary sodium to 2–3 g daily, in patients with "the clinical syndrome of heart failure," with further restriction to 2 g daily for patients with "moderate to severe heart failure." Compliance with these guidelines may be facilitated by referral to a nutritionist or by use of educational materials (see http://www.hfsa.org/hf_modules.asp). However, constant reinforcement is needed, and a simple approach may work better than detailed instruction regarding precise sodium content of specific foods. Most patients should observe the following rules:

- Avoid fast food restaurants.
- Eat in as often as possible, and when eating out, find restaurants with low sodium choices.
- Buy fresh produce, with no prior preparation, and avoid canned and packaged foods, unless they are prepared with a minimum of salt.
- Prepare foods without salt, using alternative flavorings, such as lemon or lime juice and pepper.
- Rid the kitchen/dining room table of a salt shaker.

Often patients feel that they can "cheat" on occasion, particularly on vacations. Patients should be educated that "being good" for weeks at a time may not diminish the likelihood that one or two episodes of cheating may negate all of their hard work and provoke an urgent hospitalization.

The tendency to retain fluid is driven heavily by renal tubular sodium retention, which secondarily drives water retention. The latter is further magnified by an apparent resetting of the osmolar receptors, in part mediated by excess vasopressin secretion (see Chapter 3). Thus, patients with severe heart failure are often hyponatremic, with relative excess in free water. It would be a mistake to overlook the fact that such patients, in contrast to those with the syndrome of inappropriate antidiuretic hormone, also have marked excess in total body sodium, so that restriction of both dietary sodium and free water is indicated. Fluid restriction per se may not be needed in the absence of hyponatremia. On the other hand, the presence of significant hyponatremia, variably defined across a range of serum sodium concentrations from <130 mEq/L–<135 mEq/L, contributed to by loop and thiazide diuretic therapy (coupled with intake of hypotonic fluids), warrants advice to limit free water intake. The Heart Failure Society of America 2006 Comprehensive Heart Failure Guideline[49] recommends restriction of fluid intake to 2 L daily in patients with serum sodium concentrations <130 mEq/L.

As with all patients at risk for cardiovascular events, consideration should be given to limiting cholesterol and saturated fat intake. However, the focus on this recommendation (for example, relative to attention to dietary sodium restriction) should be tailored to the needs of the individual patient. Such recommendations are more important in patients with known atherosclerotic cardiovascular disease and less important in patients with more advanced degrees of heart failure. In particular, patients with limited life expectancy and those experiencing difficulty retaining body mass should not be burdened by limitations in dietary cholesterol and fats. For diabetic patients, attention to glycemic control is the most important element to dietary management.

Advanced heart failure is often characterized by loss of body mass. Although the precise mechanisms responsible for a tendency toward cardiac cachexia remain debated (see Chapter 4),[50] contributing factors include increases in the rate of oxygen consumption, increased production of inflammatory cytokines, diminished appetite, and gastrointestinal edema with impaired absorption. Observational investigations have demonstrated a direct correlation between body mass index and prognosis in patients with heart failure.[51] Elderly patients, in particular, are prone to reduction in dietary intake. Patients should be monitored carefully for evidence of weight loss and diminished body mass. Where present, consultation with a nutritionist is warranted, with consideration of prescription of high-caloric dietary supplements. Care should be given to prescribe supplements that are low in sodium content.

Conversely, heart failure is increasingly recognized as having a strong association with morbid obesity. Although the mechanisms remain unclear, obstructive sleep apnea, hypoxemia, and pulmonary hypertension are key contributing factors. Patients with morbid obesity and heart failure should be considered for referral to obesity centers, where a multidimensional approach can be considered, including dietary and psychological counseling, tailored exercise, treatment of obstructive sleep apnea, and surgical procedures designed to reduce caloric intake or absorption.

Exercise

Recommendations regarding physical activity in patients with heart failure and in those at risk for this condition have changed radically over the past 25 years. Prior to that time, standard teaching advocated prescription of bed rest for patients with heart failure (see Chapter 1). This recommendation stemmed from the view that exercise tended to impose excess stress on the heart, thereby accelerating the progression of disease. It was bolstered by case reports and uncontrolled data demonstrating improvement in cardiac function in patients who were put to bed for prolonged time periods.

Prospective observational studies have demonstrated reduced cardiovascular risk in individuals engaged in regular exercise, compared with those who are more sedentary.[52] In addition, controlled trials performed in patients with ischemic heart disease[53] or heart failure[54] have demonstrated clinical benefits in those randomized to regular exercise training. Exercise has been shown to improve functional capacity in patients with heart failure. Furthermore, a meta-analysis has indicated a net reduction in adverse clinical outcomes, including death, among patients with heart failure randomized to exercise training across a number of controlled trials.[54] A large-scale randomized controlled trial is presently underway in an effort to confirm the benefits of exercise on clinical outcomes in patients with heart failure, using the combination of all-cause death and all-cause hospitalization as the primary endpoint.

Various mechanisms have been suggested as the basis for exercise-induced improvement in clinical outcomes in patients with heart failure. These have included benefits of exercise on blood pressure, lipid profile, body fat and insulin sensitivity, thrombogenicity, autonomic tone, and resting myocardial oxygen demand. Exercise has been shown to reverse endothelial dysfunction in patients with heart failure[55], an effect that may be mediated through effects of periodic increases in endothelial laminar shear, which induces nitric oxide production, diminishes oxidative stress, and stimulates vasodilatation. Endothelial laminar shear also alters endothelial gene expression in a manner that induces endothelial cytoskeletal remodeling. Through its impact on arterial flow patterns, exercise may improve vascular function and hemodynamics, prevent adverse vascular remodeling, and prevent coronary ischemia.

Beyond effects on the cardiovascular system, exercise has a favorable effect on the skeletal musculature, which is functionally abnormal in patients with heart failure (see Chapter 2).[56,57] Finally, exercise may have favorable psychological effects, improving patient affect and feelings of competence, self-sufficiency, and general well-being.

These findings have sparked a shift in clinical recommendations over the past two decades. The ACC/AHA 2005 Guideline Update for the Diagnosis and Management of Chronic Heart Failure in the Adult lists exercise training as a class I recommendation in patients with grade C (prior or present symptoms) heart failure.[58] The HFSA 2006 Comprehensive Heart Failure Guideline cites investigations supporting a benefit of exercise training[59] but stops short of making a specific recommendation in this regard, based on currently available data. In addition to the benefit of aerobic exercise, strength training has also been advocated. Clinical trials have used various exercise training protocols. At this time, no specific exercise training prescription can be strongly advocated over any other.

Potentially Adverse Agents

A number of substances—notably alcohol and cocaine—have been associated with myocardial injury and/or cardiomyopathy. All patients should be advised to avoid use of illicit drugs. Recommendations regarding alcohol are more problematic.

Alcoholic cardiomyopathy appears to be idiosyncratic, occurring in some patients with only moderate alcohol intake, but occurring in only a small minority of patients with a long history of heavy alcohol ingestion. Although alcohol is a mild negative inotrope, it is also a vasodilator, and some observational studies have suggested an association with reduced risk of vascular disease. It appears likely that alcohol interacts with other environmental and genetic factors to sporadically induce myocardial dysfunction. All patients with heavy alcohol consumption should be counseled regarding the many adverse health consequences. Those with cardiomyopathy should be strongly urged to permanently abstain. However, there is less agreement regarding recommendations for patients with dilated cardiomyopathy in whom clear linkage with alcohol use is absent. For such patients, the HFSA 2006 Comprehensive Heart Failure Guideline[60] recommends limitation to ≤1 standard drink per day in women and ≤2 standard drinks per day in men. All individuals should be advised not to smoke.

Cyclooxygenase (COX)-inhibiting nonsteroidal anti-inflammatory drugs (NSAIDs) should be avoided in all patients with heart failure, if at all possible. These agents, regardless of COX-2 selectivity, vasoconstrict, raise blood pressure, reduce glomerular filtration rate, and induce sodium and water retention. Depending on the nature of the pathology for which these agents might otherwise be recommended and the severity and stage of heart failure, alternatives to be considered include acetaminophen, opiates, and steroids. Where the nature of the disease and risk–benefit ratio favors use of NSAIDs, careful attention should be given to fluid management, diuretic use, and blood pressure control.

Agents that induce cardiomyopathy include the cancer chemotherapeutic agents anthracyclines and trastuzumab and the newer Tyrosine Kinase inhibitor class of agents.[61] Agents that have been implicated in exacerbating heart failure include antagonists of tumor necrosis factor alpha[62] and thiazolidinedione insulin sensitizers.[63] Risk–benefit relations should be carefully considered in using any of these agents, particularly in patients with other predisposing factors for heart failure. When prescribing these agents, consideration should be given to monitoring patient clinical status and cardiac function.

Calcium channel blockers are often considered contraindicated in patients with heart failure, due to the variable degree of negative inotropic effect of these agents.[64] An alternative concern is that vasodilator calcium channel blockers may stimulate neurohormonal responses, which may predispose to worsening cardiac function and clinical heart failure. Newer long-acting calcium channel blockers may pose less concern because slow-release preparations or slow rates of receptor association are less likely to induce reflex neurohormonal stimulation. In addition, older studies suggesting that calcium channel blockers provoke or exacerbate heart failure were performed prior to the widespread use of neurohormonal blockers, which may blunt adverse effects of calcium channel blockers. Calcium channel blockers are effective antihypertensive and anti-ischemic agents and may be useful in slowing ventricular response to atrial fibrillation. Use of these agents, where indicated for these purposes, should not be precluded in patients with heart failure who are being appropriately medically managed. It should be noted that dihydropyridine calcium channel blockers may induce lower extremity edema in the absence of heart failure, due to a regional effect on vascular permeability.

Heart Rate and Rhythm Management

Patients with heart failure generally function within a narrower-than-normal heart rate window for maintenance of cardiac output, due to limitation in stroke volume adjustment, related to impaired preload reserve, inotropic reserve, or both. Tachyarrhythmias, including sinus tachycardia, are especially deleterious as they reduce stroke volume and increase ventricular diastolic pressure and myocardial oxygen demand. Persistent tachycardia is an important stimulus—sometimes the sole cause—for progressive ventricular remodeling and dysfunction, perhaps related to associated impairment of myocyte calcium handling. A heart rate of 60 min^{-1} is an appropriate target for most patients in sinus rhythm or atrial fibrillation. For patients in sinus rhythm this target is achievable by gradual up-titration of beta blockers (see subsequent text).

For patients with atrial fibrillation, consideration should be given to restoring sinus rhythm, a goal that may require long-term antiarrhythmic drug use—usually amiodarone. The atrial contribution to ventricular filling often represents an important factor in maintaining physiologic filling pressure and cardiac output, particularly in patients with left ventricular hypertrophy, in whom relaxation is impaired and diastolic stiffness is increased. Where sinus rhythm restoration is not possible, ventricular response should be reduced to as close to 60 min^{-1} as possible, with use of beta blockers, and calcium channel blockers, such as diltiazem and/or digoxin.

Patients with atrial fibrillation and heart failure or ventricular dilation or dysfunction should be anticoagulated with warfarin, unless there is a strong contraindication.[65] Strong consideration should be given to continuation of warfarin anticoagulation indefinitely in these patients, given the high risk for reversion to atrial fibrillation, with associated risk for systemic thromboembolism.

Patients with pathologic LV dilation are prone to ventricular arrhythmias. Sudden cardiac death, mostly due to ventricular tachycardia and fibrillation, is a common mode of death in patients with heart failure and LV dilation. Antiarrhythmic agents—particularly amiodarone—often suppress ventricular arrhythmias, but their use has not been shown to reduce the frequency of sudden cardiac death.[66] Implantable cardioverter-defibrillators significantly reduce mortality rates in select patient populations (see subsequent text).

Patient Monitoring

In recent years, various forms of heart failure disease management have been found to significantly improve patient outcomes.[67,68] These programs comprise patient education, often using material developed for this purpose (see http://www.hfsa.org/hf_modules.asp), care by a nurse-educator, attention to patient compliance to dietary and medication prescription, various forms of frequent or continuous clinical monitoring, and medication—particularly diuretics given in response to early signs of fluid overload and worsening symptoms.

Monitoring systems may be as simple as a scale to track daily weight or as complex as implantable devices that monitor central hemodynamics or lung water. Some studies[69] have shown incremental benefit from daily telemonitoring of weight, vital signs, and patient symptoms, with generation of clinical alerts, compared with programs using only telephone contact. Implantable systems provide incremental information but have not yet been shown to provide significant clinical benefit, compared with less invasive forms of clinical monitoring.[70] Systems under development may eventually communicate directly with the electronic medical record.

Measurement of daily weight is a critical component of evaluation for patients prone to fluid overload.[71] Fluctuations of >2–3 pounds should alert the patient and provider to consider diuretic dose adjustment. During visits to the health care provider, in addition to vital signs, signs of heart failure and fluid status—particularly jugular venous pressure and presence of edema—should routinely be assessed. Blood chemistry should be periodically monitored, including serum concentrations of electrolytes, urea nitrogen, and creatinine. Such measurement is particularly warranted in patients experiencing fluid status fluctuation and undergoing diuretic dose adjustment, and those receiving combination therapy with ACE inhibitors, ARBs, and/or aldosterone blockers.

Measurement of natriuretic peptide concentrations—either B-type natriuretic peptide or N-terminal-pro-B-type natriuretic peptide—can be a valuable adjunct to clinical assessment of volume status and heart failure severity, particularly among patients in whom there is a disparity between symptoms and physical findings. Preliminary studies have suggested that incorporating these measurements into routine care can reduce hospitalization rates and improve clinical outcomes.[72] Firm conclusions in this regard await results of more definitive large-scale randomized controlled trials.

PHARMACOLOGIC MODALITIES

Advancement in drug therapy for chronic heart failure over the past two decades has radically altered the treatment approach and the prospects for patients. Improved clinical outcomes have mostly come through use of neurohormonal antagonists—ACE inhibitors, ARBs, beta blockers, and aldosterone receptor blockers.

Direct-Acting Diuretics

Diuretics are a mainstay of therapy for patients with heart failure prone to volume overload, despite the fact that their benefit on symptoms or clinical outcomes has never been documented by a prospective, randomized controlled trial. Symptomatic benefit to patients manifesting either acute or chronic volume overload appear self-evident to clinicians to the point where most placebo-controlled trial designs with these agents appear to be inappropriate. Observational studies have demonstrated an association between diuretic use, particularly in high doses, and both worsening renal function and adverse clinical outcomes.[73,74] However, despite appropriate attempts at covariate adjustment, it seems likely that these relationships are influenced by increased diuretic treatment in response to clinical worsening. All pharmacologic and device clinical trials with documented clinical efficacy have used diuretics as routine or widespread background therapy, so that it is difficult to be sure that similar benefits would be derived without background diuretic use.

Reduction in intravascular volume reduces capillary hydrostatic pressure, thereby diminishing transudation of fluid into the extravascular tissues of the lungs, viscera, and soft tissues. Reduced intravascular volume directly reduces ventricular filling pressures and so can be expected to decrease cardiac output. Reduced ventricular end-diastolic pressure tends to decrease cardiac output by the Starling mechanism, with the magnitude of this mechanism dependent on the steepness of the Starling curve (see Chapter 2). In patients with higher filling pressures and flattened Starling curves, there may be little change in systolic function for a given change in filling pressure. Importantly, in patients with more severe degrees of volume overload and right ventricular dilation, extramyocardial factors may result in paradoxical effects, with decreases in filling pressure associated with increased cardiac output. Such factors include functional tricuspid and mitral regurgitation, which may diminish during diuresis and drive an increase in cardiac output. Furthermore, right ventricular dilation impedes LV filling via ventricular interdependence. Diuresis, with decreased right ventricular volume, may therefore facilitate LV filling and augment cardiac output via the Starling mechanism.

Diuretics act by decreasing renal tubular sodium reabsorption, increasing sodium clearance, and secondarily removing water. Although for some patients, thiazide diuretics may be adequate, most patients with heart failure and signs and symptoms of fluid overload require more potent agents that act at the loop of Henle. Response to these agents is highly variable, owing in part to variable bioavailability of the oral agents. Although most patients can be treated effectively with furosemide, torsemide offers advantages to difficult-to-manage patients, owing to its greater and more predictable degree of bioavailability.[75] As heart failure progresses, patients may become less responsive to diuretics, often in association with worsening renal function. Options include (i) increasing diuretic dose; (ii) concomitant use of aldosterone blockers (which should be considered regardless, in the presence of worsening heart failure—see subsequent text); (iii) use of a thiazide diuretic—particularly metolazone—approximately 30 minutes prior to administering the loop diuretic. For hospitalized patients, consideration can be given to continuous furosemide infusion, as well as to concomitant use of an intravenous inotropic and/or vasodilator agent.

Diuretic initiation or dose adjustment, with marked diuresis, requires careful monitoring of electrolytes and renal function. Diuretic-induced renal functional impairment may be due partly to reduced cardiac output via the Starling mechanism. (On the other hand, renal function may actually improve following diuresis due to increased cardiac output—see previous discussion.) In addition, increased sodium delivery to the distal nephron results in compensatory effects, partly mediated by adenosine,[76] which tend to limit sodium excretion, in part by reducing glomerular filtration rate. Non–potassium-sparing diuretics, including thiazide and loop diuretics, promote potassium wasting and often require potassium replacement. Hyponatremia frequently accompanies diuretic treatment due to oral intake of hypotonic fluids. Significant hyponatremia, variably defined across a range of serum sodium concentrations from <130 mEq/L–<135 mEq/L, should be treated with fluid restriction (see previous discussion).

Angiotensin-Converting Enzyme Inhibitors

The finding that ACE inhibitors improved clinical outcomes, including survival, across a broad spectrum of patients with clinical heart failure and reduced LVEF[77,78,79,80,81] represented a major turning point in treatment of this condition, demonstrating for the first time that the natural history of this condition can be pharmacologically influenced (Fig. 6-5). These agents, initially thought to exert their benefits through vasodilatation, were found superior to other equally potent vasodilator combinations,[82] paving the way to a broader appreciation of the potential for neurohormonal modulation to impact the cardiovascular system.

In addition to reducing cardiac filling pressures and augmenting cardiac output, ACE inhibitors diminish the progression of adverse ventricular remodeling[83,84] and can even reverse this progression, diminishing LV mass and volume in patients with LV dilation. Mechanisms for ACE inhibitor cardiovascular effects include diminished production of angiotensin II and potentiation of bradykinin. These combined actions result in antihypertrophic, antiproliferative, antifibrotic, antithrombotic, and antioxidant

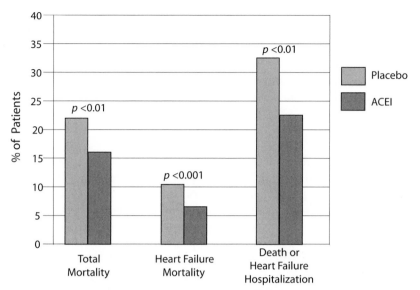

Figure 6-5: Angiotensin-converting enzyme inhibitors (ACEIs) in chronic heart failure—pooled analysis of 32 randomized trials. Modified from Garg and Yusuf (1995). JAMA 273(18):1450–1456.

effects. Portions of the clinical benefit of ACE inhibitors in patients with heart failure are likely to derive from effects on the vasculature and the kidneys. ACE inhibitors reverse vascular fibrosis and endothelial dysfunction and delay the progression of glomerulosclerosis. Each of these actions is likely to contribute to the net clinical effects of improved survival and reduced frequency of hospitalization for heart failure.

ACE inhibitors or ARBs should be initiated in all patients with reduced LVEF (generally implying LV dilation) unless clearly contraindicated (as in the presence of significant renal artery stenosis) or prior demonstration of intolerance. In patients with reduced LVEF without heart failure symptoms, ACE inhibitors prevent hospitalization for heart failure and attenuate adverse LV remodeling. They should be initiated in low doses and gradually up-titrated, monitoring blood pressure, symptoms, renal function, and electrolytes. It is generally recommended that dose up-titration continue until either dose-limiting intolerance is observed or the target dose is reached, defined as the target dose used in clinical trials, or equivalent. Examples of target doses include enalapril 10 mg twice daily and captopril 50 mg three times daily.

Most clinical trials demonstrating clinical outcome benefit by ACE inhibitors have restricted enrollment to patients with reduced LVEF ($\leq 35\%$ or $\leq 40\%$). Therefore the firmest recommendations for ACE inhibitor prescription focus on this population, as there is little clinical trial evidence on which to base a similar recommendation for patients with heart failure and preserved LVEF. However, ACE inhibitors have beneficial effects on the vasculature, which prevent cardiovascular events and the development of heart failure in patients with atherosclerotic disease and in those with cardiovascular risk factors.[85] Furthermore, experimental evidence indicates that ACE inhibitors prevent cardiovascular fibrosis and remodeling. For these reasons, ACE inhibitors should be strongly considered in patients with hypertensive cardiovascular disease (HCVD) and clinical heart failure, a group that comprises most patients with heart failure and relatively preserved LVEF (i.e., those with nondilated LV cavity).

Adverse effects of ACE inhibitors include cough, hypotension, renal impairment, and hyperkalemia. Angioedema is a rare but potentially life-threatening complication of ACE inhibitor use. Reduction in glomerular filtration rate, with a modest rise in serum creatinine concentration, is a pharmacologic effect of ACE inhibitors that does not generally imply renal injury and so does not necessarily require dose reduction or cessation of treatment. On the other hand, in the presence of renal artery stenosis, ACE inhibitors may induce a major reduction in glomerular filtration pressure and result in severe renal failure.

Angiotensin Receptor Blockers

On the assumption that ACE inhibitor benefit is based on partial inhibition of angiotensin-II production, an expectation existed that direct inhibition of the AT_1 receptor (the predominant receptor responsible for the adverse cardiovascular effects of angiotensin-II) would produce superior clinical effects. This expectation has not been borne out by clinical trials in which effects of the two classes of agents have been compared head-to-head.[86,87,88] Nevertheless, the net clinical benefit of ARBs appears to be similar to that of ACE inhibitors,[89,90] and two trials[91,92] have suggested or demonstrated incremental clinical benefit of adding an ARB to ACE inhibitor treatment. Therefore, although clinical practice guidelines still place ACE inhibitor treatment slightly higher than ARB treatment on the recommendation hierarchy, most investigators and clinicians now believe that either an ACE inhibitor or an ARB is acceptable in initiating treating patients with heart failure and reduced LVEF. One program of studies (CHARM) investigated the role of ARBs across a spectrum of uses and populations, including as an alternative to ACE inhibitors in intolerant patients,[89] as add-on treatment to an ACE inhibitor,[91] and as first-line treatment for patients with preserved LVEF[93] (Fig. 6-6; see subsequent text).

ARBs are more effective than ACE inhibitors in blocking the adverse cardiovascular effect of angiotensin II, since the latter agents are only partially effective at inhibiting the cleavage step responsible for producing this hormone from its prohormone

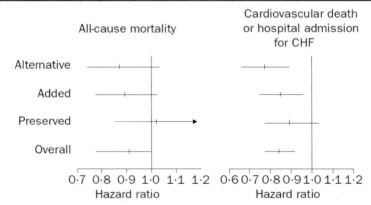

CHARM:
Candesartan Effect on Clinical Outcomes

Figure 6-6: Impact of candesartan versus placebo in patients with heart failure symptoms used as an alternative to angiotensin-converting enzyme (ACE) inhibitor treatment in intolerant patients with reduced left ventricular ejection fraction (LVEF); as add-on treatment for patients with reduced LVEF receiving ACE inhibitors; or in patients with preserved LVEF. CHF, congestive heart failure. From Pfeffer MA, Swedberg K, Granger CB, et al.; CHARM Investigators and Committees (2003). Effects of candesartan on mortality and morbidity in patients with chronic heart failure: the CHARM-Overall programme. Lancet 362(9386):759–766.

angiotensin-I (see Chapter 4). However, ACE inhibitors, but not ARBs, prevent the breakdown of bradykinin, an agent that may contribute to some of the salutary vascular effects of ACE inhibitors. It is possible that this balance of actions is responsible for the approximately equivalent net effect of the two classes of agents on clinical outcomes. The clinical benefits of ARBs are likely to be linked to their ability to prevent or reverse left ventricular remodeling and dilation,[94] as well as to the other favorable cardiovascular effects associated with inhibiting angiotensin-II, listed previously in the description of ACE inhibitor effects.

Although preference is usually given to ACE inhibitors, ARBs may be an acceptable alternative as first-line therapy in patients with reduced LVEF, with or without symptoms of heart failure. Certainly, in patients with dose-limiting cough in response to ACE inhibitors, ARBs should be substituted. ARBs can be considered for the rare patient with angioedema in response to ACE inhibitor treatment. There have been very rare cases of angioedema reported with administration of an ARB, although the incidence is far lower than that seen with ACE inhibitors. There is no evidence that ARBs produce a lower rate of the other ACE inhibitor-related adverse effects, namely hypotension, hyperkalemia, and renal insufficiency. Specifically, clinical investigation has failed to substantiate a lower rate of renal functional impairment with ARB, compared with ACE inhibitor treatment.[95]

There are conflicting findings regarding the value of adding an ARB to an ACE inhibitor. In a large-scale, three-arm investigation in a post-MI (myocardial infarction) heart failure population, patients randomized to the combination of valsartan and captopril did no better than those randomized to either drug alone.[87] In contrast, within a chronic heart failure population with continued symptoms while receiving conventional background treatment including an ACE inhibitor, patients randomized to addition of candesartan had a reduced incidence of the combined endpoint of cardiovascular death or heart failure hospitalization, compared with patients randomized to placebo.[91] Although there is debate regarding the reasons for these apparently conflicting results, it is reasonable to consider adding an ARB to ACE inhibitor treatment in persistently symptomatic patients with heart failure and reduced LVEF. Since these agents may be additive in producing adverse effects, such as hypotension, hyperkalemia, and renal insufficiency, patients should be monitored carefully following institution of this combination of agents.

As with ACE inhibitors, the data for outcome benefit with ARBs are most clear for patients with heart failure who have a reduced LVEF. One study examining candesartan effects in patients with heart failure and preserved LVEF showed a nonsignificant trend toward reduction in the combined endpoint of cardiovascular death or heart failure hospitalization.[93] Additional support for the value of ARB treatment in patients with hypertensive heart failure with preserved LVEF (nondilated LV) comes from studies performed in select non–heart failure populations. The ARB losartan achieved reduced cardiovascular (CV) events (mostly stroke) and greater regression of electrocardiographic evidence of LV hypertrophy, compared with the beta blocker atenolol, in patients with hypertension and baseline LV hypertrophy.[31] In patients with diabetes and albuminuria, the vast majority of whom were hypertensive, ARBs reduced the incidence of progressive renal insufficiency.[96,97] In one such study,[96] there was a reduced incidence of new-onset heart failure. Although these findings may be considered peripheral to the question of ARB effects in heart failure patients with preserved LVEF, for the largest proportion of these patients—those with HCVD—these studies all point to a valuable role for ARB treatment, with benefits on clinical outcomes likely to be derived from effects on the vasculature and kidneys, as well as on the heart. Additional investigations are underway to specifically address the population with heart failure and preserved LVEF. Until these results are available, it seems advisable to strongly consider ARB or ACE inhibitor treatment, at least in that predominant segment of the population with heart failure with preserved EF—that is, those with hypertensive disease.

Beta Adrenergic Blockers

We have long known that the adrenergic nervous system is up-regulated in patients with heart failure, and for many years, the presumption was held that this response is a necessary compensatory factor serving to normalize hemodynamics in the setting of an otherwise failing heart. As a result, beta adrenergic blocking agents were considered contraindicated in heart failure. Beginning in the 1970s, observational data began to be published suggesting the opposite: that beta blockade could have a salutary effect in patients with dilated cardiomyopathy.[98] Some authors believed that energy-sparing effects of beta blockers could benefit failing hearts.[99] Beginning in the mid-1990s, large-scale controlled trials displayed an improvement in clinical outcomes among patients with heart failure and reduced LVEF (dilated LV), of both ischemic and nonischemic cause, randomized to receive a beta blocker[2,3,4,100] (Fig. 6-7). These findings have created a paradigm shift in

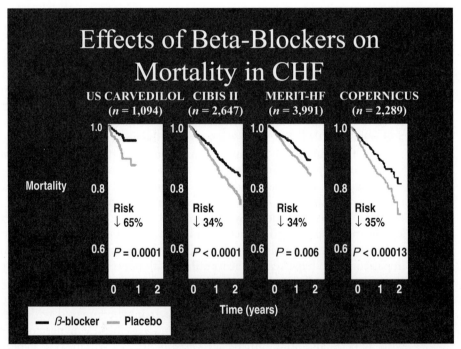

Figure 6-7: Beta blocker effects on mortality in four randomized controlled trials of patients with heart failure. From Packer M, Bristow MR, Cohn JN, et al. (1996). The effect of carvedilol on morbidity and mortality in patients with chronic heart failure. N Engl J Med 334:1349–1355; CIBIS-II Investigators and Committees (1999). The Cardiac Insufficiency Bisoprolol Study II (CIBIS II): a randomised trial. Lancet 353:9–13; MERIT-HF Study Group (1999). Effect of metoprolol CR/XL in chronic heart failure: Metoprolol CR/XL Randomised Intervention Trial in Congestive Heart Failure (MERIT-HF). Lancet 353:2001–2007; and Packer M, Coats AJ, Fowler MB, et al.; Carvedilol Prospective Randomized Cumulative Survival Study Group (2001). Effect of carvedilol on survival in severe chronic heart failure. N Engl J Med 344(22):1651–1658.

our thinking about therapeutics in heart failure, representing the strongest rationale yet for abandoning focus on agents that directly augment myocyte contractility, in favor of approaches that inhibit pathways responsible for adverse myocardial remodeling and dysfunction. Since that time, beta blockers have become a mainstay of therapy in patients with heart failure and reduced LVEF, with recommendations for consideration of cautious administration even in patients with advanced heart failure.

In the short-term, beta blockers slow heart rate, reduce myocyte contractility, and diminish the impact of persistent adrenergic stimulation on myocyte signaling pathways. Administered chronically, beta blockers restore cellular responses to physiologic adrenergic stimulation and halt or reverse adverse myocardial remodeling. In some patients with dilated cardiomyopathy, beta blocker administration for several months results in complete normalization of LV volume and EF. These findings suggest that a subset of this population has a form of adrenergic cardiomyopathy, which can be completely reversed with beta adrenergic blockade. It seems plausible that in some patients, adrenergic activity, perhaps provoked by an environmental stimulus, is sufficient to promote ventricular remodeling and dysfunction, leading to heart failure, similar to what is observed in catecholamine-induced animal models of cardiomyopathy. Excessive heart rates most likely contribute to the pathophysiology of this condition, and the energy–sparing effect of slowing the heart rate is an important contributor to the long-term salutary impact of beta blockers.

In large-scale randomized controlled trials, beta blockers reduce mortality and the frequency of hospitalization for heart failure. These observations have been made in a broad spectrum of patients with reduced LVEF, including asymptomatic patients with prior myocardial infarction and patients with both ischemic and nonischemic cardiomyopathies and symptoms ranging from mild to severe (NYHA [New York Heart Association] class II–IV) (although few patients were enrolled in these trials during a hospitalization for heart failure exacerbation).[2,3,4,100]

More than other classes of cardiovascular therapeutic agents, beta blockers are diverse in their specific actions, with variable degrees of specificity for the beta-1 receptor. That is, some agents produce balanced inhibition of the beta-1 and beta-2 receptors, and other agents also inhibit the alpha adrenergic receptor. Still other agents have a degree of intrinsic sympathomimetic activity. There is also variability in various agents' ability to cross the blood–brain barrier. For these reasons, and because of apparent variability in clinical responses, recommendations for beta blocking agents are generally restricted to those agents with demonstrated clinical outcome benefit in this condition—carvedilol, metoprolol (particularly the long-acting preparation of metoprolol succinate), and bisoprolol.

Treatment with one of these agents is recommended for most patients with heart failure and reduced LVEF. In patients who have experienced clinical exacerbation, beta blocker treatment should ordinarily be deferred until the clinical condition has stabilized. However, it is increasingly common practice to start treatment while such patients are still in the hospital. Initial doses should be low, with careful observation for signs of worsening heart failure, and with up-titration over weeks. Up-titration should continue until either the target dose (dose shown to improve clinical outcomes) is reached or further increase is deemed undesirable based on blood pressure, heart rate (e.g., ≤ 60 min^{-1}) or adverse events such as a limiting degree of light-headedness or worsening heart failure.

Aldosterone Receptor Blockers

Aldosterone secretion is up-regulated in heart failure. Adrenal secretion of aldosterone is partially under control of angiotensin-II and is partially independent of angiotensin-II, so that its secretion is not fully inhibited by ACE inhibitors and ARBs. Furthermore, aldosterone receptors are stimulated by glucocorticoids, particularly under conditions of increased oxidative stress (see Chapter 3).

Stimulation of aldosterone receptors in the kidney increases renal tubular sodium/potassium exchange, resulting in sodium retention and potassium wasting. Aldosterone receptor blockers, originally used in patients with heart failure as potassium-sparing diuretics, fell out of favor for a number of years because of the greater potency of loop diuretics and concerns regarding hyperkalemia, particularly as ACE inhibitors came into use. However, aldosterone receptors are now recognized as ubiquitous within the cardiovascular tissue, and aldosterone receptor stimulation has been found to stimulate maladaptive cardiac hypertrophy, vascular fibrosis, calcification, and inflammation, raising interest in the potential value for aldosterone receptor blockers beyond their diuretic action.

Aldosterone receptor blockers have now been shown to reduce mortality in two patient populations with reduced LVEF: patients with severe or recently severe symptoms of heart failure,[101] and patients with evidence of clinical heart failure at the time of myocardial infarction[102] (Table 6-2). In the former case, the benefits were additive to those from ACE inhibitors, and in the latter case, to both ACE inhibitors and beta blockers use. At present, addition of aldosterone receptor blockers is recommended in these two populations. Although unproven, it stands to reason that addition of aldosterone blockade can achieve improved outcomes in other populations of patients with heart failure as well. Ongoing studies are investigating potential benefits in patients with reduced LVEF and less severe symptoms and in patients with heart failure and a preserved LVEF.

Doses of aldosterone receptor blockers used in recent clinical trials (25 mg/day of spironolactone and 50 mg/day of eplerenone) are lower than those that had

TABLE 6-2				
Effects of Aldosterone Blockade on All-Cause Mortality				
	Placebo	Aldosterone blockade	Hazard ratio	Log rank p-value
EPHESUS	554/3319	478/3313	0.85 (0.75,0.96)	0.008
RALES	386/841	284/822	0.70 (0.60,0.82)	<0.001

Impact of aldosterone receptor antagonists on all-cause mortality in patients with clinical heart failure and reduced left ventricular ejection fraction (LVEF) following myocardial infarction (EPHESUS) and in patients with severe or recently severe heart failure and reduced LVEF (RALES).
From Pitt B, Remme W, Zannad F, et al.; Eplerenone Post-Acute Myocardial Infarction Heart Failure Efficacy and Survival Study Investigators (2003). Eplerenone, a selective aldosterone blocker, in patients with left ventricular dysfunction after myocardial infarction [EPHESUS]. N Engl J Med 348(14):1309–1321; and Pitt B, Zannad F, Remme WJ, et al. (1999). The effect of spironolactone on morbidity and mortality in patients with severe heart failure. Randomized Aldactone Evaluation Study Investigators [RALES]. N Engl J Med 341(10):709–717.

previously been used for diuresis. Serum potassium concentrations should be monitored after initiating therapy, particularly with background use of an ACE inhibitor and/or ARB. Particular caution should be exercised in the presence of renal insufficiency, where there may be a greater propensity to retain potassium. The additional adverse effect of gynecomastia, reported in approximately 10% of men, is not seen with the newer agent eplerenone.

Direct Vasodilators and Nitrates

An early major breakthrough in heart failure therapy came with the demonstration that the direct-acting vasodilator nitroprusside acutely improved hemodynamics in patients with heart failure,[103] producing a decrease in ventricular filling pressures and augmentation in cardiac output. Similar findings were observed with other classes of vasodilators, such as ACE inhibitors, and result from a combination of afterload reduction—due to arteriolar dilation—and preload reduction—due to venodilation.

These findings brought vasodilators into use in patients hospitalized with heart failure exacerbation to augment systemic perfusion and relieve pulmonary congestion. They also gave rise to an expectation of longer-term outcome benefit from vasodilator administration. Although this hypothesis appeared to be borne out by trials of ACE inhibitors, it became clear that clinical outcome benefits differed with different classes of vasodilators of comparable acute hemodynamic potency. ACE inhibitor benefit derives substantial contribution from nonvasodilator mechanisms (see previous discussion). The alpha blocker prazosin has no demonstrable benefit on long-term outcomes.[104] The combination of hydralazine and isosorbide dinitrate improves clinical outcomes, but across the population studied, the effect appears more modest than that of ACE inhibitors.[82] It appears that the long-term benefits observed with select vasodilator agents are derived from mechanisms distinct from vasodilatation.

The outcome and long-term symptomatic benefits of the combination of hydralazine and isosorbide dinitrate were recently confirmed in African Americans with reduced LVEF and New York Heart Association class III and IV symptoms, well-treated with ACE inhibitors or ARBs, beta blockers, and, in many cases, aldosterone receptor blockers.[42] The study population was selected because of subgroup trends from prior investigations suggesting preferential benefit from this combination of agents in African Americans. It is now speculated that the therapeutic value is derived through nitric oxide "donation," which is likely to have vasoprotective and antiproliferative effects. It is further speculated that hydralazine provides an antioxidant effect, which prevents nitric oxide degradation and attendant tachyphylaxis that may be observed with chronic nitrate administration. African Americans may have a propensity to relative vascular nitric oxide deficiency, which renders them particularly amenable to benefit from nitrate therapy. However, the hypothesis of preferential benefit in African Americans, compared with non–African Americans, has not specifically been tested.

The addition of hydralazine and isosorbide dinitrate should be considered in patients with reduced LVEF and persistent heart failure symptoms while receiving optimal treatment. Given the findings in African Americans, particular consideration should be given to implementing this treatment in this patient population. Although the benefits are not as clear in non–African Americans, this combination may be considered in these patients as well, particularly where intolerance prevents administration of ACE inhibitors or ARBs. In A-HeFT, the drugs were administered in a combination tablet, with initial doses of 37.5 mg of hydralazine hydrochloride and 20 mg of isosorbide dinitrate three times daily, and the doses doubled (two pills three times daily) if tolerated.

Intravenous vasodilators are useful agents to achieve short-term hemodynamic benefit—and thereby relieve symptoms of congestion and reduced cardiac output—in patients with exacerbation of heart failure. Consideration can be given to early use of these agents or their addition in patients who are not rapidly responding to diuretic treatment. Nitroglycerin and nitroprusside may both be used for acute hemodynamic effects, with the former producing relatively greater preload reduction and the latter relatively greater afterload reduction, although both agents have mixed effects. Nesiritide (recombinant B-type natriuretic peptide) is the one vasodilator that has been shown in a randomized controlled trial to improve symptoms in patients hospitalized with a heart failure exacerbation.[105] The key finding was improvement in dyspnea score at 3 hours. Vasodilator treatment is ideal for patients presenting with heart failure and hypertension.

For all vasodilators, there is risk of hypotension and associated systemic consequences, including renal functional impairment. They should be avoided in patients with shock and used cautiously in patients with relative hypotension—e.g., systolic blood pressure <100 mm Hg. The long-term safety of short-term vasodilator administration has not been established, and safety concerns have been raised, notably a dose-related increase in the incidence of worsening renal function with nesiritide.[106] A meta-analysis has also raised the question of excess mortality with nesiritide use,[107] although the conclusions in this regard are uncertain, and a more systematic longer-term investigation is underway. A randomized controlled trial of intermittent intravenous nesiritide in patients with severe heart failure failed to demonstrate any benefit of this strategy.[108]

Inotropic Agents and Cardiac Glycosides

During the past two decades, there has been a dramatic shift in our thinking regarding the pharmacologic approach to treating heart failure and improving its natural history, from a focus on directly alleviating the reduced myocardial contractile state to one of preventing and reversing adverse ventricular remodeling. Through this shift, our focus has moved from inotropic agents to neurohormonal blockers as the principal mode of drug treatment.

Cardiac glycosides, prescribed since the time of William Withering, (1741–1799), were long believed to exert a favorable effect on signs and symptoms of heart failure through their positive inotropic action. The mechanism is believed to result from sodium pump inhibition increasing calcium availability due to sodium/calcium exchange (see Chapter 5). More recently, consideration has been given to the favorable effect on baroreceptor sensitivity, neurohormonal activity, and heart rate as a contributing factor to the benefits derived from these agents.[109] Over the past two decades several clinical trials have documented a modest degree of digoxin-induced clinical benefit in patients with heart failure and reduced LVEF. These have included studies observing serial changes in clinical status and functional capacity in patients randomized to continuation or withdrawal of chronic oral digoxin therapy,[110,111] where worsening was observed in the group subjected to digoxin withdrawal. One large-scale outcomes trial[112] failed to demonstrate survival benefit in patients randomized to digoxin versus placebo but did demonstrate a lower rate of hospitalization for heart failure in patients with sinus rhythm randomized to receive digoxin.

Current treatment recommendations call for consideration of digoxin treatment in patients with heart failure and reduced LVEF who continue to be symptomatic despite conventional medical treatment.[113] However, it is recognized that the benefits are modest, with no survival benefit and with a narrow toxic-therapeutic ratio. Compared with prior recommendations, lower doses are presently advised, generally 0.125 mg/day. Smaller body habitus is believed to predispose to adverse effects at a given dose. The most serious adverse effects are arrhythmias, including atrioventricular block, ventricular tachycardia, and ventricular fibrillation.

More potent inotropic agents now available include drugs that increase cellular levels of cyclic AMP, which increase calcium transport across the plasma membrane by beta adrenergic receptor stimulation (e.g., dobutamine) or phosphodiesterase inhibition (e.g., amrinone and milrinone). Other drugs increase myocardial sensitivity to calcium (e.g., levosimendan). These intravenous agents, which have vasodilator as well as inotropic effects, reduce cardiac filling pressures and augment cardiac output in patients with heart failure. They are often used in patients hospitalized with severe heart failure who are not responding adequately to diuretics, and in whom systemic perfusion is considered inadequate (often evidenced by diminishing renal function and urine output). These agents are often preferred to pure vasodilators in patients with diminished blood pressure.

Serious questions have been raised regarding adverse effects and safety consequences of inotropic agents.[114,115,116] Given their vasodilator as well as inotropic effect, they may induce hypotension, particularly when administered to patients in whom cardiac filling pressures are not particularly elevated (e.g., above the mid-teens). They should never be administered unless elevation in filling pressures is certain, either through clinical assessment or through direct measurement.[117] Although the routine use of pulmonary artery catheters has not been found to improve clinical outcomes, they are valuable instruments to assess cardiac filling pressures in those patients believed to have heart failure or those with hypotension where filling pressures are uncertain based on clinical assessment.

These potent inotropic agents are proarrhythmic. They increase heart rate and thereby increase myocardial oxygen consumption and worsen energy starvation. A number of observational studies have suggested that even their short-term use is associated with excess mortality. Although there is ample rationale for this possibility, causality cannot be ascertained from these data, since these agents tend to be used in extremely ill patients. However, large-scale investigations of the orally active inotropic agents milrinone[1] and vesnarinone[118] in patients with chronic heart failure demonstrated excess mortality. Levosimendan was shown to improve clinical status during the first several days following hospitalization but at the expense of increased incidences of hypotension and both ventricular and atrial arrhythmias. Early studies suggested that use of this agent in patients hospitalized with an exacerbation of heart failure may be associated with improved survival compared to dobutamine use;[119] however, this finding was not borne out in a large-scale comparative trial, in which survival within the two patient groups was similar.[116] Although it is likely that orally active inotropic agents can improve clinical status, at least in the short-term, in patients with severe heart failure, the risk–benefit ratio has not been considered sufficient to warrant their regulatory approval. For patients with heart failure who have poor prognosis and continue to be severely symptomatic despite other treatments, it seems reasonable for the clinician and patient to consider an agent that can alleviate symptoms, even if it is associated with a shortened life expectancy.

Vasopressin Receptor Blockers

Vasopressin levels are often increased in patients with heart failure, presumably through hemodynamic signaling that overrides the plasma osmolarity, which principally regulates vasopressin secretion in the normal state (see Chapter 3). Vasopressin effects are largely mediated through the V_{1a} receptor, responsible for vasoconstriction, and the V_2 receptor, responsible for renal tubular free water reabsorption. There has been recent interest in a therapeutic role for small molecule vasopressin receptor blockers.

At the present time, selective vasopressin receptor blockade is accepted treatment for a variety of hyponatremic states, including heart failure. Administration of a vasopressin receptor blocker to patients with heart failure results in aquaresis (free water excretion) and weight loss, with associated reduction in LV filling pressure.[120,121] Compared with similar degrees of fluid removal using a loop diuretic, V_2 vasopressin receptor blockade improves rather than worsens hyponatremia, does not produce hypokalemia, and is associated with relative preservation of renal function. One trial[122] demonstrated short-term symptomatic benefit with administration of a selective V_2 vasopressin blocker beginning within 48 hours of hospitalization for worsening heart failure with clinical evidence of volume overload. Routine continuation of therapy long-term produced no effect on survival or rehospitalization for heart failure.[123] This class of agents should be useful to aid in fluid management in patients with heart failure prone to volume overload, particularly those with diuretic resistance, hyponatremia, and/or renal functional impairment. Additional research is needed to document optimal candidates for treatment and approaches to treatment, alone or in combination with natriuretic agents.

Anticoagulation

Patients with atrial fibrillation and structural heart disease should be anticoagulated with warfarin. In the absence of atrial fibrillation, use of anticoagulation in patients with heart failure leads to abnormal ventricular function is controversial. There is evidence that heart failure is a hypercoagulable state.[124,125] Observational analyses have suggested that warfarin anticoagulation is associated with reduced mortality in patients with diminished LVEF.[126] However, no randomized, controlled data presently exist to support the routine use of warfarin anticoagulation in these patients. An ongoing clinical trial is comparing the effect of warfarin versus aspirin on the incidence of death and stroke in patients with reduced LVEF.

Although aspirin is widely prescribed in patients with ischemic heart disease, on the basis of data supporting prevention of adverse coronary events in patients with known coronary artery disease, the use of aspirin in patients with heart failure is similarly controversial. There has been no prospective evaluation of the impact of aspirin treatment in heart failure patients. Some analyses have suggested an adverse interaction between aspirin and ACE inhibitors,[127] whereas others do not.[128] At this

TABLE 6-3
Categories of Devices in Heart Failure Management
• Devices to prevent/treat arrhythmias
• Devices as replacement therapy
• Devices to improve CV structure & function
• Devices to address fluid imbalance
• Devices for monitoring/disease management

point, low-dose aspirin continues to be recommended in patients with known coronary artery disease and heart failure, despite absence of specific randomized controlled data in this patient group.

A variety of newer antithrombotic agents are undergoing early clinical investigation, and these agents may, in the future, prove to have a favorable outcome impact in patients with heart failure or with LV dilation and reduced LVEF.

DEVICES

Over the past decade, a substantial amount of evidence has accumulated documenting clinical benefits derived from the appropriate use of a variety of devices in patients with heart failure (Table 6-3). Devices have been investigated and used to (i) detect and treat arrhythmia, (ii) supplement or replace cardiac output, (iii) influence underlying pathologic cardiovascular processes, (iv) correct fluid imbalance, and (v) facilitate monitoring hemodynamic status and fluid balance.

Devices That Detect and Treat Arrhythmias

Implantable cardioverter-defibrillators (ICDs) detect potentially lethal ventricular arrhythmias and correct them either by antitachycardia pacing or by delivering a shock to terminate ventricular tachycardia or fibrillation. These devices were initially used to prevent recurrence of sudden cardiac death in patients who had been resuscitated from a life-threatening ventricular arrhythmia. Since a large proportion of deaths among patients with heart failure and LV dilation occur suddenly, without preceding evidence of clinical worsening, presumably representing lethal ventricular arrhythmias, there has been considerable interest in the prophylactic use of ICDs in this population. Recent clinical trials have demonstrated reduction in all-cause mortality with ICD implant in patients with prior MI and LVEF ≤30%[129] and in both ischemic and nonischemic heart disease patients with symptoms of heart failure (NYHA class II and III) and LVEF ≤35%.[130]

Devices That Supplement or Replace Cardiac Output

Ventricular assist devices (VADs) are designed to supplement or replace cardiac output in patients with severe heart failure (Fig. 6-8). Originally designed as pulsatile pumps, transporting blood from the left ventricle to the aorta (or in the

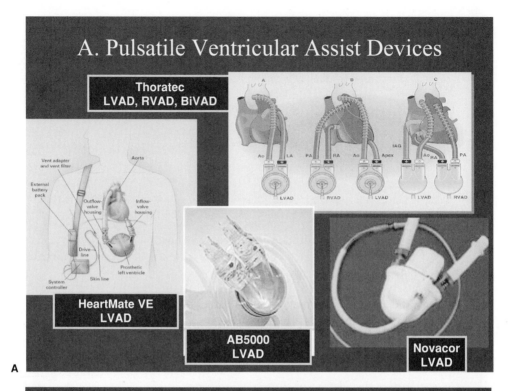

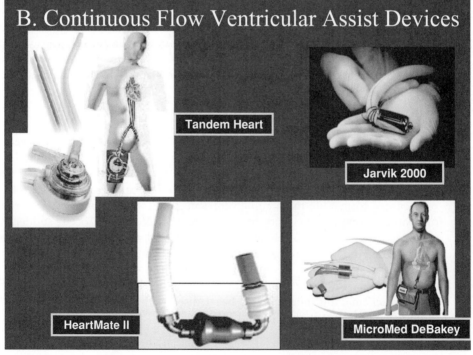

Figure 6-8: Ventricular assist devices in use and under investigation. Bi, biventricular; L, left; R, right; VAD, ventricular assist device; VE, vented-electric.

case of a right-sided VAD, from the right ventricle to the pulmonary artery), more recent designs have abandoned pulsatility and propel blood continuously, using an axial or centrifugal rotary pump. VADs have mostly been used as a bridge to transplant, maintaining life while the patient awaits a suitable heart donor. [131] There has been increasing interest in utilizing VADs in place of heart transplants (destination therapy), initially in patients who are not candidates for transplantation because of age or comorbidity. One study examined outcomes in patients with chronic severe heart failure and hemodynamic derangement randomized either to receive a left VAD or to continue on medical therapy alone.[132] Although both groups had high rates of morbidity and mortality, survival during the 2 years postrandomization was improved in the VAD group compared with the control group. Results have been criticized on the grounds that morbidity in the VAD group was high, with few patients surviving >24 months. However, outcomes with VADs have improved with improvements in device technology, patient selection, and surgical and medical care during and following implant. With newer rotary devices, trials are being designed to explore expansion of VAD destination therapy into patient populations that are somewhat less ill. As the technology advances, with improved reliability, reduced morbidity, and improved acceptability to patients, it is possible that VADs may be used as definitive (destination) treatment in broader patient populations, including those presently receiving cardiac transplant and those with somewhat less advanced disease. Additionally, percutaneously inserted devices are being used and explored (a) for short-term support until the heart recovers, (b) as a bridge to a longer-term device or transplant, or (c) during high-risk percutaneous revascularization procedures. [133,134,135,136]

There is recent evidence that VADs, through cardiac unloading, may facilitate myocardial recovery and then be removed (bridge to recovery).[137] (See subsequent text.)

Devices That Influence Underlying Pathologic Cardiovascular Processes

Just as our thinking regarding drug therapy in heart failure has evolved from a focus on treating the manifestations of heart failure (e.g., reduced cardiac contractility and fluid overload) to one of correcting underlying pathophysiological processes (e.g., neurohormonal activation and ventricular remodeling), devices are now being developed to correct the underlying disease processes, rather than merely supplementing a reduced cardiac output or shocking an arrhythmic heart into sinus rhythm.

The best current example of a device that favorably influences an underlying pathologic process is cardiac resynchronization therapy (CRT). Approximately 40% of patients with heart failure and reduced LVEF (dilated LV) have a QRS duration of $\geq$msec,[130] suggestive of a dyssynchronous (inhomogeneous) pattern of LV contraction and relaxation. Dyssynchrony may be a consequence of underlying myocardial disease, of an ischemic or nonischemic cause. It contributes to hemodynamic and clinical derangement through reducing the effectiveness and completeness of LV contraction and relaxation. Although best described in patients with LV dilation, dyssynchrony may also be an important factor influencing cardiac function and the clinical expression of heart failure in patients without LV dilation. Importantly, dyssynchrony known not to be merely a consequence of myocardial disease but also a contributing factor. Patients with intrinsic conduction disease or right ventricular (RV) pacing appear to have a higher incidence of developing ventricular dysfunction, and CRT therapy has been observed to aid in reversing adverse LV remodeling.

CRT is achieved by simultaneously pacing the left and right ventricles. The LV is paced through a lead positioned in a posterolateral LV vein via the coronary sinus. This therapy is often delivered using a combined pacing and ICD device. Although a variety of imaging approaches have been proposed to define and identify mechanical dyssynchrony, large clinical trials of CRT have mostly used the electrocardiogram as a means of identifying patients to be enrolled. CRT was initially envisioned as a means for reducing symptoms through improved cardiac performance. Indeed, early trials demonstrated improved NYHA class, health-related quality of life, and exercise capacity.[138] A number of trials have also demonstrated improvement in the natural history of heart failure with CRT, as evidenced by reversal of adverse LV remodeling, reduced hospitalization frequency, and reduced mortality, supporting a role for dyssynchrony in the pathophysiology of heart failure[139,140] (Fig. 6-9). CRT is presently approved for patients with reduced LVEF ($\leq$35%), QRS duration $\geq$120 msec, and NYHA class III or IV symptoms. Given the pathophysiologic role of dyssynchrony, trials are underway to explore expanding the CRT indication to patients with less symptomatology.

VADs, originally developed to sustain life in patients with advanced cardiac disease, are being explored for their potential to reverse underlying myocardial disease processes through extreme cardiac unloading (bridge to recovery). VAD use can be associated with reversal of the pathologic myocyte phenotype.[141] One uncontrolled

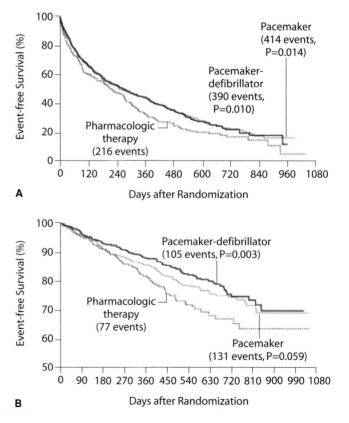

Figure 6-9: COMPANION trial results. Effects of biventricular pacing (BiVP) alone and of BiVP plus implantable defibrillator on all-cause death or hospitalization **(A)** and on all-cause death **(B)**. From Bristow MR, Saxon LA, Boehmer J, et al.; Comparison of Medical Therapy, Pacing, and Defibrillation in Heart Failure (COMPANION) Investigators (2004). Cardiac-resynchronization therapy with or without an implantable defibrillator in advanced chronic heart failure. N Engl J Med 350:2140–2150.

series demonstrated that in patients with severe LV dysfunction and clinical heart failure receiving a left VAD, coupled with administration of multiple neurohormonal antagonist and the beta-2 agonist clenbuterol (thought to induce physiologic hypertrophy), the VAD may be removed after a period of time with sustained improvement in LV function and clinical status.[137] Controlled trials are needed to better document this effect and define the potential target population.

Several additional device-based approaches are being explored to address underlying cardiovascular pathologic processes. One approach mechanically constrains cardiac enlargement. This approach has yielded some encouraging early morphologic and clinical findings,[142] but definitive demonstration of its clinical benefit requires additional investigation. Another approach provides a low level of additional aortic flow ("continuous aortic flow augmentation") on the presumption that reduced pulsatile arterial flow provokes downstream vascular and renal signals, contributing to a vicious cycle of increased cardiac load and progressive cardiac dysfunction. Early investigation has suggested improved hemodynamics, with reduced systemic vascular resistance and cardiac filling pressures, and gradually increased cardiac output.[143] Clinical application awaits results of ongoing clinical investigation. It seems likely that in the coming years, additional concepts will develop toward application of devices to address the pathophysiology of heart failure. Considerable work is presently underway to explore the application of stem cells to replace damaged or diseased myocytes.

Devices That Correct Fluid Balance

Salt and water retention and volume overload are central manifestations of heart failure and are largely responsible for hospitalizations in this condition. Diuretics represent our principal means of addressing this problem, but patients often become resistant to their effects, and treatment may be limited by renal impairment. Ultrafiltration represents a mechanical alternative to pharmacologic diuresis, traditionally reserved for the most extreme cases. Recent development of a simpler, less intrusive approach to ultrafiltration has led to an interest in broader application of such treatment. Clinical investigation has demonstrated that ultrafiltration may induce far more rapid normalization of fluid overload than is achievable through diuretics. One randomized controlled trial suggested that more routine use of ultrafiltration in patients hospitalized with worsening heart failure can reduce the incidence of subsequent rehospitalization (although the trial did not achieve its primary clinical endpoint).[144] To date it is not clear that ultrafiltration reduces the incidence of renal impairment that may be associated with aggressive diuresis. Studies are underway to test this hypothesis. Approaches are being investigated that adjust the ultrafiltration rate based on ongoing or intermittent measurement of intravascular volume or plasma refill rate. These approaches may prevent excessive rates of fluid removal and improve clinical success. At present, ultrafiltration represents a useful adjunct to treatment, at least in select patients poorly responsive to diuretics. A rationale for broader application will await additional clinical trial results.

Devices That Facilitate Monitoring Hemodynamic Status and Fluid Balance

As discussed previously, disease management has become a key component of the care of patients with heart failure. Although telephone monitoring and daily weights are mainstays of monitoring approaches, there is considerable interest in implantable devices that can provide more routine, telemetered information regarding the patient's hemodynamic and clinical status. Some hemodynamic monitoring devices are stand-alone. One such device incorporates a pressure-sensing lead in the right ventricular outflow region and estimates pulmonary artery diastolic pressure based on interrogation of the right ventricular isovolumic systolic pressure wave.[145] Others are implanted in the left atrium (transseptally) or in a pulmonary artery. ICD and pacing devices are being developed that additionally monitor pressure, to permit monitoring without an additional implantable device. Still other devices estimate lung water through measurement of pulmonary electrical impedance.[146] Each of these systems awaits definitive clinical trial evidence of significant improvement in clinical outcomes over those achievable through non–device-based approaches to clinical monitoring and management. Adverse effects associated with device implant will need to be considered in determining the net risk–benefit relationship. Device-based monitoring systems face the additional challenge of identifying optimal approaches to incorporating derived data into routine clinical decision making. Nevertheless, it is likely that the future will hold more routine application of device-based monitored information into clinical practice.

FUTURE DIRECTIONS

As we gain a deeper understanding of the cellular and molecular bases for pathologic myocyte hypertrophy and, dysfunction, and death and for interstitial fibrosis, additional treatment targets will emerge, and novel pharmacologic interventions are likely to be developed. Among the developing targets are (i) improving myocyte calcium homeostasis by correcting molecular abnormalities in the sarcoplasmic reticulum membrane, (ii) direct stimulation of cardiac myosin, (iii) targeting specific myocyte signaling pathways responsible for maladaptive hypertrophy, and (iv) reducing cardiac stiffness through targeting the pathologic extracellular matrix. Drug treatment may also increasingly be directed toward the renal and vascular contributions to the progression and clinical expression of heart failure.

Device technology is advancing rapidly, directed toward both mechanical and electrophysiologic abnormalities, as well as toward novel approaches to managing fluid overload and to monitoring changes in the patient's condition. Devices are now being developed not only to replace the function of a failed heart or to correct an aberrant heart rhythm, but also to prevent adverse remodeling, facilitate cardiac recovery, or correct underlying pathophysiologic mechanisms for the purpose of restoring normal cardiovascular function.

Where small molecule pharmacologic treatments meet their limits, gene therapy and cell-based therapies may find their role. One ongoing gene therapy approach is to increase sarcoplasmic reticular calcium ATPase as a means of restoring myocyte calcium handling and augment both relaxation and contraction. To date, myocardial cell-based therapies have shown mixed results in animal models and in small clinical trials. Approaches being investigated include injection of skeletal muscle myoblasts or pleuripotential stem cells into areas of myocardial scar. Some studies have demonstrated improved regional wall motion, although it is unclear whether these findings result from contraction of the implanted cells or associated paracrine effects. Improved cell selection, harvesting techniques, and patient selection may yield worthwhile clinical results.

Finally, there is increasing interest in the concept of personalized medicine, targeting specific treatments to specific patient groups, identified by phenotypic or genotypic characteristics. Genetic polymorphisms have already identified patient groups who appear to derive greater benefit from particular drug treatments, either because of preferential susceptibility of the biologic target to a particular drug, or because of metabolic variations that favorably influence pharmacokinetics. More powerful approaches, such as genome-wide association studies and novel informatics applied to vast databases of clinical, genomic, and proteomic information are likely to accelerate advancement in these directions.

REFERENCES

1. Packer M, Carver JR, Rodeheffer RJ, et al. Effect of oral milrinone on mortality in severe chronic heart failure. The PROMISE Study Research Group. N Engl J Med 1991;325:1468–1475.
2. Packer M, Bristow MR, Cohn JN, et al. The effect of carvedilol on morbidity and mortality in patients with chronic heart failure. N Engl J Med 1996;334:1349–1355.
3. CIBIS-II Investigators and Committees. The Cardiac Insufficiency Bisoprolol Study II (CIBIS II): a randomised trial. Lancet 1999;353:9–13.
4. MERIT-HF Study Group. Effect of metoprolol CR/XL in chronic heart failure: Metoprolol CR/XL Randomised Intervention Trial in Congestive Heart Failure (MERIT-HF). Lancet 1999;353:2001–2007.
5. Erlebacher JA, Weiss JL, Eaton LW, et al. Late effects of acute infarct dilation on heart size: a two-dimensional echocardiographic study. Am J Cardiol 1982;49:1120–1126.
6. Pfeffer MA, Pfeffer JM. Ventricular enlargement and reduced survival after myocardial infarction. Circulation 1987;75(5 Pt 2):IV93–IV97.
7. Konstam MA, Udelson JE, Anand Is, Cohn JN. Ventricular remodeling in heart failure: a credible surrogate endpoint. J Card Failure 2003;9:350–353.
8. Konstam MA. "Systolic and diastolic dysfunction" in heart failure? Time for a new paradigm. J Cardiac Fail 2003;9:1–3.
9. Francis GS, Benedict C, Johnstone DE, et al. Comparison of neuroendocrine activation in patients with left ventricular dysfunction with and without congestive heart failure. A substudy of the Studies of Left Ventricular Dysfunction (SOLVD). Circulation 1990;82;1724–1729.
10. Kraemer MD, Kubo SH, Rector TS, et al. Pulmonary and peripheral vascular factors are important determinants of peak exercise oxygen uptake in patients with heart failure. J Am Coll Cardiol. 1993;21:641–648.
11. Bonapace S, Rossi A, Cicoira M, et al. Aortic distensibility independently affects exercise tolerance in patients with dilated cardiomyopathy. Circulation 2003;107:1603–1608.
12. Treasure CB, Vita JA, Cox DA, et al. Endothelium-dependent dilation of the coronary microvasculature is impaired in dilated cardiomyopathy. Circulation 1990;81:772–779.
13. Patel AR, Kuvin JT, Pandian NG, et al. Heart failure etiology affects peripheral vascular endothelial function after cardiac transplantation. J Am Col Cardiol 2001;37:195–200.
14. Redfield MM, Edwards BS, Heublein DM, Burnett JC Jr. Restoration of renal response to atrial natriuretic factor in experimental low-output heart failure. Am J Physiol. 1989;257(4 Pt 2):R917–R923.
15. Lewis EF, Johnson PA, Johnson W, et al. Preferences for quality of life or survival expressed by patients with heart failure. J Heart Lung Transpl 2001;20:1016–1024.
16. Anand IS, MD, Florea VG, Fisher L. Surrogate end points in heart failure. J Am Coll Cardiol 2002;39:1414–1421.
17. Berger R, Huelsman M, Strecker K, et al. B-type natriuretic peptide predicts sudden death in patients with chronic heart failure. Circulation 2002;105:2392–2397.

18. Tsutamoto T, Wada A, Maeda K, et al. Attenuation of compensation of endogenous cardiac natriuretic peptide system in chronic heart failure: prognostic role of plasma brain natriuretic peptide concentration in patients with chronic symptomatic left ventricular dysfunction. Circulation 1997;96:509–516.

19. Maisel AS, Krishnaswamy P, Nowak RM, et al. Breathing Not Properly Multinational Study Investigators. Rapid measurement of B-type natriuretic peptide in the emergency diagnosis of heart failure. N Engl J Med 2002;347:161–167.

20. Moe GW, Howlett J, Januzzi JL, Zowall H; Canadian Multicenter Improved Management of Patients With Congestive Heart Failure (IMPROVE-CHF) Study Investigators. N-terminal pro-B-type natriuretic peptide testing improves the management of patients with suspected acute heart failure: primary results of the Canadian prospective randomized multicenter IMPROVE-CHF study. Circulation. 2007;115:3103–3110.

21. Wijns W, Vatner SF, Camici PG. Hibernating myocardium. N Engl J Med 1998;339: 173–181.

22. Selvanayagam JB, Jerosch-Herold M, Porto I, et al. Resting myocardial blood flow is impaired in hibernating myocardium: a magnetic resonance study of quantitative perfusion assessment. Circulation 2005;112:3289–3296.

23. Braunwald E, Kloner RA. The stunned myocardium: prolonged, postischemic ventricular dysfunction. Circulation 1982;66:1146–1149.

24. Udelson JE, Bonow RO, Dilsizian V. The historical and conceptual evolution of radionuclide assessment of myocardial viability. J Nucl Cardiol 2004;11:318–334

25. Allman KC, Shaw LJ, Hachamovitch R, Udelson JE. Myocardial viability testing and impact of revascularization on prognosis in patients with coronary artery disease and left ventricular dysfunction: A meta-analysis. J Am Coll Cardiol 2002;39:1151–1158.

26. Heart Failure Society of America: HFSA 2006 comprehensive heart failure practice guideline. J Card Failure 2006;12:e107.

27. Hochman JS, Lamas GA, Buller CE, et al. Coronary intervention for persistent occlusion after myocardial infarction. N Engl J Med 2006;355:2395–2407.

28. Levy D, Larson MG, Vasan RS, et al. The progression from hypertension to congestive heart failure. JAMA 1996;275:1557–1562.

29. Vasan RS, Larson MG, Benjamin EJ, et al. Congestive heart failure in subjects with normal versus reduced left ventricular ejection fraction: prevalence and mortality in a population-based cohort. J Am Coll Cardiol 1999;33:1948–1955.

30. Kostis JB, Davis BR, Cutler J, et al. Prevention of heart failure by antihypertensive drug treatment in older persons with isolated systolic hypertension. SHEP Cooperative Research Group. JAMA 1997;278:212–216.

31. Dahlof B, Lindholm LH, Hansson L, et al. Morbidity and mortality in the Swedish Trial in Old Patients with Hypertension (STOP-Hypertension). Lancet 1991;338: 1281–1285.

32. Fonarow GC, Adams KF, Abraham WT, et al. Risk stratification for in-hospital mortality in acutely decompensated heart failure classification and regression tree analysis. JAMA 2005;293:572–580.

33. Gheorghiade M, Abraham WT, Albert NM, et al. Systolic blood pressure at admission, clinical characteristics, and outcomes in patients hospitalized with acute heart failure. JAMA 2006;296:2217–2226.

34. Elkayam U. Nitrates in the treatment of congestive heart failure. Am J Cardiol 1996;77:41C–51C.

35. Chobanian AV, Bakris GL, Black HR, et al. The seventh report of the joint national committee on prevention, detection, evaluation, and treatment of high blood pressure: the JNC 7 report. JAMA 2003;289:2560–2572.

36. Blood Pressure Lowering Treatment Trialists' Collaboration. Effects of different blood-pressure-lowering regimens on major cardiovascular events: results of prospectively-designed overviews of randomised trials. Lancet. 2003;362:1527–1535.

37. ALLHAT Officers and Coordinators for the ALLHAT Collaborative Research Group. Major cardiovascular events in hypertensive patients randomized to doxazosin vs

chlorthalidone: the Antihypertensive and Lipid-Lowering Treatment to Prevent Heart Attack Trial (ALLHAT). JAMA 2000;283:1967–1975.

38. The ALLHAT Officers and Coordinators for the ALLHAT Collaborative Research Group. Major outcomes in high-risk hypertensive patients randomized to angiotensin-converting enzyme inhibitor or calcium channel blocker vs diuretic. The Antihypertensive and Lipid-Lowering Treatment to Prevent Heart Attack Trial (ALLHAT). The ALLHAT Officers and Coordinators for the ALLHAT Collaborative Research Group. JAMA 2002;288:2981–2997.

39. Dahlof B, Devereux RB, Kjeldsen SE, et al.; LIFE Study Group. Cardiovascular morbidity and mortality in the Losartan Intervention for Endpoint reduction in hypertension study (LIFE): a randomised trial against atenolol. Lancet 2002;359:995–1003.

40. Arnold JM, Yusuf S, Young J, et al. Prevention of heart failure in patients in the heart outcomes prevention evaluation (HOPE) study. Circulation 2003;107:1284–1290.

41. Brenner BM, Cooper ME, de Zeeuw D, et al. Effects of losartan on renal and cardiovascular outcomes in patients with type 2 diabetes and nephropathy. N Engl J Med 2001;345:861–869.

42. Taylor AL, Ziesche S, Yancy C, et al. African-American Heart Failure Trial Investigators. Combination of isosorbide dinitrate and hydralazine in blacks with heart failure. N Engl J Med 2004;351:2049–2057.

43. Kannel WB, Vasan RS, Levy D. Is the relation of systolic blood pressure to risk of cardiovascular disease continuous and graded, or are there critical values? Hypertension 2003;42:453–456.

44. Heart Failure Society of America: HFSA 2006 comprehensive heart failure practice guideline. J Card Failure 2006;12:e112.

45. Marijon E, Ou P, Celermajer DS, et al. Prevalence of rheumatic heart disease detected by echocardiographic screening. N Engl J Med 2007;357:470–476.

46. Bonow RO, Carabello BA, Kanu C, et al. ACC/AHA 2006 guidelines for the management of patients with valvular heart disease: a report of the American College of Cardiology/American Heart Association Task Force on Practice Guidelines (writing committee to revise the 1998 Guidelines for the Management of Patients With Valvular Heart Disease): developed in collaboration with the Society of Cardiovascular Anesthesiologists: endorsed by the Society for Cardiovascular Angiography and Interventions and the Society of Thoracic Surgeons. Circulation 2006;114:e84–e231.

47. Krumholz HM, Amatruda J, Smith GL, et al. Randomized trial of an education and support intervention to prevent readmission of patients with heart failure. J Am Coll Cardiol 2002;39:83–89.

48. Heart Failure Society of America. HFSA 2006 comprehensive heart failure practice guideline. J Card Failure 2006;12:e63.

49. Heart Failure Society of America. HFSA 2006 comprehensive heart failure practice guideline. J Card Failure 2006;12:e29.

50. Strassburg S, Springer J, Anker SD. Muscle wasting in cardiac cachexia. Int J Biochem Cell Biol 2005;37:1938–1947.

51. Kenchaiah S, Pocock SJ, Wang D, et al. Body mass index and prognosis in patients with chronic heart failure: insights from the Candesartan in Heart failure: Assessment of Reduction in Mortality and morbidity (CHARM) program. Circulation 2007;116:627–636.

52. Manson JE, Hu FB, Rich-Edwards JW, et al. A prospective study of walking as compared with vigorous exercise in the prevention of coronary heart disease in women. N Engl J Med 1999;341:650–658.

53. Clark AM, Hartling L, Vandermeer B, McAlister FA. Meta-analysis: secondary prevention programs for patients with coronary artery disease. Ann Intern Med 2005;143:659–672.

54. Piepoli MF, Davos C, Francis DP, Coats AJ. ExTraMATCH Collaborative. Exercise training meta-analysis of trials in patients with chronic heart failure (ExTraMATCH). BMJ 2004;328:189.

55. Linke A, Schoene N, Gielen S, et al. Endothelial dysfunction in patients with chronic heart failure: systemic effects of lower-limb exercise training. J Am Coll Cardiol 2001;37:392–397.

56. Ventura-Clapier R, Mettauer B, Bigard X. Beneficial effects of endurance training on cardiac and skeletal muscle energy metabolism in heart failure. Cardio Res 2007;73:10–18.

57. Mettauer B, Zoll J, Garnier A, Ventura-Clapier R. Heart failure: a model of cardiac and skeletal muscle energetic failure. Pflugers Archiv—Eur J Physiol 2006;452: 653–666.

58. Hunt SA, Abraham WT, Chin MH, et al. ACC/AHA 2005 Guideline Update for the Diagnosis and Management of Chronic Heart Failure in the Adult: a report of the American College of Cardiology/American Heart Association Task Force on Practice Guidelines Circulation. 2005;112:e154–e235.

59. Heart Failure Society of America: HFSA 2006 comprehensive heart failure practice guideline. J Card Failure 2006;12:e34.

60. Heart Failure Society of America: HFSA 2006 comprehensive heart failure practice guideline. J Card Failure 2006;12:e32.

61. Force T, Krause DS, Van Etten RA. Molecular mechanisms of cardiotoxicity of tyrosine kinase inhibition. Nature Reviews. Cancer 2007;7:332–344.

62. Chung ES, Packer M, Lo KH, et al.; The Anti-TNF Therapy Against Congestive Heart Failure Investigators. Randomized, double-blind, placebo-controlled, pilot trial of infliximab, a chimeric monoclonal antibody to tumor necrosis factor-alpha, in patients with moderate-to-severe heart failure: results of the anti-TNF Therapy Against Congestive Heart Failure (ATTACH) trial. Circulation 2003;107:3133–3140.

63. Macfarlane DP, Fisher M. Thiazolidinediones in patients with diabetes mellitus and heart failure : implications of emerging data. Am J Cardio Drugs 2006;6:297–304.

64. Eisenberg MJ, Brox A, Bestawros AN. Calcium channel blockers: an update. Am J Med. 2004;116:35–43.

65. Writing Committee to Revise the 2001 Guidelines for the Management of Patients With Atrial Fibrillation. ACC/AHA/ESC 2006 guidelines for the management of patients with atrial fibrillation. J Am Coll Cardiol 2006;48:854–906.

66. Bardy GH, Lee KL, Mark DB, et al. Sudden Cardiac Death in Heart Failure Trial (SCD-HeFT) Investigators. Amiodarone or an implantable cardioverter-defibrillator for congestive heart failure. N Engl J Med 2005;352:225–237.

67. Kimmelstiel C, Levine D, Perry K, et al. Randomized, controlled evaluation of short- and long-term benefits of heart failure disease management within a diverse provider network: the SPAN-CHF trial. Circulation 2004;110:1450–1455.

68. Krumholz HM, Currie PM, Riegel B, et al. American Heart Association Disease Management Taxonomy Writing Group. A taxonomy for disease management: a scientific statement from the American Heart Association Disease Management Taxonomy Writing Group. Circulation 2006;114:1432–1445.

69. Goldberg LR, Piette JD, Walsh MN, et al. WHARF Investigators. Randomized trial of a daily electronic home monitoring system in patients with advanced heart failure: the Weight Monitoring in Heart Failure (WHARF) trial. Am Heart J 2003;146: 705–712.

70. Pamboukian SV, Smallfield MC, Bourge RC. Implantable hemodynamic monitoring devices in heart failure. Curr Cardiol Rep 2006;8:187–190.

71. Heart Failure Society of America: HFSA 2006 comprehensive heart failure practice guideline. J Card Failure 2006;12:e19

72. Troughton RW, Frampton CM, Yandle TG, et al. Treatment of heart failure guided by plasma aminoterminal brain natriuretic peptide (N-BNP) concentrations. Lancet 2000;355:1126–1130.

73. Butler J, Forman DE, Abraham WT, et al. Relationship between heart failure treatment and development of worsening renal function among hospitalized patients. Am Heart J 2004;147:331–338.

74. Domanski M, Norman J, Pitt B, et al. Studies of Left Ventricular Dysfunction. Diuretic use, progressive heart failure, and death in patients in the Studies Of Left Ventricular Dysfunction (SOLVD). J Am Coll Cardiol 2003;42:705–708.

75. Murray MD, Deer MM, Ferguson JA, et al. Open-label randomized trial of torsemide compared with furosemide therapy for patients with heart failure. Am J Med 2001;111:513–520.

76. Ren Y, Arima S, Carretero OA, Ito S. Possible role of adenosine in macula densa control of glomerular hemodynamics. Kidney Intern 2002;61:169–176.

77. Swedberg K, Kjekshus J. Effects of enalapril on mortality in severe congestive heart failure: results of the Cooperative North Scandinavian Enalapril Survival Study (CONSENSUS). Am J Cardiol 1988;62:60A–66A.

78. SOLVD Investigators. Effect of enalapril on mortality and the development of heart failure in asymptomatic patients with reduced left ventricular ejection fractions. N Engl J Med 1992;327:685–691.

79. SOLVD Investigators. Effect of enalapril on survival in patients with reduced left ventricular ejection fractions and congestive heart failure. N Engl J Med 1991;325:293–302.

80. Pfeffer MA, Braunwald E, Moye LA. et al. Effect of captopril on mortality and morbidity in patients with left ventricular dysfunction after myocardial infarction. Results of the survival and ventricular enlargement trial. The SAVE Investigators. N Engl J Med 1992;327:669–677.

81. Garg R, Yusuf S. Overview of randomized trials of angiotensin-converting enzyme inhibitors on mortality and morbidity in patients with heart failure. Collaborative Group on ACE Inhibitor Trials. JAMA 1995;273:1450–1456.

82. Cohn JN, Johnson G, Ziesche S, et al. A comparison of enalapril with hydralazine-isosorbide dinitrate in the treatment of chronic congestive heart failure. N Engl J Med 1991;325:303–310.

83. Konstam MA, Rousseau MF, Kronenberg MW, et al. Effects of the angiotensin converting enzyme inhibitor, enalapril, on the long-term progression of left ventricular dysfunction in patients with heart failure. Circulation 1992;86:431–438.

84. Konstam MA, Kronenberg MW, Rousseau MF, et al., for the SOLVD Investigators. Effects of the angiotensin converting enzyme inhibitor, enalapril, on the long-term progression of left ventricular dilatation in patients with asymptomatic systolic dysfunction. Circulation 1993;88:2277–2283.

85. Yusuf S, Sleight P, Pogue J, et al. Effects of an angiotensin-converting-enzyme inhibitor, ramipril, on cardiovascular events in high-risk patients. The Heart Outcomes Prevention Evaluation Study Investigators. N Engl J Med 2000;342:145–153.

86. Pitt B, Poole-Wilson PA, Segal R, et al., on behalf of the ELITE II investigators. Randomised trial of losartan versus captopril on mortality in patients with symptomatic heart failure: the Losartan Heart Failure Survival Study—ELITE II. Lancet 2000;355:1582–1587.

87. Pfeffer MA, McMurray JJ, Velazquez EJ, et al. Valsartan in Acute Myocardial Infarction Trial Investigators. Valsartan, captopril, or both in myocardial infarction complicated by heart failure, left ventricular dysfunction, or both. N Engl J Med 2003;349:1893–1906.

88. Dickstein K, Kjekshus J. OPTIMAAL Steering Committee of the OPTIMAAL Study Group. Effects of losartan and captopril on mortality and morbidity in high-risk patients after acute myocardial infarction: the OPTIMAAL randomised trial. Optimal Trial in Myocardial Infarction with Angiotensin II Antagonist Losartan. Lancet 2002;360:752–760.

89. Granger CB, McMurray JJ, Yusuf S, et al. Effects of candesartan in patients with chronic heart failure and reduced left-ventricular systolic function intolerant to

angiotensin-converting-enzyme inhibitors: the CHARM-Alternative trial. Lancet 2003;362:772–776.

90. Pfeffer MA, Swedberg K, Granger CB, et al. Effects of candesartan on mortality and morbidity in patients with chronic heart failure: the CHARM-Overall programme. Lancet 2003;362:759–766.

91. McMurray JJ, Ostergren J, Swedberg K et al. Effects of candesartan in patients with chronic heart failure and reduced left-ventricular systolic function taking angiotensin-converting-enzyme inhibitors: the CHARM-Added trial. Lancet 2003; 362:767–771.

92. Cohn JN, Tognoni G, for the Valsartan Heart Failure Trial Investigators. A randomized trial of the angiotensin-receptor blocker valsartan in chronic heart failure. N Engl J Med 2001;345:1667–1675.

93. Yusuf S, Pfeffer MA, Swedberg K, et al. Effects of candesartan in patients with chronic heart failure and preserved left-ventricular ejection fraction: the CHARM-Preserved trial. Lancet 2003;362:777–781.

94. Konstam MA, Patten RD, Thomas I, et al. Effects of Losartan and Captopril on left ventricular volumes in elderly patients with heart failure: Results of the ELITE Ventricular Function Substudy. Am Heart J 2000;139:1081–1087.

95. Pitt B, Segal R, Martinez FA, et al. Randomised trial of losartan versus captopril in patients over 65 with heart failure (Evaluation of Losartan in the Elderly Study, ELITE) Lancet 1997;349:747–752.

96. Brenner BM, Cooper ME, de Zeeuw D, et al. Effects of losartan on renal and cardio-vascular outcomes in patients with type 2 diabetes and nephropathy. N Engl J Med 2001;345:861–869.

97. Lewis EJ, Hunsicker LG, Clarke WR, et al. Collaborative Study Group. Renoprotective effect of the angiotensin-receptor antagonist irbesartan in patients with nephropathy due to type 2 diabetes. N Engl J Med 2001;345:851–860.

98. Swedberg K, Hjalmarson A, Waagstein F, Wallentin I. Prolongation of survival in congestive cardiomyopathy by beta-receptor blockade. Lancet, 1979;1:1374–1376.

99. Katz AM. Potential deleterious effects of inotropic agents in the therapy of heart failure. Circulation 1986;73(Suppl III):184–190.

100. Packer M, Coats AJ, Fowler MB, et al. Carvedilol Prospective Randomized Cumulative Survival Study Group. Effect of carvedilol on survival in severe chronic heart failure. N Engl J Med 2001;344:1651–1658.

101. Pitt B, Zannad F, Remme WJ, et al. The effect of spironolactone on morbidity and mortality in patients with severe heart failure. Randomized Aldactone Evaluation Study Investigators. N Engl J Med 1999;341:709–717.

102. Pitt B, Remme W, Zannad F, et al. Eplerenone Post-Acute Myocardial Infarction Heart Failure Efficacy and Survival Study Investigators. Eplerenone, a selective aldosterone blocker, in patients with left ventricular dysfunction after myocardial infarction. N Engl J Med 2003;348:1309–1321.

103. Guiha NH, Cohn JN, Mikulic E, et al. Treatment of refractory heart failure with infusion of nitroprusside. N Engl J Med 1974;291:587–592.

104. Cohn JN, Archibald DG, Ziesche S, et al. Effect of vasodilator therapy on mortality in chronic congestive heart failure. Results of a Veterans Administration Cooperative Study. N Engl J Med 1986;314:1547–1552.

105. Publication Committee for the VMAC Investigators (Vasodilatation in the Management of Acute CHF). Intravenous nesiritide vs nitroglycerin for treatment of decompensated congestive heart failure: a randomized controlled trial. JAMA 2002;287: 1531–1540.

106. Sackner-Bernstein JD, Skopicki HA, Aaronson KD. Risk of worsening renal function with nesiritide in patients with acutely decompensated heart failure. Circulation 2005;111:1487–1491.

107. Sackner-Bernstein JD, Kowalski M, Fox M, Aaronson K. Short-term risk of death after treatment with nesiritide for decompensated heart failure: a pooled analysis of randomized controlled trials. JAMA 2005;293:1900–1905.

108. Yancy CW, Krum H, Massie BM, et al. The Second Follow-up Serial Infusions of Nesiritide (FUSION II) trial for advanced heart failure: study rationale and design. Am Heart J 2007;153:478–484.

109. Ferguson DW. Digitalis and neurohormonal abnormalities in heart failure and implications for therapy. Am J Cardiol 1992;69:24G–32G.

110. Packer M, Gheorghiade M, Young JB, et al. Withdrawal of digoxin from patients with chronic heart failure treated with angiotensin-converting–enzyme inhibitors. N Engl J Med 1993;329:1–7.

111. Uretsky BF, Young JB, Shahidi FE, et al. Randomized study assessing the effect of digoxin withdrawal in patients with mild to moderate chronic congestive heart failure: results of the PROVED trial. J Am Coll Cardiol 1993;22:955–962.

112. Digitalis Investigation Group. The effect of digoxin on mortality and morbidity in patients with heart failure. N Engl J Med 1997;336:525–533.

113. Heart Failure Society of America. HFSA 2006 comprehensive heart failure practice guideline. J Card Failure 2006;12:e49.

114. O'Connor CM, Gattis WA, Uretsky BF, et al. Continuous intravenous dobutamine is associated with an increased risk of death in patients with advanced heart failure: insights from the Flolan International Randomized Survival Trial (FIRST). Am Heart J 1999;138(1 Pt 1):78–86.

115. Cuffe MS, Califf RM, Adams KF Jr, et al. Outcomes of a Prospective Trial of Intravenous Milrinone for Exacerbations of Chronic Heart Failure (OPTIME-CHF) Investigators. Short-term intravenous milrinone for acute exacerbation of chronic heart failure: a randomized controlled trial. JAMA 2002;287:1541–1547.

116. Mebazaa A, Nieminen MS, Packer M, et al. Levosimendan vs dobutamine for patients with acute decompensated heart failure: the SURVIVE Randomized Trial. JAMA 2007;297:1883–1891.

117. Heart Failure Society of America. HFSA 2006 comprehensive heart failure practice guideline. J Card Failure 2006;12:e96.

118. Cohn JN, Goldstein SO, Greenberg BH, et al. A dose-dependent increase in mortality with vesnarinone among patients with severe heart failure. Vesnarinone Trial Investigators. N Engl J Med 1998;339:1810–1816.

119. Follath F, Cleland JG, Just H, et al. Steering Committee and Investigators of the Levosimendan Infusion versus Dobutamine (LIDO) Study. Efficacy and safety of intravenous levosimendan compared with dobutamine in severe low-output heart failure (the LIDO study): a randomised double-blind trial. Lancet 2002;360:196–202.

120. Udelson JE, Smith WB, Hendrix GH, et al. Acute hemodynamic effects of conivaptan, a dual V1A and V2 vasopressin receptor antagonist, in patients with advanced heart failure. Circulation 2001;104:2417–2423.

121. Gheorghiade M, Gattis WA, O'Connor CM, et al. Acute and chronic therapeutic impact of a vasopressin antagonist in congestive heart failure (ACTIV in CHF) investigators. Effects of tolvaptan, a vasopressin antagonist, in patients hospitalized with worsening heart failure: a randomized controlled trial. JAMA 2004;291:1963–1971.

122. Gheorghiade M, Konstam MA, Burnett JC, et al. Short-term clinical effects of tolvaptan, an oral vasopressin antagonist, in patients hospitalized for heart failure. The EVEREST Clinical Status Trials. JAMA 2007;297:1332–1343.

123. Konstam MA, Gheorghiade M, Burnett JC, et al. Effects of oral tolvaptan in patients hospitalized for worsening heart failure: The EVEREST Outcome Trial. JAMA 2007;297:1319–1331.

124. Sbarouni E, Bradshaw A, Andreotti F, et al. Relationship between hemostatic abnormalities and neuroendocrine activity in heart failure. Am Heart J 1994;127:607–612.

125. Yamamoto K, Ikeda U, Furuhashi K, et al. The coagulation system is activated in idiopathic cardiomyopathy. J Am Coll Cardiol 1995;25:1634–1640.

126. Al-Khadra AS, Salem DN, Rand WM, et al. Warfarin anticoagulation and survival: a cohort analysis from the studies of left ventricular dysfunction. J Am Col Cardiol 1998; 31:749–753.

127. Al-Khadra AS, Salem DN, Rand WM, et al. Effect of antiplatelet agents on survival in patients with left ventricular systolic dysfunction. J Am Col Cardiol 1998;31:419–425.

128. Teo KK, Yusuf S, Pfeffer M, et al. Effects of long-term treatment with angiotensin-converting-enzyme inhibitors in the presence or absence of aspirin: a systematic review. Lancet 2002;360:1037–1043.

129. Moss AJ, Zareba W, Hall WJ, et al. Prophylactic implantation of a defibrillator in patients with myocardial infarction and reduced ejection fraction. N Engl J Med 2002;346:877–883.

130. Bardy GH, Lee KL, Mark DB, et al. Amiodarone or an implantable cardioverter-defibrillator for congestive heart failure. N Engl J Med 2005;352:225–237.

131. Frazier OH, Rose EA, Oz MC, et al. Multicenter clinical evaluation of the HeartMate vented electric left ventricular assist system in patients awaiting heart transplantation. J Thorac Cardiovasc Surg 2001;122:1186–1195.

132. Rose EA, Gelijns AC, Moskowitz AJ, et al. Long-term use of a left ventricular assist device for end-stage heart failure. N Engl J Med 2001;345:1435–1443.

133. Thiele H, Sick P, Boudriot E, et al. Randomized comparison of intra-aortic balloon support with a percutaneous left ventricular assist device in patients with revascularized acute myocardial infarction complicated by cardiogenic shock. Eur Heart J 2005; 26:1276–1283.

134. Burkhoff D, Cohen H, Brunckhorst C, et al. A randomized multicenter clinical study to evaluate the safety and efficacy of the TandemHeart percutaneous ventricular assist device versus conventional therapy with intraaortic balloon pumping for treatment of cardiogenic shock. Am Heart J 2006;152:469.e1–e8.

135. Lee MS, Makkar RR. Percutaneous left ventricular support devices. Cardiol Clin 2006;24:265–275.

136. Henriques JP, Remmelink M, Baan J Jr, et al. Safety and feasibility of elective high-risk percutaneous coronary intervention procedures with left ventricular support of the Impella Recover LP 2.5. Am J Cardiol 2006;97:990–992.

137. Birks EJ, Tansley PD, Hardy J, et al. Left ventricular assist device and drug therapy for the reversal of heart failure. N Engl J Med 355:1873–1884.

138. Abraham WT, Fisher WG, Smith AL, et al. Multicenter InSync Randomized Clinical Evaluation. Cardiac resynchronization in chronic heart failure. N Engl J Med 2002;346:1845–1853.

139. Bristow MR, Saxon LA, Boehmer J, et al. Comparison of Medical Therapy, Pacing, and Defibrillation in Heart Failure (COMPANION) Investigators. Cardiac-resynchronization therapy with or without an implantable defibrillator in advanced chronic heart failure. N Engl J Med 2004;350:2140–2150.

140. Cleland JG, Daubert JC, Erdmann E, et al. The effect of cardiac resynchronization on morbidity and mortality in heart failure. N Engl J Med 2005;352:1539–1549.

141. Patten RD, Denofrio D, El-Zaru M, et al. Ventricular assist device therapy normalizes inducible nitric oxide synthase expression and reduces cardiomyocyte apoptosis in the failing human heart. J Am Coll Cardiol 2005;45:1419–1424.

142. Lembcke A, Wiese TH, Dushe S, et al. Effects of passive cardiac containment on left ventricular structure and function: verification by volume and flow measurements. J Heart Lung Transplant 2004;23:11–19.

143. Konstam MA, Czerska B, Böhm M, et al. Continuous aortic flow augmentation: a pilot study of hemodynamic and renal responses to a novel percutaneous intervention in decompensated heart failure. Circulation 2005;112:3107–3114.

144. Costanzo MR, Guglin ME, Saltzberg MT, et al. UNLOAD Trial Investigators. Ultrafiltration versus intravenous diuretics for patients hospitalized for acute decompensated heart failure. J Am Coll Cardiol 2007;49:675–683.

145. Magalski A, Adamson P, Gadler F, et al. Continuous ambulatory right heart pressure measurements with an implantable hemodynamic monitor: a multicenter, 12-month follow-up study of patients with chronic heart failure. Cardiac Fail 2002;8:63–70.

146. Ypenburg C, Bax JJ, van der Wall EE, et al. Intrathoracic impedance monitoring to predict decompensated heart failure. Am J Cardiol 2007;99:554–557.

CHAPTER 7

Approaches to Treatment of Patients with, or at Risk for, Heart Failure

Marvin A. Konstam • Arnold M. Katz

Numerous drug and device therapies are presently in use for management of patients with heart failure, and many more are under development (Table 7-1). In Chapter 6, we detailed the various modalities available for treating patients with heart failure. In the present chapter, we define several patient subsets, based on functional, structural, and clinical characteristics to synthesize an approach to management, drawing on the resources described in Chapter 6. Our construct of these patient subsets is based on several factors: (a) a categorization of treatment evidence according to entry criteria for clinical trials, (b) our own conceptualization of key physiologic categories of patients, (c) characterization of clinical status, and (d) approaches laid out in current clinical practice guidelines.

The division between symptomatic and asymptomatic status is important in treatment choices. For the asymptomatic patient, the strategy is principally directed toward preventing progression of the underlying cardiac disease and avoiding adverse clinical outcomes. For the symptomatic patient, these same strategies apply, but a major emphasis must be to improve health-related quality of life by relieving symptoms and improving functional status.

Many clinical trials have categorized patient clinical status based on the NYHA classification[1] (Table 7-2). Recent clinical practice guidelines have recognized limitations in NYHA classification including the frequency of shifts, in either direction, in patient classification and have adopted a broader categorization, based on a pattern of advancing cardiac and clinical functional impairment. The stages presented within the joint guideline of the American Heart Association and American College of Cardiology[2] (Fig. 7-1) are as follows: stage A, patients at high risk for heart failure in the absence of structural heart disease; stage B, asymptomatic patients with structural heart disease; stage C, patients with prior or current symptoms of heart failure; stage D, patients with advanced cardiac disease and refractory clinical heart failure. In addition to categorizing patients by the mere presence or absence of symptoms, we give special attention to treatment options and approaches for patients with advanced heart failure (stage D), characterized by severe symptoms and functional impairment despite optimal medical therapy. In addition, we focus on the patient with an exacerbation of heart failure, who may or may not have advanced disease, but for whom the immediate treatment approach should address symptom relief and restoration of a stable clinical state.

TABLE 7-1

Treatments for Heart Failure

Drugs-chronic	Drugs-acute	Devices	Surgeries/interventions
ACE inhibitors	**Diuretics**	**ICDs**	**Revascularization**
Beta blockers	**Nesiritide**	**CRT**	**Heart transplant**
ARBs	**PDE inhibitors**	**VADs**	*Mitral valve replace/repair*
Aldo blockers	**Beta agonists**	*Restraining devices*	*Ventricular reconstruction*
Hydralazine	**Nitrates**	*Aortic flow*	
Nitrates	*ET blockers*	*augmentation*	
Digoxin	*Vasopressin blockers*	*Hemofiltration*	
Diuretics	*Adenosine blockers*	*Monitoring devices*	
Vasopressin blockers	*Calcium sensitizers*		
Adenosine blockers	*Myosin activators*		
Statins			
Anticoagulants			
Erythropoietin			
analogues			

Bold: Therapies in established use.
Italic: Therapies under investigation (partial list).
ACE, angiotensin-converting enzyme; ARB, angiotensin receptor blocker; Aldo, aldosterone; CRT, cardiac resyn-chronization therapy; ET, endothelin; ICD, implantable cardioverter-defibrillator; VAD, ventricular assist device.

Categorizing Patients Based on Left Ventricular Ejection Fraction and Volumes

Chapter 2 explains the terms *systolic* and *diastolic heart failure*. Clinical trials and treatment recommendations often categorize patients based on left ventricular ejection fraction (LVEF), describing patients as having systolic or diastolic heart failure, based on whether the EF is low (e.g., ≤35% or 40%) or preserved (see Chapter 2). This focus was originally driven by an assumption of differences in pathophysiology, with low EF assumed to represent reduced contractility (systolic dysfunction) and preserved EF assumed to represent preserved contractility, and therefore by inference, predominant diastolic functional abnormalities (diastolic dysfunction).

TABLE 7-2

New York Heart Association Functional Classification

Class I	No limitation of physical activity; ordinary physical activity causes no discomfort
Class II	Slight to moderate limitation of physical activity; ordinary physical activity causes discomfort
Class III	Moderate to great limitation of physical activity; less than ordinary physical activity causes discomfort
Class IV	Unable to carry on any physical activity without discomfort

From the Criteria Committee of the New York Heart Association (1942). *Nomenclature and Criteria for Diagnosis of Diseases of the Heart.* 4th ed. 8–9. New York, New York Heart Association.

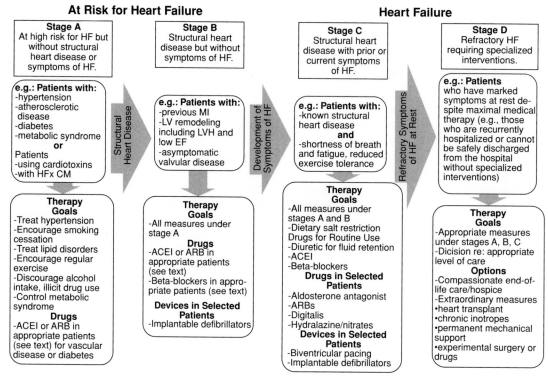

Figure 7-1: AHA/ACC Guideline classification of advancing clinical stages from risk to structural heart disease to stages of heart failure, forming a basis for treatment recommendations. From Hunt SA, Abraham WT, Chin MH, et al. ACC/AHA 2005 Guideline Update for the Diagnosis and Management of Chronic Heart Failure in the Adult: a report of the American College of Cardiology/American Heart Association Task Force on Practice Guidelines. Circulation 2005; 112(12):e154–e235.

There are a number of limitations to this conceptualization. First, in the absence of acute injury, cardiogenic shock, LV volume overload, or extremes of heart rate, LVEF is determined principally by the degree of LV remodeling with dilatation, rather than by reduced myocardial contractility.[3] Second, myocardial abnormalities in both contraction and relaxation are generally present in patients with heart failure, regardless of EF. Third, neither designation—*systolic heart failure* nor *diastolic heart failure*—identifies the underlying disease state. For patients with reduced LVEF, the causes are most commonly ischemic cardiomyopathy and idiopathic dilated cardiomyopathy. For patients with preserved LVEF, the most common cause is hypertensive cardiovascular disease (HCVD), although many other causes exist, including pericardial constriction, infiltrative cardiomyopathies, and familial hypertrophic cardiomyopathies. The recommended treatment approaches to these conditions vary substantially (though few, if any, of these recommendations are based on randomized, controlled outcome data), and the terms *systolic* and *diastolic heart failure* may mislead the clinician into assuming a single treatment approach for each of these designations. Finally, we have learned over the past two decades that clinical outcomes in patients with reduced LVEF can be improved by treatments that prevent or reverse adverse ventricular remodeling, rather than augmenting myocardial contractility.[4] The goal of improving clinical outcomes for patients with heart failure and preserved LVEF is probably better served by therapies directed toward preventing or reversing the underlying cardiac pathology—e.g., myocardial hypertrophy and fibrosis in patients with HCVD—than by focusing on functional diastolic properties per se.

Unfortunately, the vast majority of clinical trials documenting improved survival in heart failure were performed in patients with reduced LVEF. In this chapter, we divide patients according to the presence or absence of LV dilation, recognizing that reduced LVEF (see previous discussion) is principally a marker of LV remodeling with dilation. For patients without clinical heart failure, we identify both LV eccentric hypertrophy (dilation) and LV concentric hypertrophy (without dilation due mostly to long-standing hypertension) as conditions requiring treatment to prevent progression and development of clinical heart failure.

APPROACH TO THE ASYMPTOMATIC PATIENT WITH LEFT VENTRICULAR HYPERTROPHY

Hypertension is, by far, the strongest attributable risk to the development of heart failure, with a hypertensive history present in most patients with clinical heart failure, regardless of LVEF.[5] Normalization of blood pressure is, therefore, a major goal in an approach to preventing heart failure. In contrast to prior beliefs, there is now evidence of a continuum of risk across a broad spectrum of both systolic and diastolic blood pressures,[6] suggesting that even modest or intermittent hypertension should be aggressively treated.

Patients with hypertension and either electrocardiographic or echocardiographic evidence of left ventricular hypertension (LVH) deserve special mention because LVH is a risk factor for adverse cardiovascular events, independent of blood pressure.[7,8] This incremental risk may derive from linkage between the presence and degree of LVH and both the duration and magnitude of hypertension. Development of LVH may also be influenced by additional factors besides blood pressure, such as neuroendocrine activation, which may, in turn, promote atherosclerosis and vascular fibrosis. Beyond being a marker integrating both hemodynamic and nonhemodynamic factors promoting cardiovascular disease, LVH directly drives the expression of disease, generating cardiac functional impairment that promotes clinical heart failure and possibly predisposes to ischemic events.

Adequate hypertension management frequently requires use of multiple agents. Established guidelines provide ample guidance and appropriate treatment goals.[9] Chapter 6 provides further discussion of approaches to hypertensive management.

APPROACH TO CHRONIC MANAGEMENT OF THE PATIENT WITH HEART FAILURE AND A NONDILATED LEFT VENTRICLE

As in any other constellation of clinical findings, the approach to the patient with heart failure and a nondilated left ventricle must begin with consideration of the underlying cause, or at least the underlying pathophysiology. By far, the most prevalent cause of heart failure in the absence of a dilated LV cavity (usually implying preservation of LVEF) is HCVD.

Clinical trials have tended to segregate study populations merely on the basis of LVEF. The CHARM-Preserved trial showed a nonsignificant trend (Fig. 7-2) for reduction in the primary combined endpoint of cardiovascular death or heart failure–related hospitalization in patients with clinical evidence of heart failure and with LVEF >40%, randomized to the angiotensin receptor blocker (ARB) candesartan, compared with placebo.[10] For the group of patients with heart failure due to HCVD, the insight we can gain from this and similar trials is limited, since no specific cause was specified for inclusion, and patients with overt hypertension were generally excluded. In the CHARM program, patients with "persistent systolic or diastolic hypertension" were excluded,[11] and the study population for CHARM-Preserved

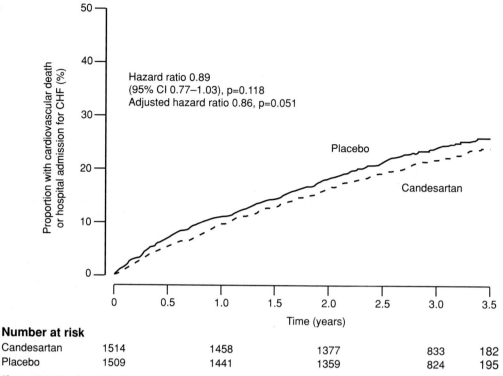

Hazard ratio 0.89
(95% CI 0.77–1.03), p=0.118
Adjusted hazard ratio 0.86, p=0.051

Number at risk

Candesartan	1514	1458	1377	833	182
Placebo	1509	1441	1359	824	195

Figure 7-2: Results of the CHARM Preserved Trial examining effects of candesartan, versus placebo in patients with heart failure in the absence of reduced LVEF. From Yusuf S, Pfeffer MA, Swedberg K, et al.; CHARM Investigators and Committees. Effects of candesartan in patients with chronic heart failure and preserved left-ventricular ejection fraction: the CHARM-Preserved Trial. Lancet 2003;362(9386):777–781.

differed substantially from the typical population with heart failure related to HCVD, in terms of age, gender distribution, and baseline blood pressure.

Figure 7-3 provides a logical approach to the differential diagnosis of a patient with heart failure and preserved LVEF.[12] Heart failure with preserved LVEF in the presence of LV dilation suggests either LV volume overload, due to mitral regurgitation, aortic regurgitation, left-to-right shunt at the left ventricular or aortic level, arterial-venous shunting, anemia, increased metabolism as occurs in thyrotoxicosis, or other forms of high-output failure. LV dilation with EF preservation is also seen in conditioned athletes, who typically have large LV stroke volumes and slow heart rates, but no heart failure. In the absence of these conditions, a preserved LVEF is associated with a nondilated LV.

In approaching the patient with heart failure and a nondilated LV, the clinician should ask the following series of questions (Fig. 7-3). First, does the patient have right heart failure and right ventricular dysfunction out of proportion to left heart failure and left ventricular dysfunction? If so, consideration should be given to pulmonary emboli, primary pulmonary hypertension, cor pulmonale, obstructive sleep apnea (see subsequent text), right ventricular infarction, right ventricular dysplasia, or primary tricuspid or pulmonary valvular dysfunction. Second, does the patient have intermittent LV ischemia or hibernating myocardium as the cause of left heart failure? Third, does the patient have mitral or aortic valvular obstruction, atrial myxoma, subvalvular or supravalvular aortic obstruction or aortic coarctation? Fourth, does the patient have constrictive or restrictive physiology, and is there

Decision Tree for Diagnosis in Patients
with Heart Failure and Preserved LVEF

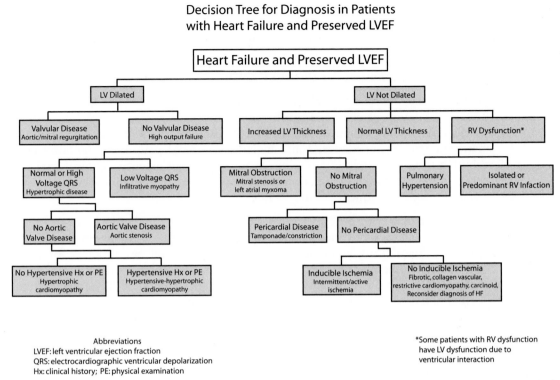

Abbreviations
LVEF: left ventricular ejection fraction
QRS: electrocardiographic ventricular depolarization
Hx: clinical history; PE: physical examination

*Some patients with RV dysfunction
have LV dysfunction due to
ventricular interaction

Figure 7-3: Decision tree for diagnosis in patients with heart failure and preserved LVEF. From Heart Failure Society of America. HFSA 2006 comprehensive heart failure practice guideline. J Card Failure 2006;12:e81.

evidence of either myocardial infiltration (suggested by increased LV thickness with normal or low QRS voltage on the electrocardiogram [ECG]) or pericardial thickening (seen on computerized tomography or magnetic resonance imaging)? Fifth, does the patient have LVH unexplained by hypertension or valvular disease, and is there a family history suggestive of hypertrophic cardiomyopathy? Finally, does the patient have long-standing hypertension? In most cases the answer to this last question will be yes, and the primary diagnosis will be HCVD (see subsequent text).

Obstructive Sleep Apnea

Special consideration should be given to the diagnosis of obstructive sleep apnea, an increasingly recognized but often-missed cause of heart failure.[13] Intermittent upper airway obstruction, with associated hypoxemia, may lead to a form of cor pulmonale, with pulmonary hypertension, right ventricular dilation and dysfunction, right heart failure, and fluid retention. It may be an occult cause of both supraventricular (including atrial fibrillation) and ventricular arrhythmias. Obstructive sleep apnea has also been associated with left heart failure, for reasons that are less clear but may include myocardial hypoxia, tachyarrhythmias, and ventricular interdependent effects. Although often associated with obesity or a thick neck, obstructive sleep apnea may be seen in patients with a normal body habitus. The patient should be questioned for snoring, nighttime sleeplessness, daytime sleepiness and frequent napping, and nightmares. The diagnosis is made by observing breathing patterns and systemic oxygenation during a sleep study. Treatment is with a continuous positive airway pressure mask during sleep. Fluid overload should be corrected with diuretics. Aggressive attempts should be made to encourage weight reduction, when warranted, including referral to an obesity center and consideration of surgical approaches.

Hypertensive Cardiovascular Disease (HCVD)

HCVD, by far the most prevalent condition in patients with heart failure without LV cavity dilation, is characterized by concentric LVH and excessive LV diastolic stiffness. Additional common factors are increased arterial stiffness, with resulting increased arterial impedance,[14] and hypertensive renal pathology, the latter contributing to urinary sodium retention. In the absence of extensive clinical trial evidence within this patient population, the following are key components of an empirical approach to treatment[3] (Table 7-3):

1. Treat hypertension, prevent/regress LVH. Hypertension should be aggressively treated. Chapter 6 provides guidance regarding blood pressure targets in the presence of clinical heart failure or cardiac dysfunction, as well as a rationale for incorporating an angiotensin-converting enzyme (ACE) inhibitor or ARB within the treatment regimen in most patients with heart failure, regardless of ejection fraction.
2. Maintain meticulous volume management. Sodium restriction should be strongly encouraged (see Chapter 6). Patients prone to fluid retention should be treated with thiazide or loop diuretics. Patients with concentric LVH and little or no cavity dilation may be particularly sensitive to shifts in volume status due to ventricular wall stiffness and preload dependency. They will require careful monitoring of body weight and renal function, often with frequent diuretic dose adjustment.
3. Maintain diastolic filling time. Preload dependence associated with concentric LVH confers increased sensitivity to inadequate filling time. These patients tolerate excessive heart rates poorly. Although there is controversy regarding the routine use of beta blockers, these agents should be considered in patients with heart failure and HCVD if heart rate is rapid (e.g., $>80–90$ min^{-1}). Consideration can also be given to the calcium channel blockers diltiazem or verapamil as additional

---

TABLE 7-3

Therapeutic Approaches in Patients with Hypertensive Cardiovascular Disease, Heart Failure, and Preserved LVEF

- Treat hypertension; prevent/regress hypertrophy
  –Anti-hypertensive treatments; particular role for ACE inhibitors/ARBs?
- Meticulous volume management
  –diuretics/Na restriction: reduce congestion without compromising forward output
- Increase diastolic filling time
  –slow heart rate; treat/prevent AF
- Improve dynamic relaxation
  –*Possible* roles of ACE inhibitors; ARBs; Ca-channel blockers
- Diminish/prevent ischemia
  –Medical treatment; revascularization

Modified from Konstam MA. "Systolic and diastolic dysfunction" in heart failure? Time for a new paradigm. J Card Failure. 2003;9:1–3. ACE, angiotensin converting enzyme; AF, atrial fibrillation; ARB, angiotensin receptor blocker.

means to lower heart rate. Consideration should be given to converting atrial fibrillation to sinus rhythm whenever feasible, and where not feasible, ventricular response should be well controlled with beta blockers, calcium channel blockers, and/or digoxin. In the absence of contraindication, patients with atrial fibrillation should be anticoagulated with warfarin.

4. Diminish/prevent ischemia. The possibility of coronary artery disease and active or inducible myocardial ischemia should be explored using noninvasive imaging and, where warranted, coronary angiography. Consideration should be given to revascularization, particularly if there is sufficient inducible ischemia to be contributing to the clinical syndrome. Medical therapy includes antiplatelet agents, beta blockers, ACE inhibitors or ARBs, nitrates, and calcium channel blockers.

Beyond these treatments, consideration has been given to drugs that may accelerate myocardial relaxation. Although most literature in this area has focused on calcium channel blockers,[15] there is evidence that ACE inhibitors and ARBs may also offer this benefit.[16] This theory has never been translated into clear-cut demonstrable clinical benefit. However, as indicated previously, there is ample rationale to treat these patients with ACE inhibitors or ARBs. Calcium channel blockers are also attractive options to control blood pressure and diminish myocardial ischemia.

APPROACH TO THE ASYMPTOMATIC PATIENT WITH LV DILATION

Increased LV volume, particularly end-systolic volume, represents a major independent risk factor for subsequent adverse clinical outcomes in patients with myocardial infarction (MI).[17,18] LV cavity dilation (generally associated with reduced LVEF—see previous discussion), regardless of etiology, constitutes stage B disease in the absence of symptomatic heart failure, according to the classification of the joint heart failure guideline of the American Heart Association and American College of Cardiology.[2] In patients with this finding, a cause should be sought, with particular consideration of ischemic heart disease. A careful history should be obtained for cocaine or excessive alcohol use and for a family history suggestive of a familial dilated cardiomyopathy.

Patients with LV dilatation require treatment designed to prevent the progression of adverse ventricular remodeling and shown to reduce the likelihood of clinical heart failure and death. They should be treated with ACE inhibitors or ARBs and with beta blockers. Each of these classes of agents can prevent or reverse LV dilatory remodeling in patients with reduced LVEF (see Chapter 6). The SOLVD prevention trial demonstrated that enalapril reduced the rate of hospitalization for heart failure among asymptomatic patients with reduced LVEF, compared with placebo.[19] Although similar data are not available with ARBs, the aggregate data from the CHARM,[20] VALIANT,[21] and Val-HeFT[22] trials suggest that benefits from ARBs are similar to those of ACE inhibitors in various populations with reduced LVEF.

The clearest evidence for benefit from beta blockers in asymptomatic patients with LV dilation and reduced LVEF comes from the CAPRICORN trial,[23] which demonstrated outcome benefits with carvedilol in such patients following MI. A similar benefit of beta blockers has not been shown in patients with LV dilatation and reduced LVEF in the absence of ischemic heart disease, but guidelines recommend beta blockers administration in this population as well, based on studies in symptomatic patients.[24] Because of variability in the pharmacology of various beta blockers, preference should be given to those agents with documented benefits in randomized clinical trials (see Chapter 6).

Use of an implantable cardioverter-defibrillator (ICD) should be considered in patients with moderate to severe reduction in LVEF who are ≥30 days after an MI. The MADIT-II trial[25] demonstrated that an ICD reduced mortality in post-MI patients with LVEF ≤30%. The benefit is more clear-cut, and guideline recommendations are stronger in patients with symptomatic heart failure than in asymptomatic patients.[2,26]

APPROACH TO CHRONIC MANAGEMENT OF THE PATIENT WITH HEART FAILURE AND A DILATED LEFT VENTRICLE

Clinical trials over the past two decades have most clearly demonstrated therapeutic benefit in patients with symptomatic heart failure, reduced LVEF, and LV chamber dilation.

Drug Therapy

Volume overload should be treated with diuretics and sodium restriction, with the addition of fluid restriction in patients prone to hyponatremia. Most symptomatic patients with reduced LVEF should be treated with ACE inhibitors and/or ARBs and with beta blockers, all of which have been demonstrated to prevent or reverse adverse ventricular remodeling and to reduce the incidence of heart failure–related hospitalization and death. Dose titration for these agents is discussed in Chapter 6. Beta blockers prescribed should be those that have demonstrated outcome benefits in randomized controlled trials. The beta blocker dose should be up-titrated gradually, observing the impact on the patient's clinical status, blood pressure, and heart rate, with the latter reduced to as close to 60 min^{-1} as possible.

Most guidelines favor ACE inhibitors over ARBs as the initial therapy, although currently available data provide little evidence for a major advantage of either class over the other. Most currently used quality measures give clinicians credit for initiating treatment with either agent. Adverse effects, such as hypotension, lightheadedness, renal functional impairment, and hyperkalemia are similar for ACE inhibitors and ARBs. However, cough and angioedema are far more common with ACE inhibitors. For this reason, ARBs should be considered for patients experiencing these symptoms. The hydralazine–isosorbide dinitrate combination should be considered in patients manifesting intolerance to both ACE inhibitors and ARBs.

For patients with persistent or recurrent symptoms despite treatment with ACE inhibitors and beta blockers, treatment options include the addition of an aldosterone receptor blocker, an ARB, the combination of hydralazine and isosorbide dinitrate, and/or digoxin. Although multiple combinations are possible, the following factors should be considered in selecting one or more appropriate choices. (Further information regarding dosing for these agents is provided in Chapter 6.)

1. Reduced mortality has been demonstrated with addition of an aldosterone blocker in patients with severe or recently severe symptoms[27] or heart failure and reduced LVEF during hospitalization for MI.[28]
2. The CHARM-Added study demonstrated reduction in the primary combined endpoint of cardiovascular death or heart failure hospitalization with the addition of candesartan to pre-existing ACE inhibitor treatment.[29]
3. There is little documentation of the safety and incremental efficacy of the combination of ACE inhibitor, ARB, and aldosterone blocker. Approximately 17% of patients in the CHARM-Added study were receiving an aldosterone receptor

blocker.[29] Use of all three agents, particularly in combination with a beta blocker, can be expected to increase the potential for clinically relevant hyperkalemia.

4. In African Americans with reduced LVEF and NYHA class III or IV symptoms who are receiving an ACE inhibitor or ARB, beta blocker, and, in many cases an aldosterone receptor blocker, addition of the combination of hydralazine and isosorbide dinitrate improved all three components of the primary composite endpoint of survival, avoidance of hospitalization for heart failure, and health-related quality of life.[30]

5. Digoxin, once the mainstay of treatment for this patient population, did not improve survival (in a population with sinus rhythm). Several studies have shown worsening of symptoms or functional status in patients on this drug who were randomized to discontinuation of digoxin treatment.[31,32] In the DIG trial, digoxin reduced the secondary endpoint of heart failure–related hospitalization.[33] However, few of these patients had received beta blockers or aldosterone blockers, so that the effects of digoxin in the presence of these now-standard treatments are uncertain.

Devices

For patients with NYHA class III and IV symptoms despite appropriate medical treatment, LVEF ≤35%, and QRS duration >120 msec, cardiac resynchronization therapy (CRT) has been shown to reduce symptoms,[34] heart failure hospitalization frequency,[35] and in one study, overall mortality.[36] CRT should be considered in this population. Its usefulness is being explored in patients with milder symptoms and functional impairment and in those with evidence of mechanical dyssynchrony, as evidenced through imaging modalities, despite a narrower QRS complex. In the United States, most patients undergoing CRT receive a device that is also an ICD, which has been found to reduce the probability of death in patients with heart failure symptoms and LVEF ≤35%.[37] Such treatments should be strongly considered in patients who fit these characteristics in the absence of substantial comorbidities. ICD implant is not warranted in patients with extensive comorbidities or in those with advanced heart failure symptoms, unless therapeutic options are available, such as CRT or heart transplant (see subsequent text), with a significant probability of improving the patient's clinical status.

APPROACH TO THE PATIENT WITH AN EXACERBATION OF HEART FAILURE

With approximately 1 million United States hospitalizations for heart failure annually,[38] an evidenced-based approach to managing patients with an exacerbation of heart failure is needed. Unfortunately, unlike acute MI, where clinical trials have identified interventions that improve clinical outcomes, there is no similar body of evidence for patients with chronic heart failure who are hospitalized with decompensation.[39] This disparity is due in part to the fact that, unlike acute MI, heart failure exacerbation is not a specific clinical-pathologic event, driven by a well-defined pathophysiologic mechanism (like acute coronary thrombosis), but instead can result from various factors (see subsequent text). Furthermore, it is not a single clinical syndrome. Rather, patients may manifest either (i) rapid accumulation of lung water (acute pulmonary edema), (ii) progressive systemic congestion, or (iii) clinical findings associated with reduced cardiac output. Pulmonary edema and systemic congestion are rarely present in the same patient, whereas systemic congestion is typically associated with signs and symptoms of reduced cardiac output. Finally, testing the impact of specific interventions has proven exceedingly difficult because these patients are inherently unstable, with many available treatment options and lack of agreement on appropriate target endpoints. For these reasons, there is a paucity of useful clinical trial evidence in patients with heart failure exacerbation, so that most guideline recommendations for managing this syndrome derive from the opinions of "experts," unsupported by solid outcome data.

Precipitating Factors

Factors that can contribute to, or precipitate, worsening heart failure include excess sodium intake, medication noncompliance, myocardial ischemia, arrhythmia, increased heart rate, elevated blood pressure, acute valve dysfunction, and pulmonary emboli. Education should be directed toward altering those factors that are under the patient's control. Most important, patients should be educated to restrict sodium intake, comply with medication prescription, and monitor and respond to changes in daily weight or clinical status. Treatment of hypertension is essential (see subsequent text). Suspicion of acute or worsening valve function should be evaluated with echocardiography. Patients with suspected pulmonary embolus should be evaluated with perfusion lung scan or computerized tomographic pulmonary angiography.

Acute myocardial ischemia should always be considered, especially in patients with a history of ischemic heart disease, symptoms suggesting angina or angina equivalent, electrocardiographic changes, and elevated serum troponin concentration. However, patients may have myocardial ischemia with none of these findings present. For this reason, once the patient's condition has been stabilized, there should be a low threshold for performing a test for inducible myocardial ischemia, such as myocardial perfusion imaging during stress or dipyridamole administration or echocardiography during stress or dobutamine administration. Computerized tomographic coronary angiography represents another screening option. If the diagnosis remains uncertain or if one or more of the previously discussed tests is consistent with acute myocardial ischemia, coronary angiography and revascularization should be strongly considered. The timing of such intervention is influenced by the patient's clinical instability, the presence of comorbidities, and the degree of suspicion of active ischemia.

Medical treatment for myocardial ischemia includes nitrates and beta blockers. The decision and timing for beta blocker therapy in patients with LV dilation and reduced LVEF must be weighed with consideration of the possibility of worsening clinical heart failure. Patients with severe heart failure, overt volume overload, and/or signs and symptoms of diminished peripheral perfusion are at greatest risk for clinical worsening with beta blocker initiation. However, most patients with an exacerbation of heart failure will tolerate gradual initiation of a beta blocker, particularly after correction of fluid overload. In an observational study, patients in whom beta blocker treatment is initiated by the time of hospital discharge show improved survival, compared to similar patients not treated at that time.[40] Additional contraindications to beta blockade are bronchospasm, symptomatic hypotension, and bradycardia. Heart failure without LV dilation and with preserved LVEF does not represent a contraindication to beta blockade. Furthermore, in patients with tachycardia, particularly where myocardial ischemia is a consideration, the value of judicious implementation of beta blockade, under careful clinical monitoring, generally outweighs the risk.

"Heart" Failure: A Cardio-Renal-Vascular Syndrome

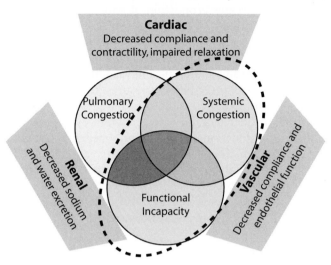

Figure 7-4: Syndromes of worsening heart failure showing the interplay between cardiac, renal, and vascular abnormalities.

The Cardio-Renal-Vascular Syndrome

Heart failure is characterized by complex cardiac, renal, and vascular interactions, mediated through both hemodynamic and neurohormonal mechanisms (see Chapters 2, 3 and 6). Increased vascular stiffness limits the ability of the intravascular space to accommodate salt and fluid loads. Endothelial dysfunction contributes to vasoconstriction and increased afterload. Renal dysfunction may limit sodium excretion and drives activation of the renin–angiotensin–aldosterone axis. ACE inhibitors, ARBs, and diuretics reduce glomerular filtration rate, and worsening renal function limits the effectiveness of diuresis. Sodium retention, vasoconstriction, or worsening of intrinsic cardiac, renal, or vascular function may trigger a vicious cycle that precipitates one of the syndromes of worsening heart failure (Fig. 7-4).

The Syndromes of Worsening Heart Failure

The vast majority of patients hospitalized because of an exacerbation of chronic heart failure have evidence of increased intravascular and extravascular fluid.[41] The vast majority also manifest dyspnea as a prominent presenting complaint. Although dyspnea is often presumed to be related to increased lung stiffness and systemic arterial hypoxemia due to elevation of pulmonary venous pressure with transudation of lung water, it may also result from reduced cardiac output with an inability to deliver sufficient oxygen to meet the body's metabolic needs, even at rest.

Patients hospitalized because of worsening chronic heart failure tend to have one of two distinct clinical syndromes, with little overlap: acute pulmonary edema (APE), or right heart failure (RHF) and systemic congestion, often associated with fatigue and lethargy, characteristic of a reduced cardiac output. The factors that predispose to one or the other of these syndromes are not fully known, though they include (a) the presence and extent of pulmonary vascular disease, predisposing to pulmonary hypertension and right heart failure while protecting against transudation of lung water; (b) left ventricular diastolic stiffness, tending to drive acute increases in pulmonary venous pressure; (c) vascular stiffness, tending to increase the volume of the central circulation. Although patients with any cause of heart failure may manifest either syndrome, patients do not tend to cross between syndromes from one hospitalization to the next. A greater proportion of patients with HCVD and a nondilated LV tend to present with APE, whereas RHF is more common in patients with LV cavity dilation and reduced LVEF due to ischemic heart disease or dilated cardiomyopathy. Patients with APE tend to have higher blood pressures, develop symptoms rapidly, and respond readily to diuretic and vasodilator treatment. In contrast, patients with RHF tend to have lower blood pressures, tend to accumulate fluid and develop worsening symptoms more insidiously, and generally require more protracted treatment to return to their baseline state. Between exacerbations, patients with APE often have little overt functional impairment, whereas those who present with RHF often show greater functional impairment between episodes of exacerbation—that is, their exacerbation tends to be more of a gradual worsening of their underlying chronic clinical condition. Unfortunately, to date, clinical trials focusing on patients with heart failure exacerbation have tended to lump these patients, rather than divide them into specific clinical syndromes.

Diagnosis and Monitoring

For patients presenting with dyspnea, the diagnosis of heart failure is often straightforward, either with clinical and radiographic evidence of pulmonary congestion (APE) or with systemic congestion (edema, ascites, and/or abdominal organomegaly) and elevated jugular venous pressure (RHF). Ventricular dysfunction shown on echocardiography supports the diagnosis. Often, however, the diagnosis is not clear, and alternative diagnoses—such as an exacerbation of lung disease—may be responsible for the patient's presentation.

Biomarkers have proved useful to aid in the diagnosis. Several studies have demonstrated the usefulness of serum assays of natriuretic peptides—notably B-type natriuretic peptide (BNP) and amino-terminal pro-B-type natriuretic peptide (NT-proBNP)—in improving diagnostic accuracy in patients presenting with acute increasing dyspnea.[42,43] Combining clinical assessment with measurement of serum concentrations of BNP or NT-proBNP improves diagnostic accuracy and facilitates the choice of appropriate treatment. Normal values render a diagnosis of heart failure exacerbation extremely unlikely. High levels provide substantial support for the diagnosis, where appropriate clinical findings are present. Caution must be practiced to avoid overinterpreting moderate or even high levels where clinical findings are discordant, since patients with cardiac dysfunction may have alternative causes of dyspnea. Normal ranges of natriuretic peptide levels tend to be higher among women, older subjects, and those with lower body mass index.[44] Obese patients tend to have lower levels for a given degree of heart failure.

Clinical assessment is the principal means for judging response to treatment of heart failure exacerbation. Patients should be monitored for resolution of peripheral, abdominal, and pulmonary extravascular fluid as well as for signs of improved peripheral perfusion. Serum levels of natriuretic peptides decline with successful treatment, particularly following relief of congestion. There is some evidence that adjusting treatment based on changes in these levels improves clinical outcomes;[45] however, advocacy for this practice must await results of larger, randomized controlled trials, which are ongoing at the time of this writing.[46] Levels of both natriuretic peptides[47] and troponin,[48] a marker of myocardial injury, are independent predictors of adverse clinical outcomes in various cardiovascular conditions, including in patients with heart failure exacerbation.

There is controversy regarding the application of pulmonary artery catheter measurements in monitoring treatment of patients hospitalized with heart failure. A number of investigations have examined the effect of *routine* invasive monitoring on clinical outcomes within intensive care units. For the most part, these trials have yielded neutral results. A recent randomized controlled trial[49] showed no benefit from routine use of invasive hemodynamic monitoring, using a pulmonary artery catheter in stable patients hospitalized with heart failure. Based on these results, routine use of invasive monitoring is not warranted. It is important to recognize that patients for whom the clinician/investigators believed such monitoring was needed were excluded from this and all other randomized trials. Hemodynamic diagnosis and monitoring using a pulmonary artery catheter should be strongly considered in patients manifesting dyspnea, hypotension, or diminished peripheral perfusion, where cardiac filling pressures cannot reasonably be estimated based on clinical grounds. Invasive hemodynamic measurement should particularly be considered in patients manifesting both dyspnea and hypoperfusion, to facilitate optimization of cardiac filling pressures.

Potent intravenous inotropic and vasodilator agents (see subsequent text) have the potential to induce hypotension and/or renal failure, and they should not be administered unless, according to the heart failure clinical practice guideline of the Heart Failure Society of America, "left heart filling pressures are known to be elevated based on direct measurement or clear clinical signs."[50] Where pulmonary artery wedge pressure is $<\sim 15$ mm Hg, intravenous inotropes or vasodilators should generally not be given. If cardiac index is also reduced substantially (e.g., <2.5 L/min/m^2), and there are clinical findings supporting hypoperfusion, consideration should be given to intravascular volume expansion.

When using invasive hemodynamic monitoring during treatment, a range of pulmonary artery wedge pressures should be identified for which the patient has adequate peripheral perfusion, without inducing pulmonary edema, and this range should be targeted during drug treatment.

Fluid Management and Basic Measures

Supplemental oxygen is indicated in most patients presenting acutely with heart failure exacerbation, particularly those with APE. Most patients require treatment to normalize intravascular and extravascular volume. Although systemic perfusion, blood pressure, and renal function must be carefully monitored during treatment, diuresis is often accompanied by improvement in cardiac output and peripheral perfusion, owing to relief of the paradoxical mechanisms (e.g., functional mitral and tricuspid regurgitation and ventricular interdependence) through which volume overload may be associated with reduced cardiac output (see Chapter 6).

Intravenous diuretics are the mainstay of treatment for patients hospitalized with volume overload. Intravenous agents are preferable over oral agents, since the rapid onset of action facilitates expeditious dose escalation (e.g., every 2–4 hours) in the event that diuresis is inadequate. Furosemide is the most commonly used agent. One approach is to initiate treatment with an intravenous dose approximately equal to patient's routine daily oral dose, with subsequent doses either maintained at that level or increased, depending on response to the prior dose.

Diuretic treatment efficacy is determined by (a) urine output; (b) the net balance between input and output; (c) changes in body weight, taking care to weigh the patient at the same time of day and under comparable conditions; and (d) resolution

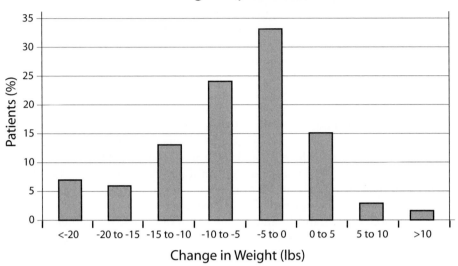

Figure 7-5: Distribution of changes in body weight during hospitalization. From Fonarow GC; ADHERE Scientific Advisory Committee. The Acute Decompensated Heart Failure National Registry (ADHERE): opportunities to improve care of patients hospitalized with acute decompensated heart failure. Rev Cardiovascr Med 2003;4(Suppl 7):S21–30.

of the clinical manifestations of extra-vascular volume overload: pulmonary rales (for patients with APE) or edema and ascites (for patients with RHF). Jugular venous pressure is an important means for judging the impact of diuresis on intravascular volume, especially in judging diuretic efficacy for patients with RHF. Although the optimal level of jugular venous pressure may vary among patients, reduction to a level <10 cm H_2O is generally a reasonable goal.

Most patients with APE show fairly brisk clinical responses to diuresis and may be stabilized and discharged within a few days. In contrast, underdiuresis represents a frequent shortcoming in the management of patients with RHF. Patients with heart failure exacerbation often show little or no change in body weight during the course of the hospitalization[51] (Fig. 7-5). A common mistake is to discharge the patient with persistent evidence of excess extravascular fluid and continued elevation of jugular venous pressure, with treatment limited by diuretic resistance, minor elevations in serum creatinine concentration, or by a desire to reduce hospital length of stay. Under such circumstances, rehospitalization within a short time is likely. In contrast, if normalization of intravascular and extravascular volume can be achieved or approached, often requiring time and patience, then cardiac output may be restored through relief of ventricular interdependence and reduction in functional valvular regurgitation (see Chapter 6). Under these conditions, a vicious cycle will have been broken, with improvement in peripheral perfusion, renal function, and diuretic sensitivity, increasing the likelihood of long-term clinical stability.

During diuretic treatment, blood pressure, signs of peripheral perfusion, renal function, and serum electrolyte concentrations should be carefully monitored. The impact of diuresis on cardiac output and on peripheral perfusion is difficult to predict. The goal is to achieve an optimal rate of decrease in intravascular volume, sufficient to cause reabsorption of extravascular fluid without decreasing peripheral perfusion. This rate varies widely among patients, with some patients tolerating <1 L of volume loss per day and others tolerating as much as 4 L. For patients with persistent volume overload, an increase in serum creatinine or urea nitrogen concentration or a drop in blood pressure is generally not an indication to decrease or halt diuresis. It may be necessary to suspend diuresis for a short time, and even to administer a small amount of fluid, followed by resumption of diuresis at a slower pace. It is likely that the optimal diuresis rate is linked to the *plasma refill rate*, the rate of fluid movement from the extravascular to the intravascular compartment.[52,53] Methodologies are being developed to provide real-time assessment of the plasma refill rate, to assist in targeting an optimal rate of diuresis.

For patients inadequately responsive to escalating doses of a loop diuretic, the following options may be considered:

1. Institution of a continuous infusion of the loop diuretic (e.g., furosemide, 5–40 mg/hr)
2. Addition of a thiazide diuretic, such as intravenous chlorothiazide (typically 500 mg) or oral metolazone (2.5–5 mg), optimally administered 30 minutes prior to administration of the loop diuretic
3. Addition of an aldosterone receptor blocker, such as spironolactone, in doses ranging from 25–100 mg daily, monitoring serum potassium levels carefully to avoid hyperkalemia
4. Addition of an intravenous vasodilator or inotropic agent (see subsequent text)
5. Institution of ultrafiltration (see Chapter 6)

Diminished peripheral perfusion and impaired renal function represent frequent obstacles to adequate diuresis. These circumstances represent appropriate indications for consideration of intravenous vasodilator and/or inotropic therapy, with the goal of sustaining a diuresis to achieve optimal fluid balance while maintaining peripheral perfusion. For patients with hypertension (see subsequent text), vasodilators (nitroglycerine, nitroprusside, or nesiritide), are the treatments of choice. For patients with lower blood pressures, these agents may also be considered in the absence of clinically relevant hypotension. However, particular care should be exercised in administering vasodilators to any patient with baseline systolic blood pressure <100 mm Hg, observing carefully for clinical evidence of diminished peripheral perfusion and renal functional impairment. Use of nesiritide, particularly at infusion rates >0.01 μg/kg/min, is associated with an increased incidence of worsening renal function.[54] For patients with either documented or anticipated intolerance to pure vasodilators, consideration should be given to a mixed inotrope/vasodilator, such as milrinone or dobutamine. Although there is concern regarding the potential adverse impact of these agents on survival (see Chapter 6), consideration of their use is warranted in patients with persistent volume overload in whom diuresis is limited by diminished peripheral perfusion and/or renal function.[50] Neither intravenous vasodilators nor inotropic agents should be used unless cardiac filling pressures are known to be elevated, based on unambiguous clinical assessment or on direct hemodynamic measurement.

Vasopressin receptor blockers are a promising treatment option for management of volume overload, particularly among patients with diuretic resistance, hyponatremia, or renal impairment, although their appropriate role is yet to be clarified. One large-scale investigation demonstrated that the oral vasopressin receptor blocker tolvaptan increased weight loss and improved dyspnea in patients recently hospitalized with worsening renal function, reduced LVEF, and evidence of volume overload with background loop diuretic administration.[55] There was no demonstrable effect on a global clinical status score, measured at 7 days, or on long-term clinical outcomes.[56]

There has been recent increase in interest for ultrafiltration due to availability of simpler systems than previously available. Clinical trials have shown that patients randomized to ultrafiltration achieve greater fluid loss than those randomized to conventional diuretic treatment, and one trial indicated a reduction in the rate of heart failure–related rehospitalization (see Chapter 6).[57] The rate of ultrafiltration should be titrated based on the same concerns mentioned previously regarding diuresis. At this time there is no evidence that ultrafiltration is safer than diuresis. It appears that greater rates of fluid removal diminish renal function, regardless of whether fluid removal is achieved through diuresis or ultrafiltration. At present ultrafiltration is generally reserved for patients who respond inadequately to diuretics. Ongoing clinical trials may shed further light on the appropriate use of ultrafiltration for patients hospitalized with heart failure and volume overload.

Blood Pressure Management

Blood pressure at the time of hospitalization correlates with clinical outcomes in patients hospitalized with heart failure exacerbation, with higher blood pressures associated with improved prognosis.[58,59] This finding probably implies differences in the nature of underlying cardiac function and in the pathophysiology of the clinical syndrome. Patients with APE tend to have higher blood pressures than those with RHF. Similarly, patients with less LV dilation and more preserved LVEF tend to have higher blood pressures than those with LV dilation and reduced LVEF. Relatively low blood pressures (even <115–120 mm Hg) at the time of presentation with heart failure exacerbation are associated with reduced in-hospital survival and probably connote greater degrees of cardiac dysfunction.

Worsening hypertension frequently precipitates worsening clinical heart failure, particularly APE, with increasing afterload causing diminished LV systolic performance and elevated filling pressures. The resulting neurohumoral response (see Chapter 3), causes vasoconstriction, tachycardia, worsening energy starvation, and worsening LV function. These factors contribute to a vicious cycle that may lead to acute pulmonary edema. Hypertension in this setting should be aggressively treated. Relief of pulmonary edema with intravenous loop diuretics may help to diminish neurohormonal stimuli, thus reducing blood pressure. However, vasodilator treatment—particularly intravenous nitroprusside or nitroglycerine—should also be considered in an effort to drive down both ventricular afterload and preload. Although there are no established treatment targets, it is reasonable to reduce systolic blood pressure to levels <130 mm Hg.

Hypotension in the setting of heart failure exacerbation generally connotes severe cardiac dysfunction and poor prognosis. Many patients with heart failure have relatively low systolic blood pressure (e.g., as low as 80–90 mm Hg) without overt evidence of hypoperfusion, so that there is no absolute numerical definition of hypotension. However, care must be exerted in managing patients with heart failure and systolic blood pressure <100 mm Hg to avoid inducing clinically relevant hypoperfusion. Clinical evidence of hypoperfusion—i.e., cool extremities, altered mentation, light-headedness, oliguria—in the setting of clinical heart failure warrants consideration of invasive hemodynamic monitoring to assist in fluid management and to optimize cardiac filling pressures. Such a goal may be defined as either a pulmonary artery wedge pressure in the range of approximately 15–20 mm Hg, or the lowest pressure that achieves adequate peripheral perfusion.

Beta blockers should not be given to patients who are hypoperfused. Vasodilator treatment must be given with caution in patients with systolic blood pressure <100 mm Hg. Great caution must be exerted in attempting such treatment in patients with any clinical evidence of hypoperfusion, observing for evidence of further decrease of peripheral perfusion and renal functional impairment. Invasive hemodynamic monitoring is generally indicated in this setting. In patients with symptomatic hypotension, where cardiac filling pressures cannot be optimized by volume management, pressor agents must be considered. Vasoconstrictors such as norepinephrine or vasopressin are effective in raising blood pressure, but tend to worsen cardiac function and raise cardiac filling pressures through increases in afterload and may also induce myocardial ischemia. Mixed inotrope/vasoconstrictors, such as high-dose dopamine, can also be effective but tend to increase heart rate as well as afterload. These changes will increase myocardial oxygen demand and so can induce ischemia and arrhythmias. More pure inotropes, such as dobutamine, have the same shortcomings, and therefore should be used sparingly. Compared with vasoconstrictor agents, dobutamine tends not to increase afterload and may reduce rather than raise cardiac filling pressures. Blood pressure may increase or decrease with dobutamine administration, but generally, blood pressure effects are modest with this agent.

Renal Function

Diminished renal function, either at baseline or during treatment, represents a strong independent predictor of adverse clinical outcomes in patients hospitalized with heart failure exacerbation. Within the *ADHERE* database, comprising patients hospitalized because of heart failure, baseline values of both creatinine and urea nitrogen serum concentrations were independent predictors of increased in-hospital mortality.[58] Increased serum creatinine concentration during treatment has been found to predict worse in-hospital and postdischarge clinical outcomes within a large administrative database.[60] It is uncertain to what extent these associations are causal in nature, though it seems plausible that abnormal renal function is both a marker and a contributor to adverse outcomes.

Worsening renal function represents a frequent limitation to diuretic treatment. Minor increases in urea nitrogen or creatinine serum concentrations should not be considered a contraindication to continued diuresis in patients with persistent volume overload. However, continued rise in these values, particularly when accompanied by other manifestations of diminished peripheral perfusion, should suggest slowing the rate of fluid removal. Alternatively, and particularly where oliguria is present, administration of a mixed inotrope/vasodilator agent should be considered (see previous discussion).

Ultrafiltration is an excellent option to reduce persistent volume overload in patients with oliguria. However, there is no evidence that ultrafiltration is associated with any lower incidence of renal impairment than diuresis, for a given rate of fluid removal. Where renal impairment is severe, consideration should be given to instituting dialysis. Hemodialysis is generally used for short-term exacerbations, whereas for longer-term treatment, patients with severe heart failure often tolerate peritoneal dialysis better than hemodialysis, because the latter can cause abrupt shifts in intravascular fluid balance.

Mechanical Circulatory Support

Where medical options have been exhausted and there is evidence of persistently diminished peripheral perfusion in the absence of severely limiting comorbidities, consideration should be given to mechanical circulatory support. This option is particularly attractive either where there is an obviously remediable contributor to the patient's clinical status, such as severe myocardial ischemia or acute severe mitral regurgitation, or where cardiac transplantation is being considered. The intra-aortic balloon pump represents a viable option for temporary support, given its ease of implant and its ability to diminish cardiac filling pressure, augment cardiac output, and increase coronary perfusion. For greater and/or longer-term support, various ventricular assist devices are available. Percutaneous options are available for rapid, short-term support[61,62,63,64] (see Chapter 6) but more sustained support requires surgical implant. Novel forms of circulatory support, such as continuous aortic flow augmentation,[65] are presently undergoing clinical evaluation.

Initiating and Maintaining a Long-Term Treatment Regimen

Initiating a long-term medical treatment plan represents an important goal during hospitalization for heart failure exacerbation. The hospital stay should be taken as an opportunity to assess the patient's medical regimen and to educate the patient and caregivers regarding diet (particularly sodium restriction), risk modification, smoking cessation, weight and clinical monitoring, and the importance of compliance with medication prescription. Medications known to improve natural history should be initiated, unless there are contraindications. Hospitalization represents an opportunity to up-titrate drug doses under close clinical and laboratory monitoring. In particular, in patients with LV dilation and reduced LVEF, ACE inhibitor and/or ARB[66] and/or aldosterone antagonist treatment should be considered (see previous discussion). Initiation of beta blocker therapy during hospitalization for heart failure exacerbation is more controversial, given the potential for these agents to worsen hemodynamics acutely. Nevertheless, strong consideration should be given to initiating beta blockers once clinical stability has been achieved, an approach that has been found to be safe. There is an advantage to initiating treatment under observation, and in-hospital treatment initiation increases the likelihood that patients will receive beta blocker therapy long-term.[40]

APPROACHES TO THE PATIENT WITH ADVANCED HEART FAILURE

Advanced heart failure may be defined as severe heart disease that is highly unlikely to be reversed, associated with severely limiting symptoms and/or diminished functional capacity; inadequately responsive to appropriate patient education, drug treatment, and device (e.g., CRT) application; often requiring repeated hospitalization; and with a markedly diminished life expectancy. Measures available for patients with advanced heart failure include implantable ventricular assist devices (VADs) or heart transplant, on the one hand, and hospice care on the other.

Recognition that the patient is in a stage of advanced heart failure should prompt the clinician to reassess the presence and adequacy of the patient's advance directives for care (see Chapter 6).[67] As treatment options become more limited and include interventions that are highly invasive, the decision regarding direction of therapy—toward a lifesaving approach or toward a palliative approach—must be tailored to both the patient's condition and his or her individual desires. The recommendation for consideration of VAD or heart transplant rests with the clinician, based on a medical assessment of prognosis with and without a device, informed by the patient's clinical status and comorbidities, and by up-to-date information regarding the risks and benefits of the various treatment options. Once the clinician determines that VAD and/or heart transplant is a reasonable option, based purely on medical grounds, it is left to the patient or health care proxy to make the final decision. The clinician has the difficult task of facilitating the patient's or health care proxy's visualization of life following such intervention, and the spectrum of possible favorable and unfavorable outcomes, to allow him or her to make an informed set of decisions.

Intravenous Drug Infusion

Continuous or intermittent intravenous infusion of an inotropic, vasodilator, or mixed inotrope/vasodilator agent may be considered as part of the medical regimen for the patient with advanced heart failure when other medical options have failed to relieve symptoms adequately, yield minimally acceptable functional status, and/or prevent recurrent hospitalization.[68] Such treatment may be part of a program of palliative care or it may be a temporizing intervention while patients undergo evaluation for further intervention, such as device implant, or await heart transplant.[69] In the latter case, given the proarrhythmic potential of inotropic agents, strong consideration should be given to ICD implant prior to hospital discharge. Milrinone is a frequent choice for such therapy. It must be stressed that such treatment should not generally be considered life-prolonging. In fact, there is evidence that inotropic agents shorten life expectancy (see Chapter 6), and represent a palatable option to improve quality of life for severely ill patients not eligible for alternative treatment options. It is possible that such treatment may prolong the lives of individual patients with low cardiac output and diminished peripheral perfusion, particularly if the proarrhythmic potential is managed with an ICD. There is also speculation that the adverse effects of these agents may be alleviated by concomitant beta blocker administration.[70] However, none of these suppositions is supported by controlled clinical trial data.

Ventricular Assist Devices and Heart Transplant

At present, decision-making regarding consideration of implantable VADs and heart transplant is generally a unified process, since both interventions are considered major and the target patient populations—patients with advanced heart failure—overlap. In the future, this decision making may diverge as newer-generation VADs and surgical techniques are shown to have less morbidity and greater patient acceptance, in which case their application may expand to patients with less advanced heart failure. As discussed in Chapter 6, VADs may be deployed as a bridge to transplant for patients who are candidates for the latter procedure but for whom survival to transplant with medical therapy alone is considered unlikely.[71] Alternatively, VADs may be considered as the definitive treatment option, or destination therapy, generally reserved for patients with advanced heart failure who are otherwise not candidates for heart transplant, due to comorbidity[72] (Fig. 7-6). The distinction between these two indications has blurred because candidacy for heart transplant is not always clear at the time of VAD implant and because VAD implant may facilitate transitioning the patient to become a viable heart transplant candidate.

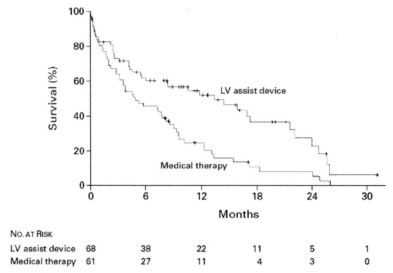

No. at Risk

LV assist device	68	38	22	11	5	1
Medical therapy	61	27	11	4	3	0

Figure 7-6: Results of the REMATCH Trial, comparing survival in patients with severe heart failure, who were not considered candidates for cardiac transplantation, randomized to receive a left ventricular assist device versus those randomized to continue medical therapy alone. From Rose EA, Gelijns AC, Moskowitz AJ, et al. Long-term use of a left ventricular assist device for end-stage heart failure. N Engl J Med 2001;345:1435–1443.

Furthermore, there is growing interest in the potential for VADs or other devices to drive or facilitate reversal of adverse ventricular remodeling and dysfunction (bridge to recovery).[73] As newer VADs are developed and tested, and greater experience is achieved, VADs may become considered reasonable alternatives to heart transplant, even among patients who are candidates for the latter procedure, or may be considered treatment options for less sick populations.

Consideration of the medical indication for recommending heart transplant or VAD entails determining the answers to three questions:

1. Is the patient's life expectancy sufficiently limited, despite optimal drug and alternative device therapy, so that such treatment may reasonably be expected to extend his or her life?
2. Is the patient's clinical status sufficiently diminished, based on symptoms, functional impairment, and/or recurrent hospitalization despite optimal drug and alternative device therapy, so that such treatment may reasonably be expected to improve his or her health-related quality of life?
3. Is it unlikely that known comorbidities will significantly detract from the expected improvement in the patient's life expectancy and health status following heart transplant or VAD implant?

For heart transplants, the decision is not based solely on the traditional risk–benefit ratio for the individual patient, but requires consideration of the risk–benefit ratio for the patient relative to that of all other patients who are candidates for the procedure. Given the limited number of transplantable organs and the high mortality rate among patients awaiting transplant, standardized criteria are established across all transplant centers to facilitate patient listing and individual organ assignment in a manner that strives for optimal use for patients with both greatest need and greatest likelihood of benefit.

There is extensive literature regarding assessing life expectancy in patients with advanced heart failure, aimed toward facilitating decision making regarding the recommendation for VAD or heart transplant.[74,75] Factors that are independently linked to the probability of mortality include the severity of cardiac remodeling (LV volumes and EF), the extent of hemodynamic derangement (particularly right atrial pressure and the presence of clinical right heart failure), and the degree of functional impairment (maximal exercise time and O_2 consumption during treadmill testing).[76] Important comorbidities that must be considered include noncardiac diseases that may limit life expectancy or functional status despite heart transplant or VAD. Significant neurologic impairment may render these procedures inadvisable. Conditions that predispose to postoperative infection must be identified and managed or avoided. For heart transplant, the presence and extent of pulmonary vascular disease must be evaluated, since excessive right ventricular afterload will cause the normal thin-walled transplanted right ventricle to fail. For VADs, conditions that increase surgical complexity, such as aortic regurgitation, must be recognized and managed or avoided. Severe right heart dysfunction or intractable ventricular arrhythmias may dictate the choice of LVAD and mandate concomitant use of a right ventricular assist device, thereby further limiting the patient's prospective lifestyle.

Following the clinician's recommendation of the medical advisability of heart transplant or VAD, the final decision rests with the patient or, where the patient is unable to make the decision, with the health care proxy. For VADs, the patient or health care proxy should be made aware of issues related to device and drive line maintenance, activity limitation, and potential morbidity including infection, thromboembolism, and device malfunction. During consideration of heart transplant, patients should be made aware of issues related to monitoring (including endomyocardial biopsy), the adverse effects and complexity of the immunosuppressive regimen, infection prophylaxis and antihypertensive drug treatment, and potential morbidity, including rejection, infection, and organ failure. Raising awareness of potential morbidity, discomfort, and required lifestyle modification must be carefully coupled with depiction of the potential life prolongation and improvement in quality of life that patients with advanced heart failure may experience following VAD implant or heart transplant.

Hospice Care

It is not necessary that every patient die in the midst of aggressive, invasive, life-prolonging efforts. Patients or health care proxies may choose hospice care when all reasonable options for life prolongation are exhausted or where the patient is known to prefer comfort and quality of life over the potential for discomfort and morbidity associated with the available treatment alternatives. A hospice approach is unfortunately less established and less frequently practiced for patients with heart failure than for patients with other conditions, such as cancer.[77,78]

It is important to present this option to patients and caregivers. Comfort measures may be delivered in the home or in specialized nursing facilities, depending on the complexity of the management regimen and the desires and capabilities of the individuals involved. Hospice should not be equated with a necessary immediate death sentence and should not be limited to patients during the last days of life. Neither should it be considered the end of all medical care. Patients may continue to live meaningful lives despite the decision to focus on comfort rather than life prolongation.

The treatment regimen should be tailored to the needs and desires of the individual patient. Indicated medications, such as ACE inhibitors and beta blockers (where tolerated), should often be continued. On the other hand, ICDs should be deactivated, and all individuals involved in the patient's care should be made aware that aggressive interventions, such as cardiopulmonary resuscitation, should not be used. Supplemental oxygen may help relieve dyspnea. Continuous intravenous inotrope/vasodilator infusion may help relieve symptoms associated with congestion and diminished peripheral perfusion and may improve patient function and self-sufficiency. On the other hand, narcotics should be liberally prescribed where alternative measures fail to provide sufficient relief of dyspnea.

FUTURE DIRECTIONS

The past two decades have seen marked acceleration in advances in therapies for patients with heart failure. The mechanisms discussed in detail in the early chapters of this book form the basis for considerable additional advances far into the future. As discussed in Chapter 6, the future holds much promise of additional strategies to prevent the development and progression of heart failure and to improve clinical outcomes for patients with this condition. During the coming decades we will become far more sophisticated in targeting treatments to specific groups of patients, defined not merely by gross cardiac morphology or function or by symptom class, but also by genomic and proteomic markers of disease susceptibility and activity. As we look back a mere 20 years, we can marvel at the advances we have made and the promise we now offer our patients. Twenty years hence, we will no doubt look back at the present times as just the beginning of the rapid expansion of our knowledge and of our ability to prevent and treat disease.

REFERENCES

1. The Criteria Committee of the New York Heart Association. *Nomenclature and Criteria for Diagnosis of Diseases of the Heart*, 4th Ed. New York, New York Heart Association. 1942; 8–9.
2. Hunt SA, Abraham WT, Chin MH, et al. ACC/AHA 2005 Guideline Update for the Diagnosis and Management of Chronic Heart Failure in the Adult: a report of the American College of Cardiology/American Heart Association Task Force on Practice Guidelines. Circulation 2005;112:e154–e235.
3. Konstam MA. "Systolic and diastolic dysfunction" in heart failure? Time for a new paradigm. J Card Failure 2003;9:1–3.
4. Konstam MA, Udelson JE, Anand Is, Cohn JN. Ventricular remodeling in heart failure: a credible surrogate endpoint. J Card Failure 2003;9:350–353.
5. Levy D, Larson MG, Vasan RS, et al. The progression from hypertension to congestive heart failure. JAMA 1996;275:1557–1562.
6. Kannel WB, Vasan RS, Levy D. Is the relation of systolic blood pressure to risk of cardiovascular disease continuous and graded, or are there critical values? Hypertension 2003;42:453–456.
7. Kannel WB, Gordon T, Castelli WP, et al. Electrocardiographic left ventricular hypertrophy and risk of coronary heart disease. The Framingham study. Ann Intern Med 1970;72:813–822.
8. Levy D, Garrison RJ, Savage DD, et al. Prognostic implications of echocardiographically determined left ventricular mass in the Framingham Heart Study. N Engl J Med 1990;322:1561–1566.

9. Chobanian AV, et al. The Seventh Report of the Joint National Committee on Prevention, Detection, Evaluation, and Treatment of High Blood Pressure: the JNC 7 report. JAMA 2003;289:2560–2572.

10. Yusuf S, Pfeffer MA, Swedberg K, et al. Effects of candesartan in patients with chronic heart failure and preserved left-ventricular ejection fraction: the CHARM-Preserved Trial. Lancet 2003;362:777–781.

11. Swedberg K, Pfeffer M, Granger C, et al. Candesartan in heart failure—assessment of reduction in mortality and morbidity (CHARM): rationale and design. Charm-Programme Investigators. J Card Failure 1999;5:276–282.

12. Heart Failure Society of America. HFSA 2006 comprehensive heart failure practice guideline. J Card Failure 2006;12:e81.

13. Parish JM, Somers VK. Obstructive sleep apnea and cardiovascular disease. Mayo Clin Proceed 2004;79:1036–1046.

14. Katz AM. *Physiology of the Heart*, 4th Ed. Philadelphia, Lippincott Williams & Wilkins. 2005;338–339.

15. Lorell BH, Paulus WJ, Grossman W, et al. Modification of abnormal left ventricular diastolic properties by nifedipine in patients with hypertrophic cardiomyopathy. Circulation 1982;65:499–507.

16. Friedrich SP, Lorell BH, Rousseau MF, et al. Intracardiac angiotensin-converting enzyme inhibition improves diastolic function in patients with left ventricular hypertrophy due to aortic stenosis. Circulation 1994;90:2761–2771.

17. St John Sutton M, Pfeffer MA, Plappert T, et al. Quantitative two-dimensional echocardiographic measurements are major predictors of adverse cardiovascular events after acute myocardial infarction. The protective effects of captopril. Circulation 1994;89:68–75.

18. Migrino RQ, Young JB, Ellis SG, et al. End-systolic volume index at 90 to 180 minutes into reperfusion therapy for acute myocardial infarction is a strong predictor of early and late mortality. The Global Utilization of Streptokinase and t-PA for Occluded Coronary Arteries (GUSTO)-I Angiographic Investigators. Circulation 1997;96:116–121.

19. SOLVD Investigators. Effect of enalapril on mortality and the development of heart failure in asymptomatic patients with reduced left ventricular ejection fractions. N Engl J Med 1992;327:685–691.

20. Granger CB, McMurray JJ, Yusuf S, et al. Effects of candesartan in patients with chronic heart failure and reduced left-ventricular systolic function intolerant to angiotensin-converting-enzyme inhibitors: the CHARM-Alternative trial [see comment]. Lancet 2003;362:772–776.

21. Pfeffer MA, McMurray JJ, Velazquez EJ, et al. Valsartan in Acute Myocardial Infarction Trial Investigators. Valsartan, captopril, or both in myocardial infarction complicated by heart failure, left ventricular dysfunction, or both. N Engl J Med 2003; 349:1893–1906.

22. Cohn JN, Tognoni G, for the Valsartan Heart Failure Trial Investigators. A randomized trial of the angiotensin-receptor blocker valsartan in chronic heart failure. N Engl J Med 2001;345:1667–1675.

23. Dargie HJ. Effect of carvedilol on outcome after myocardial infarction in patients with left-ventricular dysfunction: the CAPRICORN randomised trial [see comment]. Lancet 2001;357:1385–1390.

24. Heart Failure Society of America: HFSA 2006 comprehensive heart failure practice guideline. J Card Failure 2006;12:e27.

25. Moss AJ, Zareba W, Hall WJ, et al. Prophylactic implantation of a defibrillator in patients with myocardial infarction and reduced ejection fraction. N Engl J Med 2002; 346:877–883.

26. Heart Failure Society of America. HFSA 2006 comprehensive heart failure practice guideline. J Card Failure 2006;12:e71.

27. Pitt B, Zannad F, Remme WJ, et al. The effect of spironolactone on morbidity and mortality in patients with severe heart failure. Randomized Aldactone Evaluation Study Investigators. N Engl J Med 1999;341:709–717.

28. Pitt B, Remme W, Zannad F, et al. Eplerenone, a selective aldosterone blocker, in patients with left ventricular dysfunction after myocardial infarction. N Engl J Med 2003;348:1309–1321.

29. McMurray JJ, Ostergren J, Swedberg K, et al. Effects of candesartan in patients with chronic heart failure and reduced left-ventricular systolic function taking angiotensin-converting-enzyme inhibitors: the CHARM-Added trial. Lancet 2003;362:767–771.

30. Taylor AL, Ziesche S, Yancy C, et al. African-American Heart Failure Trial Investigators. Combination of isosorbide dinitrate and hydralazine in blacks with heart failure. N Engl J Med 2004;351:2049–2057.

31. Packer M, Gheorghiade M, Young JB, et al. Withdrawal of digoxin from patients with chronic heart failure treated with angiotensin-converting–enzyme inhibitors. N Engl J Med 1993;329:1–7.

32. Uretsky BF, Young JB, Shahidi FE, et al. Randomized study assessing the effect of digoxin withdrawal in patients with mild to moderate chronic congestive heart failure: results of the PROVED Trial. J Am Coll Cardiol 1993;22:955–962.

33. Digitalis Investigation Group. The effect of digoxin on mortality and morbidity in patients with heart failure. N Engl J Med 1997;336:525–533.

34. Abraham WT, Fisher WG, Smith AL, et al. MIRACLE Study Group. Multicenter InSync Randomized Clinical Evaluation. Cardiac resynchronization in chronic heart failure. N Engl J Med 2002;346:1845–1853.

35. Bristow MR, Saxon LA, Boehmer J, et al. Comparison of Medical Therapy, Pacing, and Defibrillation in Heart Failure (COMPANION) Investigators. Cardiac-resynchronization therapy with or without an implantable defibrillator in advanced chronic heart failure. N Engl J Med 2004;350:2140–2150.

36. Cleland JG, Daubert JC, Erdmann E, et al. Cardiac Resynchronization-Heart Failure (CARE-HF) Study Investigators. The effect of cardiac resynchronization on morbidity and mortality in heart failure. N Engl J Med 2005;352:1539–1549.

37. Bardy GH, Lee KL, Mark DB, et al. Sudden Cardiac Death in Heart Failure Trial (SCD-HeFT) Investigators. Amiodarone or an implantable cardioverter-defibrillator for congestive heart failure. N Engl J Med 2005;352:225–237.

38. Rosamond W, Flegal K, Friday G, et al. American Heart Association Statistics Committee and Stroke Statistics Subcommittee. Heart disease and stroke statistics—2007 update: a report from the American Heart Association Statistics Committee and Stroke Statistics Subcommittee. Circulation 2007;115:e69–e171.

39. Felker GM, Adams KF, Konstam MA, et al. The problem of decompensated heart failure: Nomenclature, classification, and risk stratification. Am Heart J 2003;154 (2 suppl):S18–S25.

40. Fonarow GC, Abraham WT, Albert NM, et al. OPTIMIZE-HF Investigators and Coordinators. Carvedilol use at discharge in patients hospitalized for heart failure is associated with improved survival: an analysis from Organized Program to Initiate Lifesaving Treatment in Hospitalized Patients with Heart Failure (OPTIMIZE-HF). Am Heart J 2007;153:82.e1–e11.

41. Gheorghiade M, Filippatos G, De Luca L, Burnett J. Congestion in acute heart failure syndromes: an essential target of evaluation and treatment. Am J Med 2006;119 (Suppl 1):S3–S10.

42. Maisel AS, Krishnaswamy P, Nowak RM, et al. Breathing Not Properly Multinational Study Investigators. Rapid measurement of B-type natriuretic peptide in the emergency diagnosis of heart failure. N Engl J Med 2002;347:161–167.

43. Moe GW, Howlett J, Januzzi JL, Zowall H. Canadian Multicenter Improved Management of Patients With Congestive Heart Failure (IMPROVE-CHF) Study Investigators. N-terminal pro-B-type natriuretic peptide testing improves the management of patients with suspected acute heart failure: primary results of the Canadian prospective randomized multicenter IMPROVE-CHF study. Circulation 2007;115:3103–3110.

44. Wang TJ, Larson MG, Levy D, et al. Impact of age and sex on plasma natriuretic peptide levels in healthy adults. Am J Cardiol 2002;90:254–258.

45. Troughton RW, Frampton CM, Yandle TG, et al. Treatment of heart failure guided by plasma aminoterminal brain natriuretic peptide (N-BNP) concentrations. Lancet 2000;355:1126–1130.

46. Lainchbury JG, Troughton RW, Frampton CM, et al. NTproBNP-guided drug treatment for chronic heart failure: design and methods in the BATTLESCARRED trial. Eur J Heart Fail 2006;8:532–538.

47. Konstam MA. Natriuretic peptides and cardiovascular events: more than a stretch. JAMA 2007;297:212–214.

48. Sato Y, Kita T, Takatsu Y, Kimura T. Biochemical markers of myocyte injury in heart failure. [49 refs] Heart 2004;90:1110–1113.

49. ESCAPE Investigators and ESCAPE Study Coordinators. Evaluation study of congestive heart failure and pulmonary artery catheterization effectiveness: the ESCAPE trial. JAMA 2005;294:1625–1633.

50. Heart Failure Society of America: HFSA 2006 comprehensive heart failure practice guideline. J Card Failure 2006;12:e96.

51. Fonarow GC. ADHERE Scientific Advisory Committee. The Acute Decompensated Heart Failure National Registry (ADHERE): opportunities to improve care of patients hospitalized with acute decompensated heart failure. Rev Cardiovasc Med 2003; 4 Suppl 7:S21–S30.

52. Boyle A, Sobotka PA. Redefining the therapeutic objective in decompensated heart failure: hemoconcentration as a surrogate for plasma refill rate. J Card Failure 2006; 12:247–249.

53. Marenzi G, Lauri G, Grazi M, et al. Circulatory response to fluid overload removal by extracorporeal ultrafiltration in refractory congestive heart failure. J Am Coll Cardiol 2001;38:963–968.

54. Sackner-Bernstein JD, Skopicki HA, Aaronson KD. Risk of worsening renal function with nesiritide in patients with acutely decompensated heart failure. Circulation 2005;111:1487–1491.

55. Gheorghiade M, Konstam MA, Burnett JC, et al. Short-term clinical effects of tolvaptan, an oral vasopressin antagonist, in patients hospitalized for heart failure: The EVEREST Clinical Status Trials. JAMA 2007;297:1332–1343.

56. Konstam MA, Gheorghiade M, Burnett JC, et al. Effects of oral tolvaptan in patients hospitalized for worsening heart failure: The EVEREST Outcome Trial. JAMA 2007; 297:1319–1331.

57. Costanzo MR, Guglin ME, Saltzberg MT, et al. UNLOAD Trial Investigators. Ultrafiltration versus intravenous diuretics for patients hospitalized for acute decompensated heart failure. J Am Coll Cardiol 2007;49:675–683.

58. Fonarow GC, Adams KF, Abraham WT, et al. Risk stratification for in-hospital mortality in acutely decompensated heart failure classification and regression tree analysis. JAMA 2005;293:572–580.

59. Gheorghiade M, Abraham WT, Albert NM, et al. Systolic blood pressure at admission, clinical characteristics, and outcomes in patients hospitalized with acute heart failure. JAMA 2006;296:2217–2226.

60. Krumholz HM, Chen YT, Vaccarino V, et al. Correlates and impact on outcomes of worsening renal function in patients > or =65 years of age with heart failure. Am J Cardiol 2000;85:1110–1113.

61. Thiele H, Sick P, Boudriot E, et al. Randomized comparison of intra-aortic balloon support with a percutaneous left ventricular assist device in patients with revascularized acute myocardial infarction complicated by cardiogenic shock. Eur Heart J 2005; 26:1276–1283.

62. Burkhoff D, Cohen H, Brunckhorst C, O'Neill WW. TandemHeart Investigators Group. A randomized multicenter clinical study to evaluate the safety and efficacy of the

TandemHeart percutaneous ventricular assist device versus conventional therapy with intraaortic balloon pumping for treatment of cardiogenic shock. Am Heart J 2006; 152:469.e1–e8.

63. Lee MS, Makkar RR. Percutaneous left ventricular support devices. Cardiol Clin 2006;24:265–275, vii.

64. Henriques JP, Remmelink M, Baan J Jr, et al. Safety and feasibility of elective high-risk percutaneous coronary intervention procedures with left ventricular support of the Impella Recover LP 2.5. Am J Cardiol 2006;97:990–992.

65. Konstam MA, Czerska B, Böhm M, et al. Continuous aortic flow augmentation: a pilot study of hemodynamic and renal responses to a novel percutaneous intervention in decompensated heart failure. Circulation 2005;112:3107–3114.

66. Bonow RO, Bennett S, Casey DE Jr, et al. ACC/AHA Clinical performance measures for adults with chronic heart failure: a report of the American College of Cardiology/American Heart Association Task Force on Performance Measures. Circulation 2005;112:1853–1887.

67. Heart Failure Society of America. HFSA 2006 comprehensive heart failure practice guideline. J Card Failure 2006;12:e63.

68. Young JB, Moen EK. Outpatient parenteral inotropic therapy for advanced heart failure. J Heart Lung Transplant 2000;19(8 Suppl):S49–S57.

69. Upadya S, Lee FA, Saldarriaga C, et al. Home continuous positive inotropic infusion as a bridge to cardiac transplantation in patients with end-stage heart failure. J Heart Lung Transplant 2004;23:466–472.

70. Lowes BD, Simon MA, Tsvetkova TO, Bristow MR. Inotropes in the beta-blocker era. Clin Cardiol 2000;23(3 Suppl):III11–16.

71. Frazier OH, Rose EA, Oz MC, et al. HeartMate Investigators. Multicenter clinical evaluation of the HeartMate vented electric left ventricular assist system in patients awaiting heart transplantation. J Thorac Cardiovasc Surg 2001;122:1186–1195.

72. Rose EA, Gelijns AC, Moskowitz AJ, et al. Long-term use of a left ventricular assist device for end-stage heart failure. N Engl J Med 2001;345:1435–1443.

73. Birks EJ, Tansley PD, Hardy J, et al. Left ventricular assist device and drug therapy for the reversal of heart failure. N Engl J Med 2006;355:1873–1884.

74. Costanzo MR, Augustine S, Bourge R, et al. Selection and treatment of candidates for heart transplantation. A statement for health professionals from the Committee on Heart Failure and Cardiac Transplantation of the Council on Clinical Cardiology, American Heart Association. Circulation 1995;92:3593–3612.

75. Kao W, Winkel E, Costanzo MR. Candidate evaluation and selection for heart transplantation. Curr Opin Cardiol 1995;10:159–168.

76. Lauer MS, Snader CE. Using exercise testing to prognosticate patients with heart failure. Which parameter should we measure? Cardiol Clin 2001;19:573–581.

77. Hauptman PJ, Goodlin SJ, Lopatin M, et al. Characteristics of patients hospitalized with acute decompensated heart failure who are referred for hospice care. Arch Intern Med 2007;167:1990–1997.

78. Goodlin SJ. Palliative care for end-stage heart failure. Curr Heart Fail Rep 2005; 2:155–160.

INDEX

Page numbers followed by *t* and *f* indicate tables and figures, respectively.

A

A-band, 198, 198*f*, 200, 201*f*

ACE. *See* Angiotensin-converting enzyme

Acetylcholine, 99, 102*t*. *See also* Muscarinic receptors

Acidosis
functional abnormalities in heart failure, 233–234
gap junctions and arrhythmias, 229
intracellular and sodium/hydrogen exchangers, 217, 218

Acidotic heart, 217, 218*f*

ACTH. *See* Adrenocorticotropic hormone

Actin
contractile protein in myofilaments, 162, 163*f*
contraction/relaxation in heart
actomyosin, 208
myosin interactions and role, 209
structure and role, 205
isoform shifts and hypertrophied/failing hearts, 236
myofibril in normal heart, 199
sodium/hydrogen exchangers, 218, 224*f*

α-Actinin, signaling, 163, 163*f*, 164*f*, 165, 167*f*, 169

Action potentials, cardiac, 226
alterations in failing heart, 236–237, 237*t*

Active transport, 211, 211*f*, 212, 212*f*, 215

Actomyosin, 208

Acute pulmonary edema (APE), 303, 304, 305–306, 308. *See* Fluid, retention; Heart failure, exacerbation; Pulmonary edema

Adaptor proteins, 181–183, 183*f*

Adenylyl cyclase, 98*f*, 109, 110*f*, 115

Adenosine, 102*t*

Adenosine diphosphate, see ADP

Adenosine triphosphate, see ATP

ADP, 232–233. *See also* Energy starvation

α-Adrenergic blockers, 256

α-Adrenergic receptors, 95
cardiovascular response to norepinephrine binding, 113, 114*t*, 115

G protein desensitization, 107–109
therapy with, 43

β-Adrenergic agents, 80, 81*f*

β-Adrenergic receptor agonists, 43, 81, 81*f*

β-Adrenergic receptor blockers
heart failure treatment, 247–248, 270–271
advanced, 311
asymptomatic patients with left ventricle dilatation, 299
dilated left ventricle, 301
evolving concepts, 250
exacerbation of heart failure, 302, 309
HCVD and preserved LVEF, 298
intrinsic sympathomimetic activity, 101
reversing dilatation in heart failure, 185
survival, 247
use for hypertension, 256

β-Adrenergic receptor kinase (βARK), 108, 108*f*. *See also* G protein

β-Adrenergic receptors, 111*f*, 114*t*, 115, 149

β₁-Adrenergic receptors, 95, 98*f*, 113, 114*t*, 115

β₂-Adrenergic receptors, 114*t*, 115

Adrenocorticotropic hormone (ACTH), 123

Adrenomedullin, 102*t*, 114*t*, 122

Advance directives, 259, 311

Advanced heart failure, treatment strategies, 310–314

Adverse agents, heart failure, 262–263

African Americans, 273, 301

Afterload
heart failure
exacerbation, 303, 308
hypertension etiology and pathophysiological mechanisms, 77, 77*t*
left ventricular and hypertension in development, 255
neurohormonal response, 93
hemodynamic abnormalities of forward/backward failure, 68
interplay between failing heart and peripheral circulation, 79, 80, 80*f*, 81*f*, 82*f*, 83

pumping heart, 60, 62
reduction using vasodilators, 46*f*
role in muscle performance, 54
stages in hypertrophic response, 33

Afterpolarization, 214, 229

Aging, 55, 74

Agmatine, 122

Alcohol, patients with heart failure, 262

Alcoholic cardiomyopathy, 262–263

Aldosterone
modification of cardiac function, 104
neurohormonal response in heart failure, 123
nuclear receptor activity, 102
regulatory/counterregulatory signaling responses, 97
secretion of, 124*f*

Aldosterone receptor blockers, 256, 272–273, 300–301, 307
remodeling and survival effects, 439*t*

Alkali-light chains. *See* Essential light chains

Alternative splicing, genomic DNA, 137, 137*f*. *See also* DNA, genomic

American Heart Association, stages of cardiac function, 292, 293*t*

Amino terminal pro-B-type natriuretic peptide (NT-proBNP), 304. *See also* Natriuretic peptides

ε-Amino lysyl groups, 159

Amiodarone, 264

Anaerobic glycolysis, 218

Anaerobic pathways, 231. *See also* Energy starvation

Anasarca, 3*t*, 76. *See also* Dropsy; Edema; Fluid retention

Anemia, 72

Aneurisms, 24

Angina, 253, 302

Angioedema, 267–268, 269, 300. *See also* Edema

Angiography, 253–254

Angiotensin I, 116, 117*f*

Angiotensin II
cardiovascular effects, 268
generation of active signaling peptides, 117*f*

319